HANDBOOK OF PHOBIA THERAPY

HANDBOOK OF PHOBIA THERAPY

RAPID SYMPTOM RELIEF IN ANXIETY DISORDERS

edited by
Carol Lindemann, Ph.D.

JASON ARONSON INC.
Northvale, New Jersey
London

The author gratefully acknowledges the following for permission to reprint material:

Appended tables from Amies, P. L., Gelder, M. G., and Shaw, P. M. (1983). Social phobias: A comparative clinical study. *British Journal of Psychiatry* 142:176. Reprinted by permission of the publisher.

From *Anxiety Disorders and Phobias: A Cognitive Perspective*, by Aaron T. Beck and Gary Emery with Ruth L. Greenberg. Copyright © 1985 by Aaron T. Beck, M.D., and Gary Emery, Ph.D. Reprinted by permission of Basic Books, Inc., Publishers.

Chambless, D. L. (1985). Agropahobia, in *Handbook of Clinical Behavior*, ed. M. Hersen and A. D. Bellack, pp. 49-87. New York: Plenum. Reprinted by permission of the publisher.

Foa, E. B., and Steketee, G. (1984). Behavioral treatment of obsessive-compulsive ritualizers, in *New Findings in Obsessive Compulsive Disorders*, ed. T. R. Insel, pp. 46-69. Washington, DC: American Psychiatric Press. Reprinted by permission of American Psychiatric Press.

Klosko, J. S., and Barlow, D. H. (1987). Cognitive-behavioral treatment of panic attacks. *Journal of Integrative and Eclectic Psychotherapy* 6:462-469. © 1987 Brunner/Mazel, Inc. New York. Reprinted by permission of the publisher.

Weekes, C. (1973). A practical treatment of agoraphobia. *British Medical Journal* 2:469-471. Reprinted by permission of British Medical Journal.

Copyright © 1989 by Jason Aronson Inc.

10 9 8 7 6 5 4 3 2 1

All rights reserved. Printed in the United States of America. No part of this book may be used or reproduced in any manner whatsoever without written permission from *Jason Aronson Inc.* except in the case of brief quotations in reviews for inclusion in a magazine, newspaper, or broadcast.

Library of Congress Cataloging-in-Publication Data

Handbook of phobia therapy.

   Includes index.
   1. Phobias—Treatment.   2. Panic disorders—Treatment.
I. Lindemann, Carol G.   [DNLM: 1. Phobic Disorders—
therapy—handbooks.   WM 34 H236]
RC535.H349   1989   616.85'2206   89-6535
ISBN 0-87668-866-0

Manufactured in the United States of America. Jason Aronson Inc. offers books and cassettes. For information and catalog write to Jason Aronson Inc., 230 Livingston Street, Northvale, New Jersey 07647.

IN MEMORY OF MY FATHER
Joseph S. Lindemann

Contents

Contributors xi
Preface xv
Acknowledgments xix

1 The Development of Phobia Therapy   1
   Carol Lindemann

PART I
SPECIFIC ANXIETY DISORDER

2 Diagnosing Anxiety   15
   Ira M. Lesser

3 Agoraphobia   39
   Dianne L. Chambless

4 Evaluation Anxieties   87
   Aaron T. Beck

5	Generalized Anxiety Disorder Ronald E. Coleman Carol A. Gantman	113
6	Childhood Phobias Harold S. Koplewicz	145
7	Flying Phobia T. W. Cummings	159
8	Obsessive-Compulsive Disorder Edna Foa Gail Steketee	181

PART II
TECHNIQUES

9	Cognitive-Behavioral Therapy Janet S. Klosko David H. Barlow	209
10	Psychoeducation Ronald M. Rapee Michelle Craske David H. Barlow	223
11	In Vivo Desensitization: Contextual Analysis Manuel D. Zane	237
12	In Vivo Desensitization: Anxiety Coping Techniques Jerilyn Ross	243
13	In Vivo Desensitization: Action and Talking Therapy Arthur Hardy	259
14	Imaginal Desensitization R. Reid Wilson	269
15	Breathing Control Jonathan H. Weiss	297

16	Bibliotherapy *Claire Weekes*	327
17	Marital Therapy *Steven Friedman*	339
18	Systems Therapy *Richard Platt*	365
19	Psychoanalytic Psychotherapy *Sander M. Abend*	393
20	Medication *Eric Hollander* *Donald F. Klein*	405

Index   427

Contributors

Sander M. Abend, M.D.
Private Practice
New York, NY

David H. Barlow, Ph.D.
Phobia and Anxiety Disorders
  Clinic, Center for Stress
  and Anxiety Disorders
State University of New York
  at Albany
Albany, NY

Aaron T. Beck, M.D.
University of Pennsylvania
  School of Medicine
Center for Cognitive Therapy
Philadelphia, PA

Dianne L. Chambless, Ph.D.
Agoraphobia and Anxiety
  Program
Temple University Medical
  Center
Bala Cynwyd, PA

Ronald E. Coleman, Ph.D.
Friends Hospital
Philadelphia, PA

Michelle Craske, Ph.D.
Phobia and Anxiety Disorders
  Clinic, Center for Stress
  and Anxiety Disorders
State University of New York
  at Albany
Albany, NY

Capt. T. W. Cummings
Freedom from Fear of Flying
Coral Gables, FL

Edna Foa, Ph.D.
Medical College of
  Pennsylvania at EPPI
Philadelphia, PA

xi

Steven Friedman, Ph.D.
Department of Psychiatry
State University of New York
Health Science Center at
   Brooklyn
New York, NY

Carol A. Gantman, Ph.D.
CG Associates-Psychological
   Healthcare
Bala Cynwyd, PA

Arthur Hardy, M.D.
Terrap Programs
Menlo Park, CA

Eric Hollander, M.D.
Obsessive Compulsive
   Disorder, Biological Studies
   Program
Department of Psychiatry
College of Physicians and
   Surgeons of Columbia
   University and the NYS
   Psychiatric Institute
New York, NY

Donald F. Klein, M.D.
Department of Psychiatry
College of Physicians and
   Surgeons of Columbia
   University and the NYS
   Psychiatric Institute
New York, NY

Janet S. Klosko, Ph.D.
Anxiety Disorder Clinic
New York Hospital-Cornell
   Medical Center
New York, NY

Harold S. Koplewicz, M.D.
Child and Adolescent
   Psychiatry
Long Island Jewish-Hillside
   Medical Center
Glen Oaks, NY

Ira M. Lesser, M.D.
Center for the Study and Care
   of Treatment Resistant
   Patients
Department of Psychiatry
UCLA School of Medicine
Harbor-UCLA Medical Center
Los Angeles, CA

Carol Lindemann, Ph.D.
Private Practice
New York, NY

Richard Platt, Ph.D.
Focus
Albany, NY

Ronald M. Rapee, Ph.D.
Phobia and Anxiety Disorders
   Clinic, Center for Stress
   and Anxiety Disorders
State University of New York
   at Albany
Albany, NY

Jerilyn Ross, M.A.
Roundhouse Square
  Psychiatric Center
Alexandria, VA

Gail Steketee, M.S.W.
Medical College of
  Pennsylvania at EPPI
Philadelphia, PA

Claire Weekes, M.B.E., M.D., F.R.A.C.P.
Rachel Forster Hospital
Sydney, Australia

Jonathan H. Weiss, Ph.D.
Private Practice
New York, NY

R. Reid Wilson, Ph.D.
Private Practice
Chapel Hill, NC

Manuel D. Zane, M.D.
Phobia Clinic
White Plains Hospital Medical
  Center
White Plains, NY

Preface

This book is written for the practitioner—psychologists, psychiatrists, social workers, and other mental health workers who treat anxiety disorders. The collection of chapters will provide the therapist with an orientation to the major theoretical and technical issues, and a concrete, working understanding of how a number of specific new techniques are applied.

For the psychotherapist, perhaps the most compelling aspect of these phobia treatments is their ability to rapidly bring significant improvement. The availability of (1) a set of specific interventions that can effect change in most people suffering from a specific complaint, together with (2) relatively precise knowledge of when and why to use these interventions, permanently changes one's perspective on therapy. Although many people seeking psychotherapy have general complaints, some seek therapy for specific, clearly delineated problems. For this latter group, exploratory psychotherapy often proves inefficient, and it can be argued that the patient is best served by therapy that provides rapid symptom relief.

For example, a person threatened with job loss because of phobic avoidance of a crucial segment of his job, or a person who has panic attacks and is too afraid to leave home alone may be eager for symptom relief rather than a prolonged treatment involving exploration of underlying factors. In the latter case, particularly, it is most beneficial to treat the panic disorder directly, before a consolidation of phobic avoidance and agoraphobia occurs. Psychodynamic factors can, if indicated, be explored after the crisis has abated. It is gratifying to both the therapist and patient when the therapist can say that he has treatment methods that have helped over 80% of people with similar problems.

Chapter 1 is a brief history of phobia therapy in the context of the evolutionary trends in general psychotherapy during the past fifteen years. Part I begins with Dr. Lesser's chapter on changes in the diagnostic understanding of anxiety disorders, setting the stage for the remainder of Part I, which then addresses the specific subtypes of anxiety disorder for which special techniques have been developed. Agoraphobia, certainly the most dramatic subtype, is seen most frequently. Generalized anxiety disorder, or what has been called free floating anxiety, is another common syndrome for which techniques are now available. Obsessive-compulsive disorder (to be distinguished from the obsessive-compulsive personality disorder) remains a difficult syndrome to treat. The simple phobias (those in which there is situation specific panic) are exemplified by fear of flying, and the social phobias are illustrated in the chapter on evaluation anxiety. The authors of these chapters advocate techniques that range from behavioral to psychoeducational, to an integration between dynamic and symptom-focused approaches.

Part II concentrates on technique, describing in detail components of the treatment program outlined in the first section, such as cognitive-behavioral therapy, desensitization, family therapy, hypnotherapy, psychoanalysis, and medication. The array of techniques described in this volume have certain similarities that may be helpful to bear in mind. The most consistent finding is that in any effective treatment program, the phobic person must reenter the phobic situation. The respective authors may vary in their strategies and procedures at three specific stages: how they prepare the patient to enter the phobic situation, what takes place in the situation itself, and how the experience is subsequently worked through.

Dr. Barlow and his colleagues present what is currently regarded as the most effective nonpsychopharmacological treatment. Their cognitive-behavioral therapy updates and further refines behavioral techniques and as of this writing, is considered state of the art. The components of the behavioral package are then explored in a series of chapters including psychoeducation, imaginal and in vivo desensitization, the control of hyperventilation, and anxiety coping techniques.

All of the technique chapters address, to some degree, all three phases of treatment. Some of the early programmatic approaches, such as those originated by Drs. Zane and Hardy, integrate all three aspects. Both use groups in their time-limited programs, often employing aides who are themselves former phobics. The groups first learn a body of structured information, then enter the phobic situations together with the support of others who understand their struggle. When the patient is in the phobic situation, a number of techniques help reduce the levels of anxiety. These are generally called *anxiety coping techniques*. Examples of these techniques are presented in the training manual excerpt by Jerilyn Ross. Some are developed to help the patient feel more in control when in the phobic situation. Some work by suggestion, others through changing the focus of attention. Paraprofessionals often specialize in the in vivo work. Imaginal desensitization is usually conducted in a traditional office setting as described by Reid Wilson.

The remaining chapters in Part II demonstrate broader-based techniques, often combining some behaviorism with other forms of therapy. As clinical practice has developed beyond the limits of the stricter behavioral orientation, phobia therapy has moved closer to general supportive psychotherapy, including employing some dynamic interventions. Phobia therapy is by no means synonymous with behavior therapy. Although it emerged primarily from behavior therapy, most therapists were skilled in using other therapeutic modalities before beginning to specialize in phobia therapy. They brought to the new task their experience with strategic, family, group, or psychodynamic therapy, modifying these approaches appropriately to suit the needs of the phobic patient.

With many patients, while the core of the treatment remains symptom focused, it proves impossible to ignore certain intrapsychic issues, of which resistance is a prime example, since to do so might otherwise impede progress. Furthermore, as certain patients begin to recover, they seem to want to discuss dynamic material: dreams, insight into the meaning of the symptoms, interpersonal dynamics maintaining the symptoms, and aggressive and libidinal conflicts. Many patients express a desire to know why they have experienced these problems.

Whether the future holds an increasing synthesis of techniques and levels of integration not yet imagined, is beyond our power to see at this juncture. The dramatic developments of the past two decades show no signs of leveling off. New research, broader clinical experience, and the work of innovative therapists promise many more advances. At this time, these pages represent the breadth of current methodologies available to treat this challenging group of patients.

Acknowledgments

This volume would not have been possible without the contributions of countless individuals who must remain anonymous, with whom I have worked over the years. I, and all the therapists whose papers are included in this collection, have learned from each of these people we have tried to help to overcome their problems. That wealth of clinical experience is the background of the ideas presented here. Every contributor joins me in hoping that the material here for your consideration leads to further improved skills and relief of patient suffering.

Among those whose help should be notably recognized, in addition to the authors whose papers are included in this volume, are the members and staff of the Phobia Society of America who have helped this project come to fruition. My publisher, Jay Aronson, deserves special thanks, since his firm belief in the value of this collection was a constant spur to my efforts. I am grateful to the Aronson staff, especially Dorothy Erstling, who managed this project from start to finish. I would also like to thank my colleagues at the Phobia Center of the New York Psychological Center, especially Harriet Dalin, Bess Goldenberg, and Frank Mosca. Their participation in the gradual development of these ideas over the course of the years we have worked together has been invaluable. My research assistant, Kim Finck, was greatly helpful in assembling the collection and in many other ways. Finally, a special expression of gratitude goes to my husband, Sander Abend, who has been so generous with his time and expertise as well as with his encouragement and support. His editorial judgment along with the excellence of the chapter he contributed have improved the book incalculably.

1 The Development of Phobia Therapy

Carol Lindemann

Phobia therapy is relatively new to the therapeutic field. It differs from previous therapies in several ways: (1) it focuses on a diagnostic category rather than on a theory or method, (2) it uses specific techniques that have been developed empirically, and (3) it makes symptom relief a primary goal rather than subordinating it to broader treatment goals.

Treatment of a specific diagnostic category is not new; therapeutic approaches to drug addiction and alcoholism are of that nature. Other examples are Masters and Johnson's work, from which emerged specific therapies for sexual disorders, and the treatment of eating disorders. The development of highly effective treatments for specific disorders is the primary cause of this new special syndrome orientation. Earlier, all these disorders were approached with the same general psychotherapy techniques.

This chapter traces the developments in research and theory that made possible the new approach to treating phobias.

DEPARTURE FROM FREUDIAN ORIENTATION

Freud, together with the variety of psychoanalytic schools to which his work gave rise, remains the chief source of a comprehensive general theory of psychology. Phobia therapy represents a departure from a Freudian theoretical orientation, being based primarily on pragmatic considerations of "what works." Contributors from disparate orientations—behavioral, psychopharmacological, and psychodynamic—converged in their interest in treating anxiety. This diverse group, despite considerable jostling for dominance of one contributor over another, has developed a broadly eclectic treatment orientation employing a unique blend of techniques. The initial lack of a theory that might give cohesion to this body of therapy techniques is rapidly being remedied as new information emerges.

The idea of symptom relief without attention to underlying dynamics initially evoked strong doubts among the psychodynamically oriented community. Pessimistic predictions of symptom substitution, and of psychological decompensation after symptom removal, however, turned out to be groundless. On the contrary, successful symptom removal has been found in general to lead to increased self-esteem, assertiveness, feelings of well being, and improved levels of functioning in patients who experience it. This finding has stimulated the promotion of symptom-focused psychotherapy, as well as encouraging a shift of emphasis toward discernible change through psychotherapeutic treatment.

NEW DIAGNOSTIC CLASSIFICATION OF ANXIETY DISORDERS

In a very brief period the new work in phobias and related anxiety disorders has gained such importance that it has spurred a complete revision of the diagnostic classification of anxiety in the *Diagnostic and Statistical Manual* (DSM-III and DSM-III-R).

Because panic disorder is now seen as a physiological as well as a psychological phenomenon, the research accompanying the development of this new field has been on the cutting edge of psychobiology. Anxiety, as a major component of psychological life, has always been of primary importance, but the new ability to treat the symptoms quickly and successfully has made this a hot new topic.

FREUDIAN APPROACH

Freudian theory, which provides the historical foundation for our understanding of psychopathology, must be the point of departure for a review of the new understanding of anxiety disorders. In *Studies in Hysteria* (Freud and Breuer 1895) Freud described the role of repressed traumatic memories in the development of such symptoms as hysterical paralysis and phobias. In later revisions of his theory of anxiety and symptom formation he determined that unconscious fantasies as well as actual trauma were pathogenic. His technique was to understand with the patient the unconscious conflicts connected with those experiences and fantasies, relieving the symptoms through conscious recognition and resolution of unconscious irrational elements.

Freud's goal, however, soon shifted from symptom removal, to the development of an understanding of how symptoms were formed and the elaboration of a general theory of psychopathology. His study of Little Hans (Freud 1909) still serves as a model for the psychoanalytic understanding and treatment of phobias. Little Hans had a fear of horses, and he resisted going out on the street where horses and carriages were numerous. Freud understood Hans's phobia in terms of an oedipal conflict that activated the defenses of denial, displacement, and projection. In this case, an understanding of unconscious conflicts and their resolution led to the disappearance of the symptom.

Although much of the early psychoanalytic literature emphasized oedipal conflicts in the development of phobias, more recently an equal emphasis has been placed on separation anxiety as pathogenic. For example, Frances and Dunn (1975) speak of agoraphobia as an attachment-autonomy conflict and understand the disorder in terms of object theory while minimizing the significance of infantile sexuality.

Freud discouraged symptom removal without an understanding of the intrapsychic conflicts involved because of the danger of symptom substitution. Theoretically, the symptom serves a purpose as an expression of psychic conflicts, and, as such, it plays a part in maintaining the psychic balance. If abruptly removed, it might be replaced with a less adaptive symptom. Further, as psychoanalytic theory has developed, symptoms and anxiety are seen as motivating the patient toward treatment and as indicating the areas where unconscious problems that require further exploration are to be found. Freud was fond of saying that "the better is always the enemy of the good" (Freud 1937, p. 231), meaning that too early a relief of distressing symptoms might lead patients to drop treatment before more extensive solutions were achieved. The analytic posture recommends that understanding the workings of the patient's mind be the goal, and that beneficial change be a secondary consequence of that process, albeit a desirable one.

It is not possible to take an analytic stance of trying to achieve understanding with symptom change as a byproduct, and at the same time have as a goal the rapid modification of symptoms. Further, the analytic viewpoint that phobias are based on underlying conflicts, and that avoidance of the phobic situation is a symbolic avoidance and fulfillment of the conflicted impulse, directs the therapist to look away from the patient's concrete conscious experience of distress. On the experiential level, phobics understand their avoidance to be of the terrifying feelings that are experienced in the phobic situation. The phobic claims he is reluctant to walk the street, fly on a plane, or eat in a restaurant because he fears those situations will cause panic. Only rarely does he have, or is he interested in gaining insight: he wants simply to be rid of the debilitating anxiety.

BEHAVIORIAL APPROACH

From an entirely different perspective, the behaviorists' explanation of phobic symptom formation is based on the theory of conditioned learning. The learning theorists have attacked the disease model of mental illness. Psychic pain, or symptom formation, need not be thought of as indicating an underlying dynamic cause in the psychic structure parallel to the relationship between physical pain and the underlying cause of infection, inflammation, or injury. The behaviorists have been especially interested in phobias because a phobia can be induced experimentally and then successfully treated (Watson and Rayner 1920, Jones 1924), thus serving as a perfect model of experimental psychopathology. Wolpe's *desensitization* was the first treatment based on learning theory to gain wide acceptance in the psychotherapy of phobias. The crux of the theory is *reciprocal inhibition*: "If a response antagonistic to anxiety can be made to occur in the presence of anxiety-evoking stimuli . . . the bond between these stimuli and the anxiety responses will be weakened" (Wolpe 1958, p. 71).

Desensitization, also called counterconditioning or deconditioning, is derived from classical conditioning. Pavlov's (1927) classical conditioning model, it will be remembered, is as follows: The dog is given food and salivates, the sound of the bell is presented a few seconds before the food, and the dog becomes conditioned to salivate at the sound of the bell. The application of the classical conditioning model to phobias runs as follows: A panic attack occurs, for reasons unspecified, in the elevator. The person, on the basis of a "one trial learning," becomes conditioned to have a fear response when in the elevator. Reciprocal inhibition of this response means pairing a competing response, such as relaxation, with the elevator repeatedly until the fear response is "deconditioned." In practice, this is accomplished by relaxing the patient through the Jacobson technique (Jacobson 1938) of progressively tensing and relaxing muscle groups. When the patient is fully relaxed, a hierarchy of images of feared situations is presented verbally. For example, an elevator phobic might be told to imagine, first, stepping off an elevator after a successful short ride; next, standing in an elevator with the door open. The top of the hierarchy might be imagining being stuck in a small crowded elevator. When the patient can remain fully relaxed while contemplating each feared event, the next step of the hierarchy is presented. For maximum effectiveness, where feasible, this hierarchy is then repeated in the situation itself (in vivo).

MODERN PSYCHOBIOLOGICAL APPROACH

Panic attacks are a measurable psychophysiological event. The modern history of the treatment of anxiety disorders is firmly grounded in psychobiological research and the use of psychotropic medication. Klein presented the first major breakthrough in the psychopharmacological treatment of anxiety disorders in his paper on the effective use of the tricyclic antidepressant, imipramine (Tofranil) (Klein and Fink 1962). At first this discovery raised more questions than it answered. Why did antidepressants help anxiety? Anxiety and depression theoretically were distinctly different emotions: Were they functionally the same? What was the common basis? What were the site of action and the mode of action? Some of these questions are now answered.

Separation Anxiety

In early speculations (Klein and Fink 1962) the panic reaction was explained in terms of the separation anxiety model as elaborated by Bowlby (1960). The initial reaction of infants separated from their mother is marked by crying and the increased motoric activity of anxiety, followed later on by the reduced activity and vocalization associated with states of anaclitic depression. The initial phase is thought to be genetically programmed in mammals as a search for the mother who has lost or abandoned the infant. This theory provided a teleological reason for the existence of panic in all mammals. The second phase is parallel to depression, indicating a substantial link between these two experientially different emotions. Separation anxiety as a core issue in agoraphobia has been emphasized in psychoanalytic studies (for example, Frances and Dunn 1975). The idea also spurred considerable research in separation anxiety as a component of panic disorders, but studies have not confirmed that a higher-than-expected number of agoraphobics have early separation experiences (Buglass et al. 1977). There may be, rather, individual differences in the propensity to react with separation anxiety to separation experiences (Bowlby 1973).

Blocking Panic Attacks

To return to the biochemical understanding pioneered by Klein, imipramine was thought to block panic attacks. Phobic patients on an adequate dosage reported that they felt a rising panic, just as before, but that the subsequent full-blown panic they were accustomed to experiencing no longer appeared. The hypothesized explanation derived from learning theory is that the person avoids the emotional experience of anxiety associated with being in the phobic situation, rather than the situation itself. The medication permits the phobic to enter the phobic situation without fear of panics, once he learns they are effectively blocked.

Anticipatory Anxiety

For several years hope was high that medication alone would be an effective treatment for phobias. Many medicated patients did overcome their former phobic avoidance, but a number did not. Despite assurance that they would not panic, they stubbornly refused to enter the phobic situation. A new concept to explain such cases developed: that of *anticipatory anxiety* (Klein 1964)—the anxiety experienced at the thought or other symbolic representation of the phobic situation. In the elevator phobia, for example, the thought of entering an elevator is believed to cause the person to anticipate that a panic will again occur there, and consequently anxiety begins merely by thinking of approaching an elevator. Further, the patient fears that panic might occur under circumstances in which help is not available, such as being alone and far from home, and this anticipation leads to phobic restrictions.

New Distinctions within Anxieties

The finding that imipramine blocks the panic attack, but does not affect the anticipatory anxiety, leads to the speculation that panic and anxiety are different. While they may be experienced as if they were on a continuum, the two affects are thought to differ physiologically (Klein and Fink 1962). The medications frequently found to be useful for reducing anticipatory anxiety are those in the benzodiazepine group (such as Valium). The treatment protocol that was initially developed treated the panic attacks with antidepressant medication, conjointly treating any residual avoidance attributed to anticipatory anxiety with minor tranquilizers and desensitization. Treatment for anticipatory anxiety currently relies less on tranquilizers because therapy techniques are more sophisticated. New developments in medications have changed the options for treating the anxiety disorders considerably (see Chapter 20).

Spontaneous Panic Attacks

In a further refinement, it was found that imipramine is far more effective with agorapobics than with certain simple phobics, such as animal phobics. The panic of agoraphobics often occurs spontaneously, for no apparent reason (Zitrin et al. 1975), rather than exclusively and inevitably when patients are in the phobic situation. Imipramine may be specifically effective in blocking these spontaneous attacks. The concept of a spontaneous panic attack was slow to gain acceptance, especially by clinicians who retain a preference for purely psychological, rather than biochemical explanations for psychological events. The observation of what appeared to be spontaneous attacks, however, led to the idea that some forms of panic have no external antecedent and may be purely physiological events. Klein's idea that these can be differentiated by the response to medication supports the view that they constitute specific syndromes. The terms *panic disorder* and *anxiety disorder* have now emerged in common parlance. What is treated is no longer merely a symptom, but one or another syndrome, and *phobia clinics* have become renamed *anxiety disorder clinics*.

Locating the Brain's Panic Center

The concept of the panic as a physiological discharge soon led to two new ideas: (1) there is a specific panic center in the brain; (2) despite the subjective emotional experience of panic, the event is physiological or biochemical in origin.

The panic center was hypothesized to have a physical location in the brain, and the limbic system and locus ceruleus are now identified as most likely contenders. Most important, the panic response involves deep brain structures rather than being an event of the cerebral cortex. The trigger mechanism appears to be altered in panic disorder, turning into a hair trigger, which fires more frequently or more readily. The panic response is also thought to be an innate, genetically determined discharge phenomenon, which follows a pattern that is relatively consistent for each person, although differing slightly from one individual to the next. Progress in research on the physical and biochemical mechanism of panic continues at a rapid pace, promising increasingly effective psychotropic medication.

CURRENT INTEGRATIVE APPROACH

Inherent in the assumption of the primacy of emotional-physiological discharge in the etiology of the panic attack is the idea that the phobia is not necessarily mediated by conscious or unconscious thought, nor must it necessarily have symbolic meaning or affective displacement. The panic attack *precedes* the thought. In 1890 William James had expressed a similar hypothesis. James's theory of emotionality reversed the notion that you run from a bear because you feel afraid: actually, you see the bear, you run, then you feel afraid. If the emotional experience of fear really follows, rather than precedes the physical expression of the emotion, then if you change the expression, you may change the subjective feeling of the emotional state. On a very simple observational level this theory appears to hold true. For example, the act of running out of a phobic situation makes many phobics feel more panicky. If one is able to induce the patient to remain in the phobic situation, the anxiety will often gradually diminish.

Dr. Aaron Beck's (1985) very popular new theory and therapeutic interventions, cognitive restructuring, is compatible with these ideas, although he begins from a different theoretical basis. He advocates inducing the patient to change the thought in order to change the experience. For the elevator phobic, for example, the thought "I will surely panic if I am stuck in an elevator" is more likely to produce anxiety than is the thought "I can cope with whatever emerges." Beck's elaborations on this theme together with the subtleties of technique, have rapidly penetrated the field of phobia therapy.

Skinner has asserted that the mind is a black box that can be known only indirectly through behavior. Cognitive theory has given the behaviorists a vehicle in which to emerge from the black box and investigate mental events as trial behaviors. The psychodynamic community has similarly become more accepting of behaviorism in recognition of the effectiveness of the treatment. The psychopharmacologist has become integrated into the treatment team, and conversely, begun to accept the effectiveness of phobia therapy.

In summary, the treatment of anxiety disorders embodies a highly effective group of symptom focused techniques, applied to specific diagnostic categories. It blends innovations in psychotropic medication, behavioral pragmatism, and the eclecticism of recent years. Exploration of the variety of therapeutic approaches has led to promising new ideas about the nature of anxiety and panic. Cross-fertilization is increasingly in evidence as data gathered from one approach informs and stimulates research and therapy from other vantage points.

REFERENCES

American Psychiatric Association, Committee on Nomenclature and Statistics (1980). *Diagnostic and Statistical Manual of Mental Disorders* (3rd ed.). Washington, DC: APA.

American Psychiatric Association, Committee on Nomenclature and Statistics (1987). *Diagnostic and Statistical Manual of Mental Disorders* (3rd ed. rev.). Washington, DC: APA.

Beck, A. T., and Emery, G. (1985). *Anxiety Disorders and Phobias: A Cognitive Perspective.* New York: Basic Books.

Bowlby, J. (1960). Separation anxiety. *International Journal of Psycho-Analysis* 41:89–113.

―――― (1973). *Separation.* New York: Basic Books.

Buglass, D., Clark, J., Henderson, A. S., et al. (1977). A study of agoraphobic housewives. *Psychological Medicine* 7:73–86.

Frances, A., and Dunn, P. (1975). The attachment–autonomy conflict in agoraphobia. *International Journal of Psycho-Analysis* 10:435–439.

Freud, S. (1909). Analysis of a phobia in a five-year-old boy. *Standard Edition* 10:5–149.

Freud, S. (1937). Analysis terminable and interminable. *Standard Edition* 23:209–254.

Freud, S., and Breuer, J. (1895). *Studies in Hysteria.* New York: Avon Books, 1966.

Jacobson, E. (1938). *Progressive Relaxation*. Chicago: University of Chicago Press.

James, W. (1890). *The Principles of Psychology*. New York: Henry Holt.

Jones, M. C. (1924). Elimination of children's fears. *Journal of Experimental Psychology* 7:382.

Klein, D. F. (1964). Delineation of two drug-responsive anxiety syndromes. *Psychopharmacologia* 53:397–408.

Klein, D. F., and Fink, M. (1962). Psychiatric reaction patterns to imipramine. *American Journal of Psychiatry* 119:432–438.

Pavlov, I. P. (1927). *Conditioned Reflexes*. London: Oxford University Press.

Watson, J. B., and Rayner, P. (1920). Conditioned emotional reactions. *Journal of Experimental Psychology* 3:1.

Wolpe, J. (1958). *Psychotherapy by Reciprocal Inhibition*. Stanford: Stanford University Press.

Zitrin, C. M., Klein, D. F., Lindemann, C., et al. (1975). Comparison of short-term treatment regimens in phobic patients: A preliminary report. In *Evaluation of Psychological Therapies*, ed. R. L. Spitzer and D. F. Klein, pp. 233–250. Baltimore: The Johns Hopkins Press.

PART I

Specific Anxiety Disorders

2 Diagnosing Anxiety

Dr. Lesser's scholarly introduction to diagnosis is essential to orient the new clinician to this field, as there has been considerable recent modification in the classification of anxiety disorders. The primary change is that the anxiety disorders are now clustered together as a diagnostic category; previously they were grouped mainly under the "psychoneuroses." A second change follows from this regrouping, in that the dynamic implication of "neurosis" is no longer present in the diagnostic category. Instead, the main defining characteristics are the presence of panic symptoms and of overt behaviors, such as phobic avoidance.

Diagnosing Anxiety

Ira M. Lesser

In the past two decades anxiety disorders have received increasing attention from clinicians, researchers, and the lay public. Awareness has grown that as a group, anxiety disorders constitute the most common psychiatric disorders in the population (Robins et al. 1984, Regier et al. 1988), causing considerable morbidity, but remaining vastly undertreated.

Are we, as has been suggested, living in an "age of anxiety" such that more people suffer from anxiety disorders? Are these illnesses, now christened with new names, really different from those described a century ago? Have an increase in diagnostic acumen, a new nomenclature, and an effective armamentarium of treatments all converged to bring more people into treatment? Does the DSM-III-R (American Psychiatric Association 1987), our most current diagnostic system, adequately separate out the variety of anxiety disorders—and, further, to what degree is this separation necessary for effective treatment planning? These questions need to be examined in evaluating diagnostic considerations in anxiety disorders.

This chapter provides an overview of diagnostic issues in anxiety disorders, with an emphasis on the panic disorders. It presents clinical material relevant to differentiating panic disorder from other psychiatric disorders and from medical disorders, bolstered by research findings from clinical investigations. Treatment considerations, although beyond the scope of this chapter and covered in depth elsewhere, are addressed as they are pertinent to the issues of diagnosis and subclassification.

HISTORICAL PERSPECTIVE

Clinical descriptions of anxiety attacks and phobias have been noted for centuries and display a startling similarity to each other. In the seventeenth century Robert Burton wrote in *The Anatomy of Melancholy* (1964):

> [T]his fear causeth in man, as to be red, pale, tremble, sweat; it makes sudden cold and heat to come over all the body, palpitation of the heart, syncope, etc. . . . it confounds voice and memory. . . . Many men are so amazed and astonished with fear, they know not where they are, what they say, what they do . . . and it makes their hearts ache, sad and heavy. They that live in fear, are never free, resolute, secure, never merry, but in continual pain. . . . Fear makes our imagination conceive what it list, invites the devil to come to us . . . and tyrannizeth over our phantasy more than all other afflictions, especially in the dark.

This literary and eloquent description includes most of the salient features of panic disorder, replete with symptoms of the attacks themselves, the anticipatory anxiety, and the depression that so commonly accompanies panic attacks.

Almost surely the equivalent of panic disorder, seen during the Civil War and described in cardiac terms, was Da Costa's syndrome. Patients with this syndrome were described as having precordial pains, palpitations, and giddiness, all occurring during rest or during slight exertion. Da Costa, a military physician, concluded: "It seems to me most likely that the heart has become irritable, from its overaction and frequent excitement, and that disordered innervation keeps it so" (Da Costa 1871). A focus on the physical, primarily cardiac symptoms of this disorder was maintained over the next half-century, and it was variously called *irritable heart, soldier's heart, effort syndrome, disordered action of the heart*, and *neurocirculatory asthenia*.

Descriptions of panic attacks were not confined to the medical or cardiac literature. Pierre Janet (1898) described the case of a woman who "experiences phenomena that are always identical: She senses a tightness in her throat along with a desire to cry, and feels suffocated and labored breathing as in an attack of asthma. Her stomach and lower abdomen become distended, she trembles, has palpitations, and breaks into a cold sweat, etc. Simultaneously, her thoughts become vague and seem to escape her. She is afraid of something without knowing what it is. The attack generally lasts for a short time, a half hour or so. . . ." Freud, too, gave classic descriptions of anxiety attacks, which he described as often being superimposed upon the more chronic manifestations of anxiety. He stated, "I call this syndrome 'anxiety neurosis' because all its components can be grouped around the chief symptom of anxiety" (Freud 1895).

For centuries, then, clinicians from both medicine and psychiatry have recognized the existence of dramatic episodes of anxiety that have both cognitive and physiological components. Naturally, when examined by medical practitioners, the focus and label given to the syndrome reflected the physical manifestations (e.g., irritable heart); when seen by psychiatrists, the psychological symptoms were highlighted (e.g., anxiety neurosis). Although this changing nomenclature has caused confusion over the years, the existence of such a syndrome has really never been questioned.

CURRENT DIAGNOSTIC PRACTICES

A major shift in classification of the anxiety disorders occurred with the publication of DSM-III (American Psychiatric Association 1980). The DSM-II category of "anxiety neurosis" had been quite heterogenous, with no distinctions being made between acute attacks and chronic manifestations of anxiety. Reflecting the principles governing the transition from DSM-II to DSM-III, the anxiety disorders were divided up into several disorders, eliminating the more general category of "neurosis." This change also signified a move away from reliance upon the concept of unconscious conflict as the etiological basis of anxiety. The current classification system was greatly influenced by the work of researchers in the field of anxiety, notably Donald Klein and colleagues (Klein 1964, 1980; Klein et al. 1987). Klein noted that when the antidepressant imipramine was given to extremely anxious and phobic patients, their acute episodes of anxiety dramatically lessened, although their chronic behavior pattern was barely altered. He developed the concept that these patients suffered from two phenomenologically distinct types of anxiety: acute panic attacks, and more general or chronic anxiety, which developed in anticipation of having another panic attack. Their phobic behavior and avoidance were seen as attempts to avoid further attacks by not entering situations where an attack was thought likely to occur or where, if one did occur, it would be difficult to receive help.

In DSM-III, the more acute, episodic type of anxiety was recognized as *panic disorder* (*PD*). On the other hand, patients with chronic anxiety but without panic attacks were classified as having *generalized anxiety disorder* (*GAD*). In addition, for those patients who had considerable phobic avoidance, the category *agoraphobia with panic attacks* was created and grouped with the phobic disorders. *Agoraphobia without panic attacks* also was designated as a separate category, although many researchers feel it is rare for agoraphobia to develop in the absence of a history of at least one panic attack. Completing the anxiety-disorder section are the diagnoses of *simple phobia*, *social phobia*, *obsessive-compulsive disorder*, *post-traumatic stress disorder*, and *atypical anxiety disorder*.

DSM-III-R (American Psychiatric Association 1987) has once again modified the classification of anxiety disorders (see Table 2–1), although the changes are more modest. Investigators were

TABLE 2-1 DSM-III Classification of Anxiety Disorders

Panic disorder with agoraphobia
Panic disorder without agoraphobia
Agoraphobia without history of panic disorder
Social phobia
Simple phobia
Obsessive-compulsive disorder
Post-traumatic stress disorder
Generalized anxiety disorder
Anxiety disorder NOS

---

uncomfortable with the DSM-III convention of classifying agoraphobia as part of the phobias and putting panic disorder in a separate category. Therefore, in DSM-III-R, the primacy of the panic attack, or of panic disorder, is strengthened even more, with agoraphobic symptoms being listed as consequences of the PD. Also, the clinician may now rate the severity of the avoidance behavior. Once again, there is a category for agoraphobia without panic attacks. The remaining categories stay much the same as in DSM-III, although the time criterion for GAD has been increased from one month to six months of continuous symptoms. This last change was made in hopes of further refining the diagnosis of GAD to include only those patients with chronic anxiety and eliminate cases where the anxiety may be more of a response to an external stressor.

The symptoms necessary for the diagnosis of a panic attack are listed in Table 2-2. At least four of these symptoms must be present during at least some of the attacks. As can be seen, the majority of these symptoms are physical—for example, cardiac, respiratory, neurological, or related to discharge of the sympathetic nervous system. Only two have a cognitive component: fear of dying, or fear of going crazy and losing control. To meet criteria for PD, the patient must have either four of these attacks in a four-week period, or one or more attacks followed by at least a month of persistent fear of having another attack. In addition, at least one of these attacks must occur in the absence of exposure

TABLE 2-2 Symptoms of a Panic Attack

Shortness of breath or smothering sensation
Choking sensation
Dizziness or faintness
Palpitations and/or rapid heart rate
Chest pain or discomfort
Trembling or shaking
Numbness or tingling sensation (paresthesia)
Sweating
Flushes or chills
Nausea or abdominal distress
Depersonalization or derealization
Fear of dying
Fear of going crazy or doing something uncontrolled

to a specific situation that would always cause anxiety (a "spontaneous" as opposed to a "situational" attack), and the attack must not be triggered by situations where the patient was the focus of others' attention (to differentiate PD from social phobia).

A panic attack, especially the first one, is a dramatic event, which patients recount in exquisite detail. They often will recall the exact date, time, place, and circumstance of their initial attack. For most patients, especially those who had been previously healthy, this event "occurs out of the blue" and "hits them like a ton of bricks," leaving them perplexed and worried about their health and safety. It is not clear why some patients can have recurrent panic attacks without developing overwhelming anticipatory anxiety and phobic avoidance, while others are almost immediately disabled. Certainly, one would suspect that premorbid personality factors would influence the course, but in some patients the illness seems to have a particular virulence that is difficult to explain.

Panic disorder can be subtyped according to the degree of phobic avoidance the patient experiences. This may range from none to extreme avoidance. Severe degrees of phobic avoidance may result in patients who are housebound, but this is not a necessary condition for diagnosing agoraphobia. Rather, agoraphobia is diagnosed when the phobic avoidance is so great that leaving home alone is difficult or endured with dread, companions often are necessary for travel, and activities outside of home are restricted. Indeed, these less severe, though still limiting and disabling, degrees of phobic avoidance are more common than total inability to leave home.

Although DSM-III-R is now the standard manual for psychiatric classification in the United States, some investigators find the section on anxiety disorders far from satisfactory. Sheehan and Sheehan (1982) suggested that a more clinically relevant distinction could be made by using the concepts of endogenous and exogenous anxiety. *Endogenous anxiety* refers to the spontaneous, autonomous episodes of anxiety that patients often refer to as coming totally out of the blue. For these attacks, there are no identifiable external stressors or situations that would always elicit a fear response. *Exogenous anxiety* refers to attacks that occur in response to an immediate, clear-cut, identifiable environmental stimulus. These two types of anxiety are presented as dichotomous, having a different clinical picture and a different response to treatment. For example, the endogenous anxiety responds to biological interventions, while the exogenous is more responsive to psychosocial modalities. Furthermore, "under the new scheme, distinctions between anxiety hysteria, conversion hysteria, anxiety neurosis, panic disorder, generalized anxiety, hypochondriacal neurosis, depersonalization neurosis, and psychosomatic symptoms become unnecessary and are subsumed under either of these two major categories" (Sheehan and Sheehan 1982).

In a series of papers Tyrer (1984, 1985, 1986) echoed some of Sheehan's concerns, especially regarding the indistinct boundaries and high degree of symptom overlap of the various anxiety disorders in DSM-III. As further evidence against the usefulness of the current diagnostic system, he also cited the lack of data regarding stability of diagnoses over time, the absence of clearcut differences in outcome, and the lack of treatment specific for each disorder. He proposed instead a "general neurotic syndrome," which would be diagnosed if there was a combination of symptoms of agoraphobia, panic disorder, social phobia, nonpsychotic depression, anxiety, and hypochondriasis; if at least one episode of illness occurred in the absence of external stressors; if there was an abnormal personality of the passive-dependent or anankastic type; and if there was a history of a similar syndrome in a first-degree relative. (At least three of these four criteria would have to be met.)

Foa and co-authors (1984), working from a behavioral and cognitive perspective, argued for a classification system based on the nature of the symptoms and their perceived source. Thus, they described external cues (e.g., specific situations associated with anxiety), internal cues (physiologic symptoms such as a panic attack), anticipated harm (fears of catastrophic events such as heart attacks or strokes), and degree of avoidance responses. This system would analyze behaviors functionally along these dimensions, and perhaps it would relate more closely to specific treatment interventions.

Given that the "modern" classification of anxiety disorders is only about a decade old, it seems both reasonable and healthy that blind acceptance of it is far from universal. As with classification in general, the system must be put to the test as more data and clinical material are collected regarding course, family incidence, comorbidity, stability over time, response to treatment, and biological and genetic factors.

DIFFERENTIAL DIAGNOSIS AMONG THE ANXIETY DISORDERS

Examination of classification systems makes it obvious that there are no absolute boundaries between the specific anxiety disorders, and that significant numbers of patients have components of several of these illnesses. Considerable work has been conducted to differentiate among these disorders, not only in terms of symptoms but from genetic, family-history, biologic, and treatment-response perspectives.

DSM-III utilized the concept of diagnostic hierarchies, whereby certain diagnoses would not be made if the symptoms occurred during the course of another disorder. Thus, panic disorder occurring during a major depression would not merit an independent diagnosis. However, data to support many of these hierarchies was lacking (Boyd et al. 1984), and in DSM-III-R the use of diagnostic hierarchies was largely curtailed. However, among the anxiety disorders, there remain instances where symptoms of one disorder may be subsumed by another disorder and not diagnosed independently. For instance, in the natural progression of panic disorder, a patient may have spontaneous (unexpected) panic attacks and then often develop simple phobias (where a particular stimulus always causes a fearful response), social phobias (where the individual fears being the object of others' scrutiny), obsessive thoughts about having another panic attack, and high levels of intercurrent or anticipatory anxiety. This patient would not have five separate anxiety disorders, but only PD with agoraphobia. The diagnostic criteria for the other anxiety disorders state that the symptoms are not exclusively related to the panic disorder. Thus for GAD "the focus of the worry is not about having a panic attack"; for simple phobia and for social phobia "the persistent fear is other than having a panic attack."

As noted above, the diagnosis of PD requires at least one of the panic attacks to be spontaneous, or unexpected. It can occur as a total surprise to the patient or in a situation where he may be uneasy but might or might not experience full-blown panic. This unexpected attack is distinguished from a situational panic attack, which occurs in the context of a situation that invariably causes the anxiety. In fact, this distinction forms the core of the current system of classification. Though at times easy to make, it depends to some degree upon the patient's powers of observation and attribution. There is little in the way of physiological data to support the distinction (although, of course, it is very difficult to study the physiological responses of an "unexpected" event). Investigations are under way to test the hypotheses that the spontaneous attack will respond preferentially to medication, while the situational attack may need the addition of behavioral psychotherapy for an adequate response, and that resolution of the spontaneous attacks should occur prior to that of the situational ones.

A number of investigators have sought to clarify the clinical distinctions among the separate anxiety disorders. Noyes et al. (1987) divided patients with PD into those with no phobic avoidance, limited avoidance, and extensive avoidance (agoraphobia). Apart from the obvious difference in phobic symptoms, there were very few meaningful clinical or demographic differences among the groups. The group with the most extensive phobic symptoms was judged to be most severely ill. These investigators concluded that patients with PD suffer from one illness, regardless of the degree of phobic avoidance. Similar findings were reported (Thyer et al. 1985) where the only symptom differences between patients with agoraphobia and those with panic disorder and no avoidance were in phobic anxiety, paranoid ideation, and interpersonal sensitivity. Agoraphobic patients also reported more alcohol intake and had fewer periods of remission. Thyer and Himle (1987) compared panic-attack symptoms of patients with PD to symptoms reported by patients with simple phobias on exposure to their feared stimulus. They reported that the intensity of symptoms was significantly greater in the PD group and that there was a different pattern of symptoms between the groups—that is, the groups shared only 30% of the variance in symptom rankings.

A recent study (Steketee et al. 1987) compared characteristics of patients with obsessive-compulsive disorder (OCD) with patients having other anxiety disorders. OCD patients demonstrated not only more obsessionality, but also more depression and interpersonal discomfort, as well as more childhood psychiatric symptoms than any other group. Cameron and co-authors

(1986) also reported that the OCD group differed most from those with the other anxiety disorders. Symptom-severity profiles were similar in patients with PD, agoraphobia, and GAD and were more severe than those seen in the other anxiety disorders. On the other hand, social and simple phobias had relatively distinct symptom patterns.

In sum, there is reasonable agreement that grouping the anxiety disorders together has merit, but within this group several disorders share considerable symptom overlap. This has clearly been shown between PD and obsessive-compulsive symptoms (Mellman and Uhde 1987) and between PD, agoraphobia, and GAD (Uhde et al. 1984, Barlow et al. 1986). Using response to treatment as a validating criterion for diagnostic distinctions is potentially misleading, but there is a possible differential treatment response among the various disorders. Simple and social phobias traditionally have been treated in a behavioral paradigm with little use of medications (although recent work on social phobia suggests medications may have a role [Liebowitz et al. 1985]); PD with or without avoidance behavior responds well to antidepressant medications and to some benzodiazepines; GAD responds to benzodiazepines and perhaps to some antidepressants; and OCD responds poorly to most modalities, though perhaps responding best to the antidepressant, clomipramine. Because the etiology of each of these disorders remains enigmatic, it is unlikely that a definite resolution of these complex relationships is at hand.

DIFFERENTIATION OF PANIC DISORDER FROM OTHER PSYCHIATRIC DISORDERS

Despite its myriad symptoms, in its pure form there should be little problem distinguishing panic disorder from other psychiatric illnesses. Certainly, patients with PD, though extremely anxious, do not display psychotic symptoms nor have a formal thought disorder. However, as Klein (1980) pointed out, it was only 25 years ago that "in the feckless habit of the time, they were then labeled schizophrenic because they had marked social impairment and severe symptoms." If there is a marked degree of phobic avoidance, the patient's overt behavior may appear similar to that of the patient with paranoid delusions. This distinction can be made by ascertaining the reasons for their not leaving home. Patients with PD fear having a panic attack outside of their home or their "safety zone"; this is in marked contrast to having a delusional belief about external forces causing them harm. The patient with PD often fears losing control or doing something "crazy," but there is not the actual fragmentation of the self as seen in schizophrenic disorders. Severely agoraphobic individuals may not function much better than a schizophrenic patient, but the symptoms and the explanation of their behavior should allow for distinguishing between these disorders.

As noted above, a number of nonpsychotic diagnoses, especially those in the somatoform group, share symptoms with PD. Patients with recurrent panic attacks and high levels of intercurrent anxiety may experience multiple physical symptoms in a variety of body systems, making the diagnosis of somatization disorder a possibility. Indeed, historically, the diagnosis of hysteria might have been applied to many of these patients. Alternatively, the patients may focus upon one symptom, such as palpitations or dizziness, with a tenacious conviction that there is something terribly wrong. In this case, confusion with hypochondriasis may occur. The important element to focus upon is not the presence of physical symptoms, but the crescendolike, dramatic anxiety of panic attack, which typically is not present in either of these somatoform disorders.

Depersonalization experiences are noted by some patients during a panic attack, although this is not one of the more common symptoms. If present, it occurs only during an attack and is accompanied by a host of other, more typical symptoms as detailed above. If the depersonalization is the sole or the most prominent symptom, then one could consider depersonalization disorder in the differential diagnosis. DSM-III explicitly states that depersonalization disorder should not be diagnosed in the context of panic disorder with or without agoraphobia.

The relationship of PD to depression is perplexing. Views range from their being variants of the same illness to their being separate illnesses altogether (Stavrakaki and Vargo 1986, Lesser 1988). Part of this confusion stems from their shared comorbidity. It has been estimated that two-thirds of patients with panic disorder will have an episode of major depression sometime during their life (Breier et al. 1986), with from 30% to 50% of patients developing a major depression after the onset of their panic disorder (secondary depression) (Lesser et al. 1988a).

A number of studies using discrimination-function and principal-component analyses (Gurney et al. 1972, Roth et al. 1972, Schapira et al. 1972, Mountjoy and Roth 1982) have reported that major depression and anxiety disorders can be differentiated by symptom picture. The symptoms that discriminated best between the two were (for depression) diurnal variation, early morning awakening, and psychomotor retardation and (for anxiety disorders) panic attacks, agoraphobia, depersonalization, derealization, and perceptual distortions.

In clinical practice, it may be quite easy to make the distinction. Some patients are quite adamant that they are not depressed, and they have none of the typical symptoms associated with depressive illness. Other patients who admit to having depressive symptoms will state clearly, "I am depressed because I have these attacks, and I can't go places that I used to. If it weren't for the fears, I would not be depressed." These patients with secondary depressions may have a syndrome more akin to demoralization. In many patients the nature of the depression is more strongly colored by the symptoms of the anxiety disorder (e.g., agitation, sleep disturbance, somatization) than by the mood-disturbance symptoms (Lesser et al. 1988b).

On the other hand, differentiation in some patients may be very difficult if the patient sees the time course of panic and depressive symptoms as being the same or as overlapping to such a degree that no temporal sequencing is possible. When the two coexist, and the depression is severe, the patient may have a more severe and protracted course of the panic disorder (Clancy et al. 1978, Van Valkenberg et al. 1984). However, secondary depressions of moderate severity are not necessarily a poor prognostic sign for the successful pharmacologic treatment of the panic disorder (Lesser et al. 1988). Even if the diagnosis cannot be made with absolute certainty, it is of some comfort that the antidepressants used to treat major depressions also are effective in panic disorder (Sheehan et al. 1980, Pohl et al. 1982, Lydiard and Ballenger 1988), and there are data showing that alprazolam is effective in treating panic disorder even when the patient has a secondary depression (Lesser et al. 1988).

Panic attacks are not diagnostic symptoms of any specific personality disorders, yet they may be a component of the clinical picture seen with some personality disorders. For example, Grunhaus and Birmaher (1985) discussed how in patients with borderline personality disorders, anxiety of panic proportions may be at the core of their pathology, and their symptom picture often includes multiple phobias.

Careful and systematic study of the personality styles or disorders associated with PD has begun only recently. As in the study of personality in depression, it has been shown that in patients with PD and agoraphobia, a broad range of personality measures are influenced by the presence of the anxiety itself (Reich et al. 1986). Thus, highly anxious people may respond to questions about long-term personality functioning differently after their anxiety has abated. This makes it difficult to assess premorbid personality styles during an active phase of illness. Nevertheless, studies have reported that among PD patients with phobic avoidance, dependent personality disorders were more prevalent (approximately 40%) than in patients with PD and no avoidance (Reich et al. 1987). The investigators correctly note that it was not possible to state whether the dependent behavior preceded the PD or was a result of it, though they cite the earlier work of others that suggests dependent traits do predispose to the development of anxiety disorders.

DIFFERENTIATION OF PANIC DISORDER FROM MEDICAL DISORDERS

It should be obvious from the foregoing that the multitude of physical symptoms accompanying PD make distinctions from actual physical disease a necessary and potentially difficult component of the total workup of these patients. Indeed, typical patients will make many visits to emergency rooms and to their primary-care physician before seeking help in the mental-health sector. Since the symptoms of anxiety mimic those seen in many medical diseases, some of which are quite serious (Hall 1980), patients often undergo many repeated diagnostic tests. The specific medical illnesses and suggested diagnostic workups have been detailed elsewhere (Dietch 1981, Katon 1986, Raj and Sheehan 1987) and will only be reviewed briefly here.

Some medical conditions actually cause symptoms of anxiety and panic; when treated, the panic attacks abate. This was officially recognized only recently in DSM-III-R with the designation of a new category, *organic anxiety disorder*. This diagnosis should be used when either recurrent panic attacks and/or generalized anxiety occur in the context of an illness or of substance use that is known to be associated with anxiety. Examples of such illnesses are hyperthyroidism, Cushing's syndrome (excess production of the hormone cortisol), pheochromocytoma (a tumor of the adrenal glands producing adrenalin), and hypoglycemia. Stimulant drugs such as amphetamines, cocaine, and caffeine, when taken in excess, also can produce a picture of panic attacks. The use of other mind-altering drugs (LSD, marijuana) can lead to episodes of acute anxiety or panic attacks, but there is no evidence that they cause anxiety symptoms in the direct manner that stimulants and caffeine do.

A large number of additional diseases cause isolated symptoms or clusters of symptoms that are prominent in PD. Symptoms referable to the cardiovascular system are probably most frequently reported by patients (Marks and Lader 1973, Katon

1986). These symptoms include palpitations, rapid heart rate, heaviness in the chest, and chest pain often radiating to the arms. Patients often think they are having a heart attack or that their heart cannot possibly continue to beat in this manner for very long. Examples of cardiac illnesses that share some symptoms with panic attacks are numerous. Cardiac arrhythmias, disturbances in the rate and rhythm of the heartbeat, can present in a similar fashion to a panic attack. Episodes of chest pain on the basis of coronary artery dysfunction (angina) also can mimic an acute panic attack, especially since panic attacks often are precipitated by exercise.

The association between the mitral valve prolapse syndrome (MVPS) and PD has been complex, and its status remains unresolved. In MVPS there is an anatomic abnormality of the heart's mitral valve. It often is present and asymptomatic in many healthy individuals. However, when severe, it may cause a syndrome characterized by palpitations, rapid heart rate, chest pain, anxiety, and fatigue. The diagnosis is usually made after clinical examination and echocardiographic studies of the heart. Many investigators (Ven Katesh et al. 1980, Liberthson et al. 1986) but not all (Shear et al. 1984) have noted that when compared to normal controls, there was a higher percentage of patients with PD who had MVP. Because MVP may place patients at increased risk for several additional medical complications, it is important to evaluate patients for its presence. However, patients with PD respond to medications in a similar fashion whether or not they have MVP (Gorman et al. 1981).

Complaints referable to the respiratory system, such as shortness of breath, rapid breathing (hyperventilation), and a feeling of "air hunger," also are frequent in patients with panic attacks. An illness such as asthma that presents in dramatic, episodic attacks and is associated with considerable anxiety can be confused with a panic attack. Other respiratory conditions to be alert for are chronic obstructive lung disease and recurrent pulmonary emboli, whereby small clotlike particles become lodged in lung tissue, thereby decreasing the ability of the lung to properly oxygenate the blood.

Because multiple hormones act on target organs, including the brain, there is a complex interplay between hormonal status and behavior. Dysregulations of the thyroid, parathyroid (important in the regulation of calcium), and adrenal glands and of the pancreas all have been associated with episodes of panic. However, in large studies of patients with PD, few abnormalities were found in thyroid function (Fishman et al. 1985, Lesser et al. 1987), and no cases were reported of hypoglycemia (Gorman et al. 1984, Uhde et al. 1984). Although the diagnosis of premenstrual syndrome is controversial, many women with PD note an increase in the number and severity of their panic attacks premenstrually.

Neurologic symptoms also are commonly seen in panic attacks. Patients often have episodes of dizziness, lightheadedness or a giddy feeling, perceptual distortions, headaches, and paresthesia (a feeling of pins and needles in the extremities). Some of these symptoms may be the result of hyperventilation, but others may be associated with actual neurologic disease such as inner-ear dysfunctions (Meniere's disease, acute labyrinthitis) or brain tumors. Panic attacks may share some symptoms with epilepsy, especially partial complex seizures or temporal-lobe seizures. However, as in other illnesses mentioned above, this is not a common cause of panic attacks.

Because many of the illnesses discussed here are serious and require specific treatment, they must be considered in the differential diagnosis. On the other hand, not every patient needs to have sophisticated medical investigations for each one. Indeed, the clinician must walk a fine line between, on the one hand, conducting appropriate medical evaluations and, on the other, reinforcing the view that the patient has a medical illness and that further testing will ultimately lead to the "answer."

A minimum medical workup should include a careful history with emphasis upon use of medications, drugs, and caffeine; a physical examination; baseline laboratory studies to assess anemia, electrolyte and calcium disturbances, and thyroid function; and an electrocardiogram. If suspicions are aroused about specific disease processes, more specialized diagnostic tests can be obtained, such as 24-hour cardiac monitoring, electroencephalograms, and glucose tolerance tests.

CONCLUSION

Anxiety disorders are very commonly seen in the general population, in medical practices, and in the mental-health setting. They have been recognized and well described for years, though they have undergone extensive changes in nomenclature. According to Spitzer and Williams (1985), the purposes of classification in mental health are communication, control (the ability to either prevent the occurrence or modify the course of the disorder), and comprehension (understanding the causes of the disorder). When compared to previous systems, our current system certainly goes a long way toward reaching these goals. Whether the panic/chronic anxiety distinction and the current separation of the remaining disorders successfully fulfills these expectations must await further findings from research and from clinical practice.

REFERENCES

American Psychiatric Association (1980). *Diagnostic and Statistical Manual of Mental Disorders* (3rd ed.). Washington, DC: APA.
American Psychiatric Association (1987). *Diagnostic and Statistical Manual of Mental Disorders* (3rd ed. rev.). Washington, DC: APA.
Barlow, D. H., DiNardo, P. A., Vermilyea, B. B., et al. (1986). Comorbidity and depression among the anxiety disorders: Issues in diagnosis and classification. *Journal of Nervous and Mental Disease* 174:63-72.

Boyd, J. H., Burke, J. D., Gruenberg, E., et al. (1984). The exclusion criteria of DSM-III: A study of the co-occurrence of hierarchy-free syndromes. *Archives of General Psychiatry* 41:983-989.

Breier, A., Charney, D. S., and Heninger, G. R. (1986). Agoraphobia with panic attacks: Development, diagnostic stability, and course of illness. *Archives of General Psychiatry* 43:1029-1036.

Burton, R. (1964). *The Anatomy of Melancholy.* London: Dent.

Cameron, O. G., Thyer, B. A., Nesse, R. M., and Curtis, G. C. (1986). Symptom profiles of patients with DSM-III anxiety disorders. *American Journal of Psychiatry* 143:1132-1137.

Clancy, J., Noyes, R., Hoenk, P. R., and Slymen, D. J. (1978). Secondary depression in anxiety neurosis. *Journal of Nervous and Mental Diseases* 166:846-850.

Da Costa, J. M. (1871). On irritable heart: A clinical study of a form of functional cardiac disorder and its consequences. *American Journal of Medical Science* 61:17-52.

Dietch, J. T. (1981). Diagnosis of organic anxiety disorders. *Psychosomatics* 22:661-669.

Fishman, S. M., Sheehan, D. V., and Carr, D. B. (1985). Thyroid dysfunction in panic disorder. *Journal of Clinical Psychiatry* 46:422-423.

Foa, E. B., Steketee, G., and Young, M. C. (1984). Agoraphobia: Phenomenological aspects, associated characteristics and theoretical considerations. *Clinical Psychology Review* 4:431-457.

Freud, S. (1895). On the grounds for detaching a particular syndrome from neurasthenia under the description "anxiety neurosis." *Standard Edition* 3:87-115.

Gorman, J. M., Fyer, A. J., Glicklich, J., et al. (1981). Mitral valve prolapse and panic disorders: Effect of imipramine. In *Anxiety: New Research and Changing Concepts,* ed. D. F. Klein and J. G. Rabkin, pp. 317-326. New York: Raven Press.

Gorman, J. M., Martinez, J. M., Liebowitz, M. R., et al. (1984). Hypoglycemia and panic attacks. *American Journal of Psychiatry* 141:101-102.

Grunhaus, L., and Birmaher, B. (1985). The clinical spectrum of panic attacks. *Journal of Clinical Psychopharmacology* 5:93-99.

Gurney, C., Roth, M., Garside, R. F., et al. (1972). Studies in the classification of affective disorders: The relationship between anxiety states and depressive illness—II. *British Journal of Psychiatry* 121:162–166.

Hall, R. C. W. (1980). *Psychiatric Presentations of Medical Illness: Somatopsychic Disorders.* New York: Spectrum Publications, Inc.

Janet, P., and Raymon, F. (1898). *Les Nevroses et Idées Fixes.* 2 vols. Paris: Felix Alcan.

Katon, W. (1986). Panic disorder: Epidemiology, diagnosis, and treatment in primary care. *Journal of Clinical Psychiatry* 47 (Suppl. 10):21–27.

Klein, D. F. (1964). Delineation of two drug-responsive anxiety syndromes. *Psychopharmacologia* 5:397–408.

Klein, D. F. (1980). Anxiety reconceptualized. *Comprehensive Psychiatry* 21:411–427.

Klein, D. F., Ross, D. C., and Cohen, P. (1987). Panic and avoidance in agoraphobia: Application of path analysis to treatment studies. *Archives of General Psychiatry* 44:377–385.

Lesser, I. M. (1988). The relationship between panic disorder and depression. *Journal of Anxiety Disorders* 2:3–15.

Lesser, I. M., Rubin, R. T., Lydiard, R. B., et al. (1987). Past and current thyroid function in subjects with panic disorder. *Journal of Clinical Psychiatry* 48:473–476.

Lesser, I. M., Rubin, R. T., Pecknold, J. C., et al. (1988a). Secondary depression in panic disorder and agoraphobia: Frequency, severity, and response to treatment. *Archives of General Psychiatry* 45:437–443.

Lesser, I. M., Rubin, R. T., Rifkin, A., et al. (1988b). Secondary depression in panic disorder and agoraphobia, II. Dimensions of depressive symptomatology and their response to treatment. *Journal of Affective Disorders.*

Liberthson, R., Sheehan, D. V., King, M. E., and Weyman, A. E. (1986). The prevalence of mitral valve prolapse in patients with panic disorder. *American Journal of Psychiatry* 143:511–515.

Liebowitz, M. R., Gorman, J. M., Fyer, A. J., and Klein, D. F. (1985). Social phobia: Review of a neglected anxiety disorder. *Archives of General Psychiatry* 42:729–736.

Lydiard, R. B., and Ballenger, J. C. (1988). Panic-related disorders: Evidence for efficacy of antidepressants. *Journal of Anxiety Disorders* 2:77–94.

Marks, I., and Lader, M. (1973). Anxiety states (anxiety neurosis): A review. *Journal of Nervous and Mental Diseases* 156:3-18.

Mellman, T. A., and Uhde, T. W. (1987). Obsessive-compulsive symptoms in panic disorders. *American Journal of Psychiatry* 144:1573-1576.

Mountjoy, C. Q., and Roth, M. (1982). Studies in the relationship between depressive disorders and anxiety states. 2. Clinical items. *Journal of Affective Disorders* 4:149-161.

Noyes, R., Clancy, J., and Garvey, M. J. (1987). Is agoraphobia a variant of panic disorder or a separate illness? *Journal of Anxiety Disorders* 1:3-13.

Pohl, R., Berchou, R., and Rainey, J. M. (1982). Tricyclic antidepressants and monoamine oxidase inhibitors in the treatment of agoraphobia. *Journal of Clinical Psychopharmacology* 2:399-407.

Raj, A., and Sheehan, D. V. (1987). Medical evaluation of panic attacks. *Journal of Clinical Psychiatry* 48:309-313.

Regier, D. A., Boyd, J. H., Burke, J. D., et al. (1988). One-month prevalence of mental disorders in the United States. *Archives of General Psychiatry* 45:977-986.

Reich, J., Noyes, R., Coryell, W., and O'Gorman, T. W. (1986). The effect of state anxiety on personality measurement. *American Journal of Psychiatry* 143:760-763.

Reich, J., Noyes, R., and Troughton, E. (1987). Dependent personality disorder associated with phobic avoidance in patients with panic disorder. *American Journal of Psychiatry* 144:323-326.

Roth, M., Gurney, C., Garside, R. F., and Kerr, T. A. (1972). Studies in the classification of affective disorders: The relationship between anxiety states and depressive illness—I. *British Journal of Psychiatry* 121:147-161.

Robins, L. N., Helzer, J. E., Weissman, M. M., et al. (1984). Lifetime prevalence of specific psychiatric disorders in three sites. *Archives of General Psychiatry* 41:949-958.

Schapira, K., Roth, M., Kerr, T. A., and Gurney, C. (1972). The prognosis of affective disorders: The differentiation of anxiety states from depressive illnesses. *British Journal of Psychiatry* 121:175-181.

Shear, M. K., Devereux, R. B., Kramer-Fox, R., et al. (1984). Low prevalence of mitral valve prolapse in patients with panic disorder. *American Journal of Psychiatry* 141:302-303.

Sheehan, D. V., Ballenger, J., and Jacobsen, G. (1980). Treatment of endogenous anxiety with phobic, hysterical and hypochondriacal symptoms. *Archives of General Psychiatry* 37:51-59.

Sheehan, D. V., and Sheehan, K. H. (1982). The classification of anxiety and hysterical states. II. Toward a more heuristic classification. *Journal of Clinical Psychopharmacology* 2:386-393.

Spitzer, R. L., and Williams, J. B. W. (1985). Classification of mental disorders. In *Comprehensive Textbook of Psychiatry/IV*, vol. 1, ed. H. I. Kaplan and B. J. Sadock, 4th ed., pp. 591-613. Baltimore: Williams & Wilkins.

Stavrakaki, C., and Vargo, B. (1986). The relationship of anxiety and depression: A review of the literature. *British Journal of Psychiatry* 149:7-16.

Steketee, G., Grayson, J. B., and Foa, E. B. (1987). A comparison of characteristics of obsessive-compulsive disorder and other anxiety disorders. *Journal of Anxiety Disorders* 1:325-335.

Thyer, B. A., and Himle, J. (1987). Phobic anxiety and panic anxiety: How do they differ? *Journal of Anxiety Disorders* 1:59-67.

Thyer, B. A., Himle, J., Curtis, G. C., et al. (1985). A comparison of panic disorder and agoraphobia with panic attacks. *Comprehensive Psychiatry* 26:208-214.

Tyrer, P. (1984). Classification of anxiety. *British Journal of Psychiatry* 144:78-83.

Tyrer, P. (1985). Neurosis divisible? *Lancet* i:685-688.

Tyrer, P. (1986). Classification of anxiety disorders: A critique of DSM-III. *Journal of Affective Disorders* 11:99-104.

Uhde, T. W., Vittone, B. J., and Post, R. M. (1985). Glucose tolerance testing in panic disorder. *American Journal of Psychiatry* 141:1461-1463.

Van Valkenburg, C., Akiskal, H. S., Puzantian, V., and Rosenthal, T. (1984). Anxious depressions: Clinical, family history, and naturalistic outcome—comparisons with panic and major depressive disorders. *Journal of Affective Disorders* 6:67-82.

Ven Katesh, A., Pauls, D. L., Crowe, R., et al. (1980). Mitral valve prolapse in anxiety neurosis (panic disorder). *American Heart Journal* 100:302-305.

3 Agoraphobia

Dianne Chambless, one of the foremost researchers and clinicians in the field, developed in collaboration with her colleague of many years, Alan Goldstein, some of the basic concepts and theory that still dominate today's literature. This chapter is a summary of the main points of the program at Temple University Medical Center. In this integrative approach, note the emphasis on family therapy, group experience, and mixing a Gestalt and psychodynamic approach with the more behavioral techniques, such as in vivo exposure.

One of their important contributions to the effective treatment of phobias was coining the term *fear of fear syndrome* as it applies to agoraphobia (Goldstein and Chambless 1978). The phrase refers to their concept that it is neither an underlying psychodynamic conflict, nor the phobic situation per se, that is feared. Rather, patients come to fear the anxiety syndrome that will be evoked when the trigger situation is approached. This simple phrase had surprisingly far-reaching consequences in the development of phobia therapy. Desensitization hierarchies (for example, approaching a supermarket, entering a supermarket, standing in line to pay) may not always be effective in diminishing a phobia, because the avoidance may be primarily of the patient's internal experience of physiological arousal in anxiety. This observation has helped to bring the more strictly behaviorally oriented practitioners to adopt more readily the cognitive-behavioral approach, expanding the therapeutic goals to more closely resemble those shared by the general psychotherapy community.

Agoraphobia

Dianne L. Chambless

INTRODUCTION

The advances in the treatment of agoraphobia since 1970 and the adoption of the new techniques by practitioners stand as a gratifying example of the potential benefits to be gained from persisting with clinical research, difficult though it be. By 1981 Barlow and Wolfe were able to report that across treatment centers 65% to 75% of agoraphobic clients were found to improve with fairly brief behavioral treatment. Prior to the advent of active therapies for this problem, agoraphobia tended to be a lifelong disabling disorder, from which Roberts (1964) found only 24% to recover with standard interventions. There was enough known about agoraphobia by 1984 to fill an entire volume; in fact, two had been written on the subject for professional audiences (Chambless and Goldstein 1982, Mathews et al. 1981). Because all of this material cannot be compacted into one chapter, the focus here will be on those aspects of our knowledge most pertinent to service providers. The reader expecting to practice heavily in this area or to perform research on this topic would do well to consult these more extensive works.

Agoraphobia is most briefly described as a fear and avoidance of public places and of being away from home, based on the anticipation of experiencing noxious levels of anxiety or panic attacks. Within this general framework, people with this fear are found to avoid a wide variety of situations: public conveyances, shops, restaurants, theaters, journeys away from home, standing in lines, being in elevators, and even being home alone are common triggers for anxiety. There are two underlying, related themes. The agoraphobic fears any situation where one is confined with restricted freedom of movement or possibility for escape, whether by physical constraint or social convention. Consequently, she or he may avoid visits to the dentist, social engagements (the more formal, the more anxiety provoking), and elevators. Agoraphobia is not, therefore, the opposite of claustrophobia, as the dictionary would lead one to believe. In fact, on the average, these clients are more afraid of enclosed than of open spaces.

Agoraphobics fear that their anxiety levels will rise to panic in these situations and that they will be unable to escape. Their goal may be simply to escape the noxious situation or, commonly, to reach a situation where they feel safe. This introduces the second theme, which involves not so much the fear of being someplace in particular, but the fear of being away from people and places that give the agoraphobic person a relative sense of security. Thus, many agoraphobics are able to function much better if accompanied by a trusted companion, typically a spouse or other family member, but possibly any responsible figure, or if they remain in, or close to, their homes or other familiar places. There are variations on the safety theme. For example, intensely hypochondriacal agoraphobics may feel relatively safe anywhere near a hospital or doctor's office.

Recalling these themes of being trapped and of being alone and cut off from support and security is most helpful in understanding an agoraphobic's idiosyncratic reactions. For example, some clients consistently feel trapped whenever presented with something that must be done. One woman became persistently panicky in her last trimester of an unwanted pregnancy because she then had no choice. She had to go through with the delivery. This sort of client may react adversely to being pushed strongly in treatment. A second client felt alone, "dead, cut off from the world," whenever she closed her eyes. Consequently, she had difficulty at the beauty parlor, not because she felt trapped, as many clients do, but because so many procedures required that she close her eyes to avoid damage from chemicals. Coping strategies for her symptoms had to be altered accordingly. Hence, although it is certainly crucial to obtain a list of the places clients avoid, it is also extremely important to remember that an agoraphobic's fears generalize not just along physical lines but also along cognitive ones.

Agoraphobic people vary widely in the size of their safety zones and in the degree to which a companion limits their anxiety. There is also considerable variability in the degree to which a particular agoraphobic is symptomatic on a given day or during a particular year. Some can vary from being almost asymptomatic to being housebound within a month (Buglass et al. 1977), and some report having periods of remission over a number of years (Marks 1970). This changeability bewilders and often frustrates not only the agoraphobic but also those in her or his life. These fluctuations in avoidance are generally based on the agoraphobic's perception of the likelihood of panic at a given time. Commonly, agoraphobics begin the day by monitoring their levels of anxiety and make or alter decisions about their activities accordingly. Panic attacks are quite variable in occurrence, and agoraphobic people may have periods of years without frequent panic and gradually begin to do more. However, when a series of panics is once again experienced, often associated with increased stress, a rapid acceleration in avoidance typically follows.

The problem of panic is, thus, central to the understanding of agoraphobia. Under conditions of extreme fear, most phobic clients report the symptoms of panic, which include rapid heartbeat, chest pain, difficulty with breathing, dizziness, faintness, a sense of unreality, shaking, numbness or tingling in the extremities, and an urge to urinate or defecate. Particular symptoms are salient for different people. For the agoraphobic person the panic is accompanied by an intense urge to flee, a sense of doom, and thoughts of impending catastrophe. These attacks are all the more frightening in the case of agoraphobia, for, contrary to specific phobias, agoraphobic panic is rather unpredictable in nature, often striking without warning, seemingly without reason, and engendering a sense of helplessness. This erratic course of panic has led some to believe that these attacks reflect an endogenous disturbance, best treated with psychotropic medication (e.g., Sheehan et al. 1980). I find it more useful to conceive of panic as a reaction some people are prone to have when under stress, just as others might develop hypertension, ulcers, or migraines. There is increasingly good evidence that the panic reaction is familial in origin and more likely to develop in female family members (Crowe et al. 1983). Whatever its origin, the unpredictability of panic leads the agoraphobic to think of no place as being completely safe and to discount occasions when, on a sortie into the external world, the expected panic did not occur. The avoidance behavior thus is negatively reinforced on an intermittent basis and is, consequently, all the more resistant to alteration.

Panic attacks are highly noxious unconditioned stimuli. Places, thoughts, and feelings associated with panic quickly become anxiety-provoking themselves. Consequently, although agoraphobia has been described as a fear of fear (Goldstein and Chambless 1978), fear of many intense sensations that share component responses with panic may develop. Often, agoraphobics become fearful of anger, worrying that being upset will drive them to panic, and even of intense, presumably pleasant, sensations such as profound relaxation or orgasm because of the sense of loss of control accompanying these events. Almost all become hyperalert to the physiological sensations associated with their attacks and focus on these sensations, monitoring their bodies for any increase in these signs, and spiraling into panic or fleeing when the dreaded signals are detected. Finally, the agoraphobic's assessment of the possible consequences of panic is an important component of the phobic response. Almost all believe that some catastrophe will result. There are two general categories of these catastrophes: physiological events such as having a heart attack, fainting, and vomiting; and social/behavioral events such as losing control, screaming, babbling, and becoming insane. During the panic state, most strongly believe these events are imminent. When calm, fewer hold these beliefs fixedly despite all medical and psychological reassurance, but the majority continue to have some concerns that spring back to full force when anxiety next increases. These doubts about mental and physical integrity are pervasively demoralizing and serve to drive the agoraphobic's anxiety quickly higher when the thoughts occur.

In summary, we can see that although panic attacks may initially strike "out of the blue" as a nonspecific response to stress, the agoraphobic's response to the panic serves to perpetuate the stress and to make the likelihood of continued attacks all the higher.

Whether community samples or clinical populations are studied, agoraphobia is found to be about four times more prevalent in women than men (reviewed by Chambless 1982, Weissman 1983). In recent community studies reviewed by Weissman, generally two to four out of 100 women were diagnosed as agoraphobic. The problem is most likely to begin in late adolescence and young adulthood (Marks 1970), although many clients report having had similar feelings for circumscribed periods during childhood, often taking the form of school phobia or panic attacks without subsequent phobic complications.

Any number of stressors have been listed as the final precipitants of panic attacks. These stressors do not necessarily have any particular attributes but most often they relate to the themes of being trapped and/or alone. Late adolescent onset generally is related to separation issues such as leaving home, going to college, taking a job, and leaving behind childhood. Onset in the twenties may pertain to moving away from parental attachments into adult relationships. For example, one client, raised in a conservative Catholic home, had decided that as she approached 30 she would like to move out of her parents' home and share an apartment with her boyfriend. In the months of frantic quarrels that followed, her mother threatened that the client would cause her to have a nervous breakdown by such wicked behavior. The client remained in the parental home but became agoraphobic, feeling trapped but unable to break the bond with her mother. A final example of this issue is the young married woman with children who is unhappy with her relationship but feels trapped in her marriage. She feels unable to leave owing to her own fears of being alone and most often also owing to the very real difficulties a female, single parent faces: inadequate child support, economic discrimination, poor vocational training, and isolation with the burdens of raising children alone. Women may be particularly prone to agoraphobia because they are shaped to be more emotionally dependent on relationships than are men and because of their economic dependence on men. (For a more complete discussion of these issues see Chambless 1982.) Other common precipitants include bereavement and moving (both again involving separation), physical illness or surgery, and the assumption of new responsibilities such as those brought on by a promotion. Similar events may exacerbate the symptoms of one who is already agoraphobic.

Even once we have added in the ingredient of a familial predisposition to have panic attacks when under stress, we have not solved the problem of the onset of agoraphobia, because not everyone who develops panic attacks becomes phobic. In part this may reflect modeling, because families of agoraphobics are more likely to have all sorts of phobias than are families of probands with panic disorder (Harris et al. 1983). Elsewhere (Chambless and Goldstein 1981, Goldstein and Chambless 1978) we have argued that other important contributing factors are (a) a tendency to misattribute the source of panic, looking to physical situations or some disease process as the cause of distress rather than the pertinent stressors; (b) a vulnerability to separation whether through overprotection, neglect, or childhood separation trauma, which is related to (c) a sense of being inadequate to care for oneself and function as an autonomous adult. All of these characteristics point to important therapeutic issues to be resolved in the treatment of an agoraphobic client.

Associated Problems

Part of the complexity of treating agoraphobics should be apparent from the list of problem areas requiring attention that has been presented so far. There are, however, additional complicating factors that need to be addressed. Only the most common will be touched on here (see Chambless 1982 for a more complete treatment). Depression is so often associated with agoraphobia that there have been attempts, now largely abandoned, to categorize this disorder as *atypical depression*. The great majority of these clients are mildly to moderately severely depressed. Depression is frequently part of the initial sense of being abandoned, helpless, and overwhelmed that the person is already undergoing when the panic attacks begin or recur. Once panic attacks have begun and avoidance behavior is established, even if the external crisis is resolved, depression is still likely, now a result of the agoraphobic symptoms. Not only is the distress associated with panic related to increased depression, avoidance is strongly related to higher levels of depression. Being dysfunctional when faced with the most mundane task, like grocery shopping, is destructive to self-esteem. Moreover, the restrictions of being agoraphobic cut one off from many of the most powerful reinforcers in our society: social contact, avocational interests, and career advancement.

Agoraphobics are characterized by very high levels of chronic anxiety. Many report having always been "high strung," which fits with a prevalent familial pattern of anxiety problems as well as phobias (Harris et al. 1983). Their tension no doubt increases their tendency to develop panic attacks. This propensity to be a "worrier" may be associated with their tendency toward hypochondriasis, which is particularly pronounced in the men. Their anxiety and avoidance are typically increased by even mild illnesses, and they often "catastrophize" that any physical symptom is a sign of impending major, perhaps fatal, illness. Although they may, if able to reach and wait in a physician's office or emergency room, seek repeated assurance about their health, they are generally loath to accept medical treatment, being terrified that the prescribed medication will drive them out of control or cause life-threatening side effects.

Finally, a significant problem for the great majority of agoraphobics is social anxiety, which is generally related to a strong fear of others' negative evaluations. It has been previously noted that interpersonal relationships are extremely important to these clients. They are easily distressed by loss of approval or even temporary withdrawal of affection and are greatly disturbed at being the target of another's anger. As a result, they are often unassertive, particularly in intimate relationships, and allow themselves to be manipulated or bullied. These tendencies are worsened by the development of agoraphobia, in that the increased dependency associated with the disorder causes them to fear offending significant others even more. In addition, the associated loss of self-esteem increases their sense of inadequacy in interpersonal situations, and their fears that their anxiety will be noticed by others (it generally is not) may cause them to avoid formerly satisfying social contacts.

Treatment Planning

It is difficult to discuss treatment planning without alluding to treatment approaches. Consequently, some techniques will be briefly mentioned in this section; more detailed explanations will follow in the treatment section. There are several central decisions to be made at this juncture: what kind of treatment is needed for the phobias; how urgent the need for intervention is;

what other issues, if any, must be addressed for the resolution of the phobias; and whether any physical or emotional factors contraindictate treatment.

By this time we have diagnosed the client as agoraphobic, but this includes a range of clients from those who do not avoid but are fearful to those who are totally housebound. Not surprisingly, different treatment approaches are advisable according to the severity of the case. Clients who are not avoidant and those who are mildly avoidant may not require treatment with therapist-assisted in vivo exposure. In these cases, training in anxiety- and panic-management techniques coupled with clear instructions for self-directed exposure may be adequate. When clients are more severely avoidant, individual or group in vivo exposure is advisable. Those who avoid many situations can be placed in a group and treated more economically in that fashion. If a client is very avoidant of only a few situations, it is important to determine whether he or she will be able to get adequate practice on those items in a group situation. Otherwise, individual treatment is more efficient. A common example is the client who has most difficulty with driving, where individualized attention is often necessary.

In the case of a complex agoraphobia, the phobic symptoms seem only a part of a wide range of problems the person faces. The phobia is intertwined with personal, interpersonal, and situational difficulties in a way that makes treatment much more difficult. Excerpts from the intake session of Ms. H. will be used to illustrate some of the issues besides the agoraphobia that come to light and that require attention. Ms. H. is a 50-year-old married woman with three children who range in age from 16 to 21. She is middle-class, college-educated, and holds a job requiring presentations to groups. During the 10 years she has been agoraphobic, work has been a safe place for her, but in the 2 months before intake she has been distressed to see her panic attacks (three in the last 7 days) spread to her job. She fears passing out, acting foolish and losing control, and the body sensations concerning dizziness, wobbly legs, sweating, and heart palpitations.

She is moderately socially phobic, extremely anxious, and moderately depressed.

> C: All the time, I'm so extremely embarrassed about it [*her symptoms*]. [*Client describes how competitive her workplace is, how she fears discovery and dismissal because of her problem.*]
> T: What a terrible pressure to be under, to feel like you have to hide all the time.
> C: Right, right, right. I'm in a panic all the time that they will find out. I don't know if the "they" is really my colleagues, or if the "they" is the world. Or if the "they" is the people who told me when I was young that I must always be wonderful.
> T: Yeah.
> C: And my house is always spotless, and every assignment I get, God knows how long I work. So . . . there is your perfection [*referring again to the article she read*].
> T: Uh huh. So as hard as you work you're not perfect enough 'cause you have this problem. [*Client tells how her employers questioned whether she should get a long-term contract for her job because she lacked the appropriate degree. She has gotten much worse since then, even though ultimately the decision was made to retain her.*]
> T: Just having it questioned was very traumatic for you.
> C: Just finding me less than perfect, that was a very bad situation.
> T: So, what you're afraid of is passing out and embarrassing yourself in front of these people whose criticism you fear?
> C: I'm afraid . . . I'm afraid to walk on the street, too.
> T: Uh huh, even people you don't know, you'd be embarrassed.
> C: I . . . I don't even know what it is I'm afraid of all the time. I couldn't go anywhere this summer because I was . . . just like . . . a rag [*after her job was questioned*]. The night [*after the issue of possibly terminating client was raised*] I was driving home from a ballet class, it was about 9:30–10 o'clock at

night, and I was on the road and all of a sudden I couldn't drive. I just couldn't drive.
T: You were really frozen, huh.
C: I was . . . like that [*demonstrates*].
T: Uh huh.
C: And I drove in pieces. Finally I made it to a shopping center near home, and this psychologist who was seeing me said, "What a treat!"; my husband jogged to the shopping center to rescue me. I mean, I want Dave to show me. . . . There is my, I forget what they call it, the uh, the . . .
T: Secondary gain?
C: Secondary gain, yeah. He drives me. Wonderful.
T: Uh huh. So that's a way that he can show he cares for you. And he has trouble doing that in other ways?
C: Yeah, he, uh, he's . . . I mean . . . he's an extremely loyal man. He just doesn't know how to give love. [*Client rapidly begins talking about symptoms again, and client and therapist explore the extent of them. She forces herself to go a number of places alone in her safety zone but otherwise must be accompanied. Also explored are issues that have increased her anxiety, such as a child who has a birth defect and feeling alone in America as a foreigner.*]
C: But, also there are a lot of times when I feel like just saying the hell with it. I'm staying home.
T: Yeah.
C: I just went out [*to come to the appointment*] in the midst of a real bad attack. What happened was Sunday we decided to come here on a dry run to see where it was. And it was just incredible. I got such a terrible attack. And I don't know if it was coming here, I guess . . . because this morning I was also shaking coming in [*client drove with husband following behind and leaving her at my office*] 'cause there were a lot of painful things that we mentioned.
T: Yeah. How is it for you also to meet a new person and to be

talking with a new person about your life? Is that difficult for you?

C: Yeah. You are also very young.

T: How old are you now?

C: Fifty, 51 next December.

T: And you have a sense of really becoming older now that you haven't had before? What's changed, do you think?

C: Uh, I think the children leaving home.

T: It feels like a real marker for you?

C: Yeah.

T: Uh huh. What's it like for you with them gone?

C: It's more lonely. It's a hell of a lot easier, physically, to take care of the house.

T: Yeah.

C: There's almost a Dr. Jekyll, Mr. Hyde kind of situation, because when I am feeling "normal" I do reach out for people a lot. And, uh, basically, I . . . I . . . I . . . I want people all the time. My husband is an extreme loner.

T: Yeah.

C: And I think he's the stronger of the two of us, and I think that's why I had to invent my tyranny. And, uh, after living years with someone who, I'll say, "Let's have a dinner party," and he'll say, "What for?" And then I'd have to sit down and show him that we owe many invitations, and then he'd be willing to consider it. In other words, uh . . .

T: It's not enough that you want people around.

C: Yes, it's hard for me to now know what I am like any more because I have adjusted so much. Where I come from, it's always outgoing. My parents used to go out at least three, four times a week. And you come to the suburbs, and if you're lucky, you go out once a week, so I . . . I, there's so many adjustments that I have made that sometimes I don't know the real me, and what I really wanted, or what I want now.

T: That's true; in long-term relationships you do change.

C: Right.

T: Um, you adjust to the other person, you develop different patterns. How long have you been married now?
C: Twenty-six years.
T: How did you happen to marry someone so different from you in so many ways?
C: [*Laughing*] I don't know. I was 27, and at that time the pressure on me, on a woman, to marry was much stronger.
T: You were well overdue by that point.
C: Oh, boy, I mean, I was just a total failure. And I met him, and he wanted to marry me. That was it. I think I really fell in love later. I was rather hoping to take him back home, but he wouldn't, I guess he couldn't, take off, also. And that was that.
T: How are things between you now?
C: Good. He went recently. . . . See, that may well be the fruit of my tyranny, or my sickness. Went twice to the opera with me. Normally he wouldn't.
T: You mean he went because you couldn't go alone?
C: He went because he realizes that we are doing an awful lot of things his way. He's uh, extremely tight with money, and uh, I'm more inclined to go out and spend money, and he, uh . . .
T: So there are a number of conflicts around affection and spending time with people and spending money and just kind of going out. What are the parts that sustain you and keep you together all these years?
C: [*Laughing*] I'm not sure. I love him. And he loves me very much. Uh, there's a certain dependence. Uh.

Although Ms. H. describes her marriage as good, her own report during the interview indicates there are significant problem areas. From prior therapists, Ms. H. has learned to see her phobia as an attempt to manipulate her husband for more attention. There may be some truth to this, but such an explanation is only partially correct and has served to further diminish Ms. H.'s self-esteem. This analysis overlooks the loneliness the client feels within this marriage and the positive relationship of marital dissatisfaction to the incidence of panic attacks. Fear of the attacks is the more proximal factor related to her avoidance behavior. The loneliness theme is continued with her feelings about living in the United States and about her children's leaving home. Clearly, couples therapy is of top priority in this case. It is quite likely that if Mr. H. were asked by the therapist to come in for sessions to help his wife rather than because he needed therapy himself, he would be willing to come.

As is common for agoraphobic clients, when Ms. H. touched on sensitive issues during intake she dropped them quickly and began describing or experiencing her anxiety symptoms, illustrating the cognitive set where symptom focus rather than problem solving predominates. This is also well depicted in the scene she describes where, riding in the car with her husband, she suddenly has a severe panic attack under circumstances where she is ordinarily comfortable. She first attaches her panic to riding in the car and, with continued discussion, begins to see the relationship between her anxiety and her own feelings. Continued work on her attentional set and attribution needs to be part of her therapy as well.

Finally, the excerpt demonstrates a theme that pervaded the session with this client: her perfectionism and extreme sensitivity to criticism. On the one hand, she was very proud of her accomplishments, whereas on the other she was terrified of someone's finding fault with her work. Although she was ultimately granted a long-term contract, the idea that anyone questioned renewing her contract had so unsettled her that she had begun a severe downward spiral and could hardly face her colleagues. Losing some of her physical attractiveness in aging made her very jealous and uneasy around younger women, and having a brain-damaged child who could never be an academic star was excruciating. These concerns also served to keep Ms. H. highly chronically anxious and thus more likely to panic and be avoidant.

Comprehensive treatment of such cases will require concurrent focus on these problems as well as the agoraphobic symptoms. This is not to suggest that one cannot treat agoraphobia without addressing every problem such clients face. Rather, it is important to look at the web of relationships among problems and to treat those that feed into anxiety and other phobic symptoms.

Finally, factors that contraindicate the proposed treatment program need to be considered. If group treatment is planned, the usual considerations apply as to whether a client can function appropriately in a group. Clients with severe social phobia may be unable to make use of a group, or worse, they may be further sensitized in such a setting. Clients who became housebound at an early age may be so unsocialized as to need extensive individual work before they are ready for group. Chronic physical illness may require alterations in the treatment plan; the energy required for an ordinary in vivo exposure program may be lacking, and a gentler, shaping approach is called for. Consultation with the client's physician is highly advisable in these cases. Most often, the physician will encourage pushing the client much harder than the latter thinks is physically healthy, but there are exceptions.

Finally the therapist needs to assess whether additional problems faced by the client are so severe as to preclude a therapeutic response to an exposure-based treatment. Severe depression is one such case. In this situation, the client may fail to habituate to phobic situations and also may be so distraught as to have difficulty cooperating with a demanding treatment program. Because most agoraphobics are depressed and their depression usually lifts with treatment, it is a judgment call as to when the depression must be addressed first. Similarly, crises that prevent the client's devoting time and attention to the treatment program may well require postponement of treatment.

A last problem is substance abuse. About 1 of 20 agoraphobics applying for treatment has a serious, current alcohol-abuse problem. A smaller number may be addicted to other substances, such as high doses of minor tranquilizers. Exposure treatment has not been effective, in my experience, as long as the substance abuse continues. It does present a tricky problem, in that most agoraphobics are afraid of being away from home and trapped in an inpatient facility for detoxification and treatment and swear that, if only their anxiety could be reduced, they would stop drinking or taking drugs. For similar reasons, Alcoholics Anonymous meetings are likely to be anathema to these clients. Central-nervous-system depressants make change so difficult, however, that I find reducing their anxiety first to be impossible and require these clients to get treatment initially for the substance abuse.

TREATMENT TECHNIQUES

In Vivo Exposure

The keystone to treatment of agoraphobia is in vivo exposure: the deliberate practice in reality of those things a client has been avoiding. In extensive empirical validation, this treatment has been found to lead to at least 50% improvement on avoidance behavior in 60% to 70% of the agoraphobic clients treated (Jannson and Öst 1982). Exposure works not only to increase approach behavior but also to decrease subjective anxiety, panic attacks, and the depression associated with agoraphobic restrictions. This approach is coupled with an explanation of how anxiety works in the phobic situation: that anxiety will rise to some maximum point and then decrease. If one stays in the phobic situation until a decrease occurs, on subsequent occasions the anxiety response will be weaker and shorter lived, until the fear is largely overcome. Clients are reassured that none of their feared catastrophes will occur if they remain until habituation, rather than fleeing as is their wont. In vivo exposure has come to replace systematic desensitization with agoraphobic clients, as the latter has not proved to be a powerful intervention with this population (reviewed by Goldstein and Chambless 1978).

Exposure has been carried out in a number of different ways: a flooding approach where the client is pushed into highly anxiety-provoking situations from the start, a shaping approach where the client retreats every time anxiety begins to rise and then enters the situation again, and a graduated approach where a rough hierarchy is used, but the client is encouraged to enter and remain in situations that are anxiety provoking and to increase task difficulty as soon as possible. All three approaches have been effective in research trials (reviewed by Emmelkamp 1982). However, in practice it is very difficult to persuade clients to adopt the flooding approach, as well as it is unnecessarily painful for them, and the shaping approach is slow and unwieldy to apply in situations where free access to come and go many times is not feasible (e.g., a concert or restaurant). Consequently, when the term *in vivo exposure* is used, it typically refers to graduated exposure, with individual therapists varying in how quickly they urge clients to challenge difficult situations.

In over a decade of research on in vivo exposure with agoraphobia, a number of important parameters have been discerned (see Emmelkamp 1982). First, exposure needs to be long and continuous. Many clients attempt to enter their phobic situation, at least on occasion, and question why they have not improved if this technique is effective. The answer is that they usually leave the situation as quickly as possible and before habituation has occurred and that they avoid returning to it for as long as they possibly can. Not only are prolonged sessions required, but repeated sessions are also necessary because of spontaneous recovery of anxiety. An exposure session typically lasts from 1½ to 2 hours. If a shorter time must be used, then the hierarchy should be approached in finer gradations so that high levels of anxiety are not generated. As massed practice (every day) is more effective than spaced practice (every week), sessions should be scheduled as frequently as possible. It is very difficult to make progress if sessions are less frequent than once weekly, unless the client is assiduous about homework practice sessions.

Feedback about performance over a number of efforts in a

similar situation is important. As clients can do more with successive trials, this information serves to reinforce progress and to let the client see concretely the beneficial effects of exposure. The therapist's assistance in making tasks more manageable and promoting mastery is also of significant benefit, undercutting much of what is often seen as client resistance but is in fact a reflection of high anxiety. These therapist behaviors include breaking particularly difficult tasks into small steps, breaking up defensive postures such as freezing, and accompanying the client on early trials (Williams et al. 1984). Clients' sense that they have mastered the situation (not merely that they have done it) is strongly related to their predilection to try that task again.

There are a number of ways that exposure treatments can be delivered. Overall, clients seem to do as well in group as in individual treatment provided the staff/client ratio is not too low. Exposure can be carried out by the therapist, or the client may be given careful homework instructions instead. Good studies comparing the effectiveness of these approaches are lacking; however, it is clear that progress can be made with treatment manuals and explicit weekly contracts for self-directed exposure. Therapist-assisted exposure is more rapid, but some workers in the field (e.g., Hafner 1982) think this rapidity may be detrimental in the stress it may place on a family system that has adjusted to the agoraphobia. Nevertheless, highly avoidant clients may be unwilling to change their behavior without the reassurance of the therapist's presence, and the rapidity of change with therapist-assisted treatment is reinforcing and builds confidence in one's ability to overcome the phobia. Ultimately, however, clients must begin to practice alone. The cost of therapist-assisted exposure treatment may be reduced through the use of paraprofessional workers. Relatively inexperienced people can provide beneficial treatment as long as they are closely supervised.

Treatment may be home based or clinic based. Mathews et al. (1981) have devised a program to deliver treatment economically in the home through the use of treatment manuals for the clients and a few visits by the therapist to make sure the treatment plan is being appropriately followed. This is particularly advantageous for this population whose ability to reach treatment facilities is limited. Mathews and co-authors have also constructed a manual for spouses of agoraphobic clients who may be enlisted to assist in the exposure process. In two studies, treatment has been found to be equally effective whether or not the spouse was included (Boisvert et al. 1983, Cobb et al. 1983). Barlow and colleagues (1984), however, found a small positive effect of including the spouse in exposure homework for couples who were maritally distressed. The benefit seemed to be in helping the spouse become more understanding of the agoraphobic symptoms and more supportive. Nevertheless, the use of the spouse as an exposure co-therapist should be carefully considered, lest the therapist inadvertently reinforce the client's dependence on significant others. Perhaps because ongoing support is beneficial, clients who are treated in groups according to the neighborhood they live in seem to do somewhat better in treatment (Sinnott et al. 1981). If all else fails, treatment can be provided with manuals through the mail with phone or letter contacts to monitor homework assignments. This sort of treatment may be all that is possible for clients living in remote areas. It is, unfortunately, of limited effectiveness and may have no impact on the severely housebound.

In some situations, it may be difficult to carry out an in vivo exposure program because it is not feasible to practice the target behavior frequently (e.g., long trips away from home), too expensive to do (e.g., traveling in airplanes), or the precise conditions are hard to arrange at will (e.g., driving in a snowstorm at rush hour). At these times, imaginal exposure may be employed, following the same parameters as for in vivo exposure, if the client can imagine clearly and experiences the anxiety response with imagery. There is some disagreement in the literature as to how effective imaginal exposure is when compared to in vivo exposure (see Emmelkamp 1982). The effects of in vivo seem to be more consistent; indeed, imaginal exposure may work in an indirect fashion by potentiating self-directed in vivo exposure.

As a result, it seems wise to use the in vivo approach when possible. There are additional advantages. In vivo work obviates the need for training clients in imagery, with which some clients have great difficulty. Moreover, it can be quite difficult to monitor avoidance in imagery (e.g., the client loses the image and cannot retrieve it), making it harder to ensure prolonged, continuous exposure.

Panic-Management Strategies

The central importance of panic attacks and the fear of fear to the development and maintenance of agoraphobia has already been emphasized. Exposure serves to mobilize clients, but if they continue to experience panic attacks, treatment gains will often be reversed. Thus, it should come as no surprise that clients with higher frequencies of panic pretreatment tend to fare worse. Two approaches to this problem have developed: psychotherapeutic interventions and psychopharmacological ones.

Psychotherapeutic Strategies

Coping with Panic

A number of interventions have been devised for handling panic when it begins to occur. Among them are cognitive restructuring, paradoxical intention, and attention manipulation.

In *cognitive restructuring*, the clients' maladaptive thoughts about anxiety are systematically challenged. This includes educating the clients about the nature of anxiety (this is basic to all exposure approaches) and training clients to provide reassurance to themselves, when anxious, that anxiety is not in fact life threatening, that they will not lose control, faint, become insane, and so forth.

Agoraphobics are usually convinced that their anxiety is apparent to all and that they are not only feeling strange but acting strangely. Thus, in the case of Ms. H., the client was convinced she wobbled terribly when walking in the open, and Ms. H. was very concerned that others would notice. In reality, neither had a noticeable change in gait. Unless clients are so convinced of the danger of falling that they hug the walls when walking, actual changes in appearance are confined to those who hyperventilate so much as to blur vision and cause dizziness. Repeated feedback while the client is anxious and thinks the symptoms are apparent helps to correct these misperceptions.

Another important cognition to challenge is the impression that anxiety is all-pervasive and forever. Agoraphobics tend to remember the worst part of an excursion as how it was the entire time and to fear if they do not leave a situation where they are anxious the anxiety will go on and on. For this reason, as well as for the therapist's information in assessing progress, it is very useful to teach them to rate their anxiety on a 0-100 scale ranging from calm to panic. There is often some resistance to doing this, as clients fear they will become more anxious if they think about how they are feeling. Once they learn to do it, however, they are generally surprised to see how brief a period of time they were actually very uncomfortable, how often the anticipation was actually worse than the doing, and how their anxiety levels typically declined after some time, even though they did not flee.

Agoraphobics tend to believe that anxiety or tension is an abnormal state, that they should be perfectly calm at all times, in all situations. It is certainly true that they experience an abnormal amount of anxiety compared to most people in, for example, stores. However, their expectation that everyone else is completely calm and their assessment that something is terribly wrong if they feel low levels of tension in such places is erroneous and maladaptive. These beliefs increase fear of fear and avoidance. An important task for the therapist is to consistently communicate that some anxiety is a normal part of life, that anxiety may be unpleasant but not terrible, and that anxiety is to be confronted and mastered, not avoided. For example, an upcoming event, such as a trip the client is dreading, should be reframed as an opportunity for practicing new skills. Anxiety experienced during exposure sessions, similarly, is not failure but is a chance to learn that dreaded consequences will not befall one and is an occasion to see oneself mastering the unpleasant feelings.

A somewhat different approach that may be used in combination with cognitive restructuring is *attention manipulation*. Agoraphobics, as has been noted, heighten their anxiety response by focusing on it and catastrophizing about it. Their attention is concentrated on the threatening aspects of a situation or of their feelings, and their thoughts are preoccupied with how they will behave, will feel, or will be harmed. Consequently, they are out of touch with the complete present reality and are fantasizing about a future, much more unpleasant time. Needless to say, this is not a reassuring approach to one's anxiety. Zane (1978) has emphasized the importance of keeping the client in the present as a way of cutting into this anxiety spiral and has suggested a number of useful techniques (see Chapter 11). One is having clients broaden their present awareness by focusing on concrete nonthreatening aspects of the situation that they have been excluding from awareness: the sound of the therapist's voice, the colors and textures of objects around them, and the sense of their feet touching the floor. This is not to be confused with distraction, which is countertherapeutic. With distraction, clients attempt to avoid realizing where they are and how they feel by fantasizing being elsewhere, engaging in endless conversation, or always carrying a book or magazine to read. The idea is not to deny one's anxiety but to also be aware of the total context, which is much more than anxiety and which is not filled with danger. Because the present situation is never dangerous in the way the client fears, only the fantasized future situation, the continued practice of having clients cut off future-oriented thoughts (e.g., "I better get out of here, or I'll faint") and concentrate on present ones (e.g., "I'm tense, but I'm conscious. I can tell because I see this, and I feel that") reduces the anxiety response considerably. This takes much practice and vigilance on the client's part. When approaching a threatening task or when discussing doing one, the therapist can anticipate the client in imagining future catastrophe, ask "where the client is," and call the client back to the present. After many repetitions, the process is internalized. Some clients find it useful to aid the thought-stopping by wearing a rubber band on the wrist, snapping it to help break up a concentration on the negative, and then concentrating on the present.

A rather different approach but one that is well in keeping with the overall message that anxiety is not threatening is *paradoxical intention* (see Chambless and Goldstein 1980). Clients are asked to exaggerate or to deliberately try to bring on their feared anxiety symptom or consequence. The woman afraid of wobbling is asked to wobble; the person embarrassed by sweating to sweat buckets; and the man with shaking hands to shake them like leaves. The client fearful of rapid heartbeat is asked to concentrate on his or her heart and to speed it up even faster, and the woman afraid of fainting is asked to faint while the therapist is there to catch her. The client fearful of insanity is urged to take the opportunity to go insane with a therapist who will handle the situation. In the case of symptoms under voluntary control (for example, trembling hands) the therapist may model the exaggerated behavior.

Paradoxical intention serves several purposes. First, it communicates that the therapist is not worried about the client's symptoms and does not believe that something awful will happen. Second, it helps the client break into the cycle of fighting anxiety and becoming even more tense from the effort. The client learns that nothing terrible happens even when one does not struggle to dampen the anxiety. In this way, paradoxical intention is a more active variation on Weekes's (1976) suggestion that one "float with anxiety" rather than fight it (see Chapter 16). The active aspect of paradoxical intention is easier for many clients than the passive approach of floating. Third, it injects a note of humor into the therapy that in itself counteracts anxiety. This can be used particularly effectively in a group where clients can play with their symptoms and gain distance from them by labeling various group members according to their predominant symptom (e.g., *The Choker*).

It is of the utmost importance that this approach only be used with compassion, lest the client think the therapist does not understand how painful and frightening the symptoms are. It is not necessary to use paradoxical intention in a manipulative fashion, that is, without explaining the purposes of the technique to the client as well as the reasons it seems to work. This is an extremely effective technique with most symptoms but is commonly frightening for clients to attempt, as they fear that the dreaded catastrophe just might befall them. Consequently, it is easiest to use attention manipulation first, resorting to paradoxical intention if it fails. Symptoms that do not respond well to being focused on directly are dizziness, nausea, and feelings of unreality. Such sensations may be increased by focusing on them. If the client cannot in fact vomit on command (I have never had a client be frightened of nausea who could in fact vomit at will), the appropriate paradoxical instruction is "go ahead and vomit." The dizzy client may be encouraged to faint if this is a feared catastrophe. Focusing on present stimuli is usually more productive for feelings of unreality than is paradoxical intention, but if necessary the client can be instructed to float as far away from the situation as possible, see how that feels, and then when that is comfortable, to return. Dizziness, numbness in the extremities, problems with breathing, and feelings of unreality primarily result from hyperventilation. Thus, it is only necessary to use other coping techniques if proper breathing has been established but the symptoms continue.

A final coping technique is *proper breathing*. Agoraphobics generate or exacerbate a number of their symptoms through hyperventilation. Others may stop breathing for short periods at times of great anxiety. Under less anxiety-provoking situations, most still breathe in a shallow, rapid fashion rather than from the diaphragm. A calming breathing pattern is to take slow, even breaths from the diaphragm. In learning this technique, it helps to place one hand on the diaphragm and another on the chest, seeking to keep the latter stationary while the former rises with inhalation and falls with exhalation. Some clients may have to practice this technique initially in a supine position before they can accomplish it sitting and standing. Clients are requested to practice several times daily for about 5 to 10 minutes and to monitor their breathing when entering an anxiety-provoking situation. The therapist also should watch for maladaptive breathing during exposure sessions and prompt the client to use the new method. Should the client become very frightened and begin to hyperventilate, she or he should be instructed to close the mouth and breathe only through the nose, as it is very difficult to hyperventilate without gasping for air. Clients who return from a task reporting they are unable to get their breath have often been hyperventilating. The instruction to blow out all air in the lungs before attempting to breathe again not only has a paradoxical effect but also helps correct overoxygenation.

Empirical research on cognitive restructuring and paradoxical intention indicates that, combined with homework instructions, these techniques are effective in the treatment of mildly to moderately avoidant agoraphobic clients (Mavissakalian et al. 1983). The former works more slowly but eventually is as effective as the latter. In the treatment of more severely avoidant clients, Emmelkamp and his colleagues failed to find any positive effects of adding cognitive restructuring to therapist-directed in vivo exposure (see Emmelkamp 1982). Research using paradoxical intention plus exposure versus the exposure alone is still in progress. Based on my experience in using in vivo exposure without cognitive restructuring or other coping techniques, I would interpret Emmelkamp's findings in the following way: Once clients manage to enter and stay in their phobic situations for an adequate length of time, they do just as well on the whole, regardless of the addition of cognitive restructuring. Getting them to enter and remain in the phobic situations without some promise of relief through coping strategies (even if this ultimately turns out to be superstitious belief) is very difficult. Thus, training in panic management cuts down on avoidance during treatment and on dropouts. I also think it is difficult to test these coping mechanisms in group designs, because different strategies work for different clients, making it nonproductive to use a prepackaged intervention.

Reducing the Propensity to Panic

It has been noted that agoraphobics are highly chronically anxious people. This high daily tension level keeps the agoraphobic in a state of excitation from which the anxiety may easily escalate into panic. A sudden loud noise may be a sufficient trigger. Once clients become more mobile and less anxious in anticipation of encountering a phobic situation, they are ready to turn their attention to treatment directed at lowering this chronic tension. Anxiety-management training has proved effective with these clients in reducing the frequency of panic attacks as well as the severity of anxious mood (Jannoun et al. 1982). Clients are first trained in progressive relaxation and cognitive restructuring, if this has not been previously taught during exposure. Because becoming profoundly relaxed may be frightening to some clients (see Heide and Borkovec 1984), the therapist may have to proceed slowly with relaxation training. Once they have acquired these skills, the next step is practicing the application of these techniques, as they imagine situations of all sorts that make them feel tense. In the third step, clients apply their skills throughout the day in situations where they feel uncomfortable as a coping skill. Anxiety-management training differs from systematic desensitization in that it is not a technique to use in a therapist's office with a particular hierarchy but is a skill for use in the daily environment, whatever the distressing stimuli, to cope with (not eliminate) anxiety. Some clients also seem to benefit from exercise programs and training in problem-solving strategies as other ways to reduce tension.

A final strategy involves training clients to identify accurately the type of emotion they are experiencing and the source of their distress. As has been earlier explained, many types of intense affect may come to be interpreted by agoraphobics as anxiety. Moreover, when anxious about other events in his life, the agoraphobic may label the source of his or her anxiety to be the shopping mall or expressway, rather than attending to the actual distressing event. Probing for the antecedents of panic can be done retrospectively in the therapist's office or during in vivo exposure sessions. In the case of Ms. H., we saw that when she discussed her unhappiness with her spouse, she consistently switched to a focus on her anxiety symptoms. With the therapist's persistently bringing her back to the topic of what was happening when she panicked under unusual circumstances (riding in the city with her husband was usually a "safe" activity), she was able to identify part of her distress as being attributable to her loneliness in the marriage.

Clients can be trained to keep records of panic attacks that seem to occur out of the blue and to identify sources of discomfort that are most often interpersonal. Often they will draw a blank and have much more difficulty than Ms. H. It may be necessary to ask for a brief review of the day's events, and especially contacts with people the therapist knows to be troublesome to the client, before the pertinent events come to light. One client, for example, came to a session having panicked severely during the week, losing all the progress she had made during several previous weeks on her driving. She denied any problems during the week. When pressed to recall how long she felt strong and positive about her changes (the state in which she left the prior session), she eventually pinpointed a conversation with her husband, with whom she had a difficult relationship. He was quite controlling and rigid in his expectations for her in general. Observing her progress, her spouse announced that because she was getting better, they could now start on the family that he wanted but that the client definitely did not want. The client reported feeling trapped, condemned by him as a failure if she remained agoraphobic but subject to relentless pressure to meet his expectations if she improved. Subsequent to this conversation, she became panicky again driving short distances and lost motivation to continue practicing. It was important that she see that her anxiety was an understandable response to what seemed to be irresolvable conflict rather than a property of driving and that she needed to find ways of dealing with her anger and resentment in her relationship.

It is easier to intervene if this attribution training can be done in the in vivo session itself. The therapist can then more readily identify feelings being mislabeled as *anxiety*. A client was working on riding subways without the therapist, who waited at the end of the line. She returned to meet the therapist, eyes brimming with tears and face full of sorrow. Left without the opportunity of escape when she had parted from the therapist at the other end of the line, she found that beyond the panic was a feeling she found even more difficult and fought to reject: a sense of overwhelming isolation and sorrow. Although this was hard for her to experience, she ceased to fear panic and began to confront her terrible loneliness and her history of abandonments in her therapy. Staying in touch with core feelings and aware of causes of distress seems to be highly effective in reducing so-called *spontaneous panic attacks*. Anxiety-management training is still advisable, however, for reducing the chronic generalized anxiety levels.

Psychopharmacological Intervention

A very different approach to the control of panic is the use of psychotropic medication. A considerable amount of research has been conducted on the effects of various medications on clients who have panic attacks, including those with agoraphobia (see review by Liebowitz and Klein 1982). Major tranquilizers, such as the phenothiazines, seem to exacerbate the symptoms, whereas minor tranquilizers help control the chronic anxiety for a time but seldom adequately control panic. Nevertheless, most clients with agoraphobia have a long history of minor-tranquilizer use. Typically, they avoid large amounts of these drugs but take them when panicky or when forced to confront a difficult situation. A few, however, become addicted.

As the role of the tricyclic antidepressants in controlling panic has received considerable publicity in recent, years, more and more agoraphobic clients have had experience with these drugs. Monoamine oxidase (MAO) inhibitors (e.g., Nardil) have similar effects but are not widely used in the United States because of potentially serious side effects. These drugs have a therapeutic effect in the treatment of agoraphobia. The results of various treatment centers vary as to whether they add to the effects of in vivo exposure. Data from the most carefully conducted research indicate the answer is "no," but that these drugs combined with education and systematically followed homework instructions do constitute an effective treatment in the absence of therapist-assisted exposure (Mavissakalian and Michelson 1983). Agoraphobic clients have often had bad experiences with a tricyclic because the drug was prescribed by a physician unfamiliar with its use in anxiety disorders rather than depression. Agoraphobic people are extremely sensitive to and frightened by the drug's side effects (e.g., heart palpitations, hand tremors) and many become very agitated and discontinue the medication unless they are built up slowly on the drug in 10- or 25-mg increments. Paradoxical effects of the drug are common, making it rather difficult to know if the client is agitated because the dosage is too high or too low. The most common therapeutic dose of imipramine (Tofranil) is 150 mg daily. However, about one-fourth of agoraphobic people have been found to be so sensitive to the drug that they reach a therapeutic level on as little as 75 mg. Clients are continued on the medication for about a year, once good results are reached, before withdrawal is attempted. If panic attacks begin again, the drug is reintroduced.

Propranolol (Inderal), a beta-adrenergic blocker often used to control high blood pressure, has been tested on agoraphobic clients with mixed results. It seems to effectively control some of the physical sensations of anxiety (e.g., rapid heartbeat, trembling hands) but to be ineffective for the psychological aspects.

For clients whose main concern is rapid heartbeat, however, the drug may be quite beneficial. It is sometimes combined with imipramine to reduce the noxious heart palpitations some clients have with that drug, is often used with paroxysmal tachycardia, and is increasingly prescribed to clients with mitral valve prolapse. Consequently, it is beneficial to be aware of the drug and its effects.

Finally, a highly touted new drug has appeared on the scene that is said to have antipanic properties—alprazolam (Xanax). As its name would suggest, it is closely akin to diazepam (Valium). From its chemical properties, it is difficult to discern why this drug should be more effective than Valium with panic. Moreover, the same potential for abuse and for decreasing effectiveness of the drug over the space of a few months would seem to apply to this new compound. Nevertheless, it is being eagerly received, for it is much more difficult to get clients adjusted on the tricyclics and to get them to stay on them than it is to take a drug that has an immediate sedating effect and fewer unpleasant side effects. The drug may have potential as a short-term treatment for panic attacks during a limited period of stress (although its effectiveness needs to be demonstrated in controlled trials, which are currently being conducted), but it does not seem appropriate for long-term use with a chronic disorder such as agoraphobia.

There are drawbacks as well as benefits to the use of these drugs. The long-term disadvantage to tricyclics, MAO inhibitors, and propranolol is the tendency for relapse once the drug is withdrawn. Anecdotally, this is the case for alprazolam as well. This is understandable in that the clients have learned no other ways of controlling their panic and attribute their improvements to the drug. Furthermore, there is about a 20% initial refusal rate by clients who are afraid of ill effects from the drug or loss of control associated with a foreign substance in the body (see Telch et al. 1983). In addition, with the tricyclics, the drug class of the most documented effectiveness, there is an average of a 40% dropout rate due to side effects. Last, agoraphobia most often begins in women of childbearing years, and none of these drugs is considered safe to take during pregnancy. Moreover, the long-term risk of damaging side effects remains unknown.

For all of these reasons, I do not see pharmacotherapy as the first-line treatment of choice, unless there is urgent need for rapid control of frequent panic. Nevertheless, it may be the only effective treatment for agoraphobic people isolated in areas where behavioral treatment is not available or for those who cannot obtain treatment at a fee they can afford. I do describe pharmacotherapy as an alternative to clients applying for treatment, but it is unusual that they opt for trying this approach first. If a client has not made substantial progress in 3 to 6 months of behavior therapy despite genuine efforts on her or his part, we discuss the use of medication again at that time. At times, the medication makes a dramatic difference. Unfortunately, the same factors that predict poor response to exposure (high depression and high frequency of panic) also predict poor results with imipramine (Zitrin et al. 1980).

The Process of Treatment

Throughout this chapter, I have emphasized the multiple problems clients with complex agoraphobia bring into treatment. Because many therapeutic strategies and techniques not specific to the treatment of agoraphobia are required for comprehensive treatment, I will most often, in this section, have space only to point out the problems that need to be addressed and how they are likely to occur.

The client's depression interacts with his or her response to treatment, requiring the therapist to intervene when maladaptive behavior common to depressed clients surfaces. For example, it is common for a client to downplay or ignore gains made during a session unless the therapist encourages the client to recognize and acknowledge them by verbalizing them to the group or to the therapist. Similarly, clients lose track of the progress they have made and persist in thinking they have not changed over the weeks of treatment. Having them keep records of progress is helpful, particularly in the face of the setbacks that are bound to occur. Because losing ground after a particularly bad panic attack is such a common event, we encourage clients to make sure to have a setback while they are still in treatment. This does not prevent them from feeling helpless when the relapse occurs, but, when reminded of what we told them, they do bounce back more quickly. Clients often are distressed because their expectations of therapy were unrealistic; they hoped the anxiety would be "cured." We stress the importance of viewing therapy not as a cure but as a way to learn to cope. It is an unusual client who never has a panic attack again after termination.

As clients change in treatment and as they learn to identify sources of tension and unhappiness in their lives, they need therapy focused on the other identified problem areas as well. Because these problems often interfere with exposure treatment if ignored, it is preferable to conduct this treatment concurrently with the exposure work (see Chambless and Goldstein 1981 for an extensive description of this format). Many therapists have been caught in the trap of trying to resolve the other issues first and then turn to the exposure. This is a road to nowhere, in that the client is generally unwilling, and indeed unable, to focus on other problem areas while so distressed by phobias and panic. Moreover, until awareness is developed through treatment, the client may be unaware that there is a connection between other life events and agoraphobia. Certainly, multiple sessions weekly are costly; however, if desirable, costs may be held down through using trained paraprofessionals for the exposure work (see Zane and Seif 1983).

The most common problem that emerges is the agoraphobic person's difficulty in recognizing and expressing feelings and needs in significant personal relationships. Communications training is important, but the larger proportion of the work lies in helping the person to sort out what she or he wants or feels and to believe that she or he is entitled to these feelings and their expression. Gestalt therapy techniques are often extremely useful in this way. Because of the agoraphobic's extreme sensitivity to others' reactions, desensitization to anger and withdrawal may be required.

Couples or family sessions are almost always desirable in the treatment of agoraphobia, if only to provide the significant others with information about how to support the agoraphobic person through the change process. Commonly, however, the work needs to go beyond simple information. After prolonged agoraphobia, couples and families may interact extensively around the symptoms and need help finding healthier ways to relate as the client improves. Most importantly, the agoraphobic person's sense of being trapped and/or alone is generally, at least in part, a reflection of how she or he feels in these intimate relationships. Assisting the couple or family in developing mutually supportive relationships that also allow individuation is a central therapeutic task.

Rehabilitation counseling may be required for clients who have been out of the work force for a prolonged period owing to their phobias. Vocational counseling is also important for the female client who is considering entering the work force after caring for young children. Some sort of meaningful involvement outside the home is particularly important for these clients, not only to help them stay mobile but also to give them a sense of connection with the external world. It is particularly beneficial for them to know they could be financially self-sustaining, as this fosters their feeling more powerful in their marital relationship.

I have emphasized the importance of separation and threats of separation in the history of agoraphobic clients. Many times, these clients have unresolved grief reactions that surface when they are alone and that spur their avoidance of this situation. Others may have images of especially painful memories, such as those reported by Ms. H., who stayed awake as a child at night monitoring her mother's breathing and watching the hospital door to see if her father was among the wounded. Psychological resolution of these issues is vitally important if the fears of being alone are to be overcome. Imaginal flooding may be used to expose the client to these images and memories within the safe context of the therapist's office. Repeated exposure sessions are necessary in this case, just as they are for the phobic stimuli. Examples of this sort of treatment have been provided by Chambless and Goldstein (1980, 1981) and Ramsey (1977). A study by Mawson and colleagues (1981) has demonstrated the empirical effectiveness of this approach, sometimes called *guided mourning* when bereavement is concerned.

This multifaceted approach to treatment, combining work on associated problems with exposure, results in improvement in a broader group of clients. With this approach, clients who fare poorly with exposure alone (those starting treatment with higher depression and marital dissatisfaction and a greater frequency of panic attacks) have an equally good chance of responding well to treatment (Chambless et al. 1986). Furthermore, a higher rate of overall improvement is noted. On broad ranges of agoraphobic avoidance, only a 39% overall improvement rate has been reported (Agoraphobia factor on the Fear Survey Schedule, Hafner and Ross 1983) with exposure alone, whereas this multitherapeutic approach results in a 55.5% improvement rate on the even broader Mobility Inventory.

TREATMENT LIMITATIONS

Although great strides have been made in the behavioral treatment of agoraphobia, there remains a notable proportion of clients who do not improve with treatment. Using an intensive approach to treatment, combining exposure with attention to the other problems that have been described, we (Chambless et al., 1986) still find 14% of clients to be treatment failures (i.e., they improve less than 25% on measures of phobic avoidance and panic attacks). With less-than-optimal treatment, the failure rate is even higher. As has been noted, at a group level the addition of pharmacotherapy seems to add little to the effectiveness of behavior therapy, although it might make some difference for individual clients. The broader approach to treatment advocated here does negate the effects of statistically documented predictors of failure with treatment by exposure and pharmacotherapy. Nonetheless, there are several common problems that crop up and remain unresolved.

The first is that of the client who is enmeshed in personally destructive relationships and who refuses to acknowledge and work on these problems in therapy or is unwilling to consider leaving a relationship in which the other will not bend. A second problem is that of the client who refuses to take any responsibility for his or her improvement. This client, despite every direct or indirect effort on the therapist's part, does not do homework assignments and is generally unwilling to tolerate even moderate levels of discomfort during treatment, expecting the therapist to magically remove all obstacles. Usually these clients have been very spoiled and babied in their families of origin and are often wealthy, so that they can lead comfortable lives within their restrictions. Yet a third problem is exemplified by those clients who fixedly believe that some catastrophe will befall them from a panic attack and who are therefore unwilling to take risks during treatment. Although some of these clients have seemed to be of low intelligence, this is not the case for all. The most puzzling problem of all is that of the occasional client who works hard in treatment but, despite repeated exposure sessions, does not show the predictable pattern of within- and across-session habituation (see Foa and Chambless 1978). Fortunately, these are clients who seem to respond well to medication.

In working with clients in less fortunate circumstances, the problems are multiplied. Not only must the frequency and comprehensiveness of treatment be reduced in most facilities, but also the client's life circumstances serve to keep her or his anxiety level extremely high, fostering panic attacks and inhibiting inhibition. Thus, social problems such as poverty, unemployment, inadequate housing, poor medical care, drug abuse by one's children, and so forth all have a profound impact on the client's emotional status but can hardly be resolved by the behavior therapist. Time and time again, these clients struggle to improve in therapy, only to be knocked flat by the next crisis in their lives. Moreover, poverty-level clients often attend treatment irregularly and follow through poorly on homework instructions. Data reviewed by Weissman (1983) indicate that agoraphobic people are disproportionately likely to be poorly educated and minority-group members. These clients are not represented in most research trials. Consequently, the improvement rates for exposure are undoubtedly an overestimate for this group. Cognitive coping strategies that were devised in interaction with educated, verbal clients may also be less useful for lower-class clients.

Complex Agoraphobia

Treatment of a case of complex agoraphobia is considerably more demanding and multifaceted than is the case with simple agoraphobia, as will be illustrated by the case of Ms. J. This client first sought treatment for agoraphobia of 4 years' duration at age 22. Ms. J. was a secretary with a high-school education. She came from a blue-collar family, was single, and lived with her parents and two brothers. An older brother was married and out of the household. Ms. J. described her mother as a very nervous person and her father as a weekend alcoholic who physically abused his wife but not his children. One of the client's brothers had severe learning disabilities; another had psychotic episodes, occasionally attempted suicide, and had been arrested for criminal acts. Ms. J. was the good child who was protective of her parents, caused no trouble, and was, she thought, consequently, ignored.

Ms. J. was very close to her mother as a young child but lost her when the latter began evening shift work, thus leaving the house when the client was just returning from school. Ms. J. reported feeling extremely isolated and abandoned, particularly because she feared her father—his angry outbursts and his overly affectionate behavior when intoxicated. The family's attention seemed primarily focused on the troublesome brothers. When Ms. J. was about 13 years old, her mother became a member of a fundamentalist religious group and involved the client in this religion as well. Feeling this to be her only connection with her mother, Ms. J. became very involved in this church, which taught that members were not to associate with people outside the faith and that all nonmembers were eternally damned. Controls over sexual behavior were particularly rigid. As Ms. J. approached adulthood, it became time for her to be confirmed as a full member of the church. She had considerable qualms about this, as she secretly disagreed with many of the teachings. Nevertheless, the church was her sole social system and her bridge to her mother. Also, she truly feared that leaving the church, whose members would no longer be allowed to speak to her, would result in her damnation. It was in this climate that the client began having panic attacks while traveling to her job in downtown Philadelphia from the semirural area where she lived. Unable to overcome the attacks, she relinquished her job and also began avoiding trapped situations in general: public transportation, elevators, restaurants, and beauty parlors. In addition, she became afraid of being more than 30 minutes from her home. She was confirmed in the church and found a position close to home.

Before being referred to me, Ms. J. had been in individual psychotherapy for about 9 months and had irregularly attended an in vivo exposure group for about 6 months. During that time, she had begun to examine herself and her needs and to separate from the church temporarily despite condemnation by her mother. She was involved in a fairly positive relationship with a man who was not a church member. Sexual contact with her boyfriend was greatly limited by sexual phobias as well as continued confusion about the morality of extramarital sexual relationships. It appeared that her exposure group was composed of clients who were much more limited; consequently, most group time was devoted to situations like shopping malls with which the client had little difficulty. Being extremely unassertive, she had never complained to the exposure-group therapist. Moreover, during the exposure-group treatment the client actually became even more socially phobic than before treatment. Group exercises used by the therapist to foster support and intimacy were instead sensitizing to this very shy client, who was phobic of physical contact.

Ms. J. began treatment with me when the former therapist moved away. She was somewhat agitated, feeling angry and abandoned, but quickly formed a relationship with me. Her financial situation and the long distance from her home (her boyfriend had to bring her) to the clinic precluded more than one session weekly. Because the exposure group had not been helpful, we agreed she would drop group and have weekly individual sessions. Identified treatment targets were increasing her mobility, reducing her social anxiety, clarifying her feelings about church and family, and resolving her conflicts about her relationship with her boyfriend. Sexuality and intimacy in general were difficult issues for her.

Initially, homework assignments were used for in vivo exposure, with the client being accompanied by her boyfriend, who was very willing to be helpful. The pair worked on beauty parlors and riding trains, although their attempts were more sporadic than desirable. This approach was taken because the client strongly needed treatment for the other target areas and because her work schedule and distant location made arranging therapist-assisted exposure sessions quite difficult. As Ms. J. conquered a situation in her boyfriend's company, she next attempted to do it on her own. This step required forceful persuasion, not only because of her fearfulness but also because of this couple's pattern of spending every available moment together. When the client seemed stuck on a plateau, occasional therapist-assisted in vivo sessions (a total of six over 9 months) were interspersed with homework assignments. These were particularly needed for train trips to unfamiliar suburbs or cities. Although more such sessions would have been desirable and would have led to quicker and more extensive change, substantial changes were apparent. Some residual avoidance of public transportation remained, and Ms. J. gave high ratings to forms of transport that she had not had occasion to attempt—boats and airplanes. She became completely mobile when traveling by automobile and was able to regularly make the 90-minute drive to the clinic alone and to take trips with friends.

In work on the other related issues, one focus was on exploring the client's values and helping her to clarify her own beliefs versus the teachings of the church. Readings about ethics and values were also suggested. Ms. J. found these both frightening and important to her, as she struggled between her desire to follow her own conscience and her fear of being damned and cut off from the fellowship of the church. Although unable to make a permanent break from the church, she decided she could not follow its teachings and became more assertive when members questioned or criticized her behavior. In particular, she decided she wanted to have a sexual relationship with her boyfriend. Discussion, readings, homework assignments, and films for desensitization were used to help reduce her anxiety about sexual activity and her intense discomfort with her body.

A central issue for Ms. J., as for almost all agoraphobics, was being alone. Although she never complained of this problem, it became clear to her as treatment progressed that she could not tolerate being alone, even to the extent of being in her room with the door closed while other family members were downstairs. Thus, although she felt increasingly stifled by her relationship with her boyfriend, she spent all her evenings with him and developed no other internal or external resources. Through homework assignments, halting and difficult progress was made on spending time in her room alone, reading, and seeking friends to socialize with. During evenings alone in her room, she became fully aware of her sense of isolation in her family and in the world in general without the church and had a number of episodes of severe panic. Anger at her parents became an important issue at this time. The client resolved to obtain her own apartment but, frightened of doing so, she precipitously moved in with her boyfriend instead. Once she had done so, she felt even more suffocated by the relationship and angry at her boyfriend for his clinging behavior. With great difficulty, she became more assertive about spending time apart from him, but this was a continual struggle.

Assertiveness training was also important in working on Ms. J.'s relationships with other people, whom she cut out of her life if ever they hurt her feelings. Through homework assignments, she began to speak more to her co-workers rather than isolating herself, to take evening classes to broaden her contacts, and to develop her interests by becoming a volunteer at a social service agency. She also began to explore career options other than her secretarial position, which she found boring and poorly paid.

After 8 months of working with Ms. J., I accepted a position in another city and let her know I would be leaving in 3 months' time. Our therapeutic relationship had been a particularly close one, and Ms. J. became extremely panicky, agitated, and severely depressed in response to this impending change. Over a number of sessions she was gradually able to express some anger at my abandoning her but continued to deteriorate, developing problems with eating, sleeping, and had suicidal impulses. Eventually, she barely spoke during her sessions; rather she sobbed for most of the hour. After a month with no movement toward resolution, we decided it might help if Ms. J. began to form a connection at that time with the therapist who would see her on my departure. She approached her new therapist, a particularly warm and supportive woman, with considerable hostility but eventually decided to trust her and to meet with her regularly. Daily telephone contact was maintained with the new therapist until her suicidal impulses subsided. Ms. J. and I also continued to meet during this period to deal with her anger and grief.

The crisis continued for several months after I moved. Ms. J. and I exchanged letters and had occasional telephone contact as well. With her new therapist, she was gradually able to explore how this situation opened up her feelings about her mother's earlier abandonment of her and her decision at that time never to care for anyone again. She struggled extremely hard not to end our relationship by cutting me off as she had all others. Through this process, the client began to open up once again to her family and to re-establish an affectionate relationship with her mother. Her letters to me became less frequent and contact with me less painful.

In her continued therapy, Ms. J. has had no further in vivo exposure but at 18-month follow-up had maintained her gains on mobility, cognitions, and fear of body sensations. During this treatment, she has continued to work on autonomy, intimacy, and sexuality. She moved to her own apartment, established closer relationships with her parents, and continued to build social contacts and friendships. At this time, she reports that her life seems enough in order that she can devote some of her treatment time to making further gains on mobility.

CONCLUSION

In reading the behavioral research literature on the treatment of agoraphobia, one has the impression that all these clients need is a few sessions of exposure to resolve their problems. This is sometimes the case, but more often, however, agoraphobics have a host of problems that the practitioner will need to address for comprehensive treatment of the whole person. In practice, most clients require 6 to 18 months of treatment, although the exposure part of treatment is generally over in the first 3 to 6 months. Thus, unless the therapist strictly delimits the treatment program to covering only phobic avoidance behavior, a broad range of skills is required for treating these clients. This makes treatment challenging and seldom boring for the therapist.

Because agoraphobics react so strongly to the tenor of interpersonal relationships, it is particularly important that the therapists be warm, accepting figures who are also able to be firm and insistent in a treatment that is often frightening. Additionally, the therapist needs to have a high frustration tolerance for missed appointments and noncompliance. Too many are ready to write these clients off as not being motivated or ready for treatment, when they are, in fact, most often simply being what they are, that is, phobic. The therapist, consequently, has to take an active and directive role, especially in the early part of treatment. Although this role is a familiar, comfortable role to behavior therapists, it may be initially awkward to those approaching this work from different theoretical perspectives.

Working with agoraphobic clients can be the most rewarding task I know of, in that one has the opportunity to help someone make dramatic changes in her or his life. The clarity of change or failure with agoraphobic clients provides concrete feedback of efficacy that is often lacking in our profession. The failures are still too many, but the successes are truly gratifying.

ACKNOWLEDGMENTS

The author wishes to thank Alan Goldstein and the clients and staff of the Agoraphobia and Anxiety Program of Temple University Medical School for their contributions to the ideas and information presented in this chapter.

REFERENCES

American Psychiatric Association (1980). *Diagnostic and Statistical Manual of Mental Disorders* (3rd ed.). Washington, DC: APA.

Barlow, D. H., O'Brien, G. T., and Last, C. G. (1984). Couples treatment of agoraphobia. *Behavior Therapy* 15:41–58.

Barlow, D. H., and Wolfe, B. E. (1981). Behavioral approaches to anxiety disorders: a report on the NIMH-SUNY, Albany Research Conference. *Journal of Consulting and Clinical Psychology* 49:448–454.

Boisvert, J. M., Marchand, A., and Gaudette, G. (1983). *Group treatment of agoraphobia with or without partners.* Paper presented at the meeting of the Association for the Advancement of Behavior Therapy, Washington, DC, December.

Buglass, D., Clarke, J., and Henderson, A. S., et al. (1977). A study of agoraphobic housewives. *Psychological Medicine* 7:73-86.

Chambless, D. L. (1982). Characteristics of agoraphobics. In *Agoraphobia: Multiple Perspectives on Theory and Treatment*, ed. D. L. Chambless and A. J. Goldstein, pp. 1-18. New York: Wiley.

Chambless, D. L., and Goldstein, A. J. (1980). Agoraphobia. In *Handbook of Behavioral Interventions*, ed. A. J. Goldstein and E. B. Foa, pp. 322-415. New York: Wiley.

────── (1981). Clinical treatment of agoraphobia. In *Phobia Psychological and Pharmacological Treatment*, ed. M. Mavissakalian and D. Barlow, pp. 103-144. New York: Guilford Press.

Chambless, D. L., and Goldstein, A. J., eds. (1982). *Agoraphobia: Multiple Perspectives on Theory and Treatment.* New York: Wiley.

Chambless, D. L., Goldstein, A. J., and Gallagher, R., et al. (1986). A multitherapeutic approach to the treatment of agoraphobia. *Psychotherapy* 23.

Cobb, J. P., Mathews, A. M., Childs-Clarke, A., and Blowers, C. M. (1983). *The Spouse as Co-therapist in the Treatment of Agoraphobia.* Manuscript submitted for publication.

Crowe, R. R., Noyes, R., and Pauls, D. L., et al. (1983). A family study of panic disorder. *Archives of General Psychiatry* 40:1065-1069.

Emmelkamp, P. M. G. (1982). In vivo exposure treatment of agoraphobia. In *Agoraphobia: Multiple Perspectives on Theory and Treatment*, ed. D. L. Chambless and A. J. Goldstein, pp. 43-75. New York: Wiley.

Foa, E. B., and Chambless, D. L. (1978). Habituation of subjective anxiety during flooding in imagery. *Behaviour Research and Therapy* 16:391-399.

Goldstein, A. J., and Chambless, D. L. (1978). A reanalysis of agoraphobia. *Behavior Therapy* 9:47-59.

Hafner, R. J. (1982). The marital context of agoraphobia. In *Agoraphobia: Multiple Perspectives on Theory and Treatment*, ed. D. L. Chambless and A. J. Goldstein, pp. 77-117. New York: Wiley.

Hafner, R. J., and Ross, M. W. (1983). Predicting the outcome of behaviour therapy for agoraphobia. *Behaviour Research and Therapy* 21:375-382.

Harris, E. L., Noyes, R., Jr., and Crowe, R. R., et al. (1983). Family study of agoraphobia. *Archives of General Psychiatry* 40:1061-1064.

Heide, F. J., and Borkovec, T. D. (1984). Relaxation-induced anxiety: Mechanisms and theoretical implications. *Behaviour Research and Therapy* 22:1-12.

Jannoun, L., Oppenheimer, C., and Gelder, M. (1982). A self-help treatment program for anxiety state patients. *Behavior Therapy* 13:103-111.

Jansson, L., and Öst, L. G. (1982). Behavioral treatments for agoraphobia: an evaluative review. *Clinical Psychology Review* 2:311-336.

Liebowitz, M. R., and Klein, D. F. (1982). Agoraphobia: Clinical features, pathophysiology, and treatment. In *Agoraphobia: Multiple Perspectives on Theory and Treatment*, ed. D. L. Chambless and A. J. Goldstein pp. 153-181. New York: Wiley.

Marks, I. M. (1970). Agoraphobic syndrome (phobic anxiety state). *Archives of General Psychiatry* 23:538-553.

Marks, I. M., and Mathews, A. M. (1979). Brief standard self-rating scale for phobic patients. *Behaviour Research and Therapy* 17:263-267.

Mathews, A. M., Gelder, M. G., and Johnston, D. W. (1981). *Agoraphobia: Nature and Treatment*. New York: Guilford Press.

Mavissakalian, M., Michelson, L., and Greenwald, D., et al. (1983). Cognitive-behavioral treatment of agoraphobia: Paradoxical intention vs. self-statement training. *Behaviour Research and Therapy* 21:75-86.

Mawson, D., Marks, I. M., and Ramm, L., et al. (1981). Guided mourning for morbid grief: a controlled study. *British Journal of Psychiatry* 138:185-193.

Ramsey, R. W. (1977). Behavioural approaches to bereavement. *Behaviour Research and Therapy* 15:131-135.

Roberts, A. H. (1964). Housebound housewives: a follow-up study of phobic anxiety states. *British Journal of Psychiatry* 110:191-197.

Selzer, M. L. (1971). Michigan alcoholism screening test. *American Journal of Psychiatry* 127:89-64.

Sheehan, D. V., Ballenger, J., and Jacobsen, G. (1980). Treatment of endogenous anxiety with phobic, hysterical and hypochondriacal symptoms. *Archives of General Psychiatry* 37:51-59.

Sinnott, A., Jones, R. B., and Scott-Fordham, A., et al. (1981). Augmentation of *in vivo* exposure treatment for agoraphobia by the formation of neighborhood self-help groups. *Behaviour Research and Therapy* 19:339-347.

Telch, M. J., Tearman, B. H., and Taylor, C. B. (1983). Antidepressant medication in the treatment of agoraphobia: a critical review. *Behaviour Research and Therapy* 21:505-517.

Weekes, C. (1976). *Simple Effective Treatment for Agoraphobia.* New York: Hawthorn.

Weissman, M. M. (1983). *The epidemiology of anxiety disorders: rates, risks, and familial patterns.* Paper presented at the National Institute of Mental Health Conference on Anxiety and Anxiety Disorders, Tuxedo, NY, September.

Williams, S. L., Dooseman, G., and Kleifield, E. (1984). Comparative effectiveness of mastery and exposure treatments for intractable phobias. *Journal of Consulting & Clinical Psychology* 52:505-518.

Zane, M. D. (1978). Contextual analysis and treatment of phobic behavior as it changes. *American Journal of Psychotherapy* 32:338-356.

Zane, M. D., and Seif, M. N. (1983). Agoraphobia: Contextual analysis and treatment. In *Agoraphobia: Multiple Perspectives on Theory and Treatment*, ed. D. L. Chambless and A. J. Goldstein, pp. 119-152. New York: Wiley.

Zitrin, C. M., Klein, D. F., and Woerner, M. G. (1980). Treatment of agoraphobia with group exposure in vivo and imipramine. *Archives of General Psychiatry* 37:63-72.

4 Evaluation Anxieties

Dr. Aaron Beck is well known for the extraordinary impact his work on cognitive therapy has had on the current reconceptualization of psychotherapy. His central thesis is that cognition, or how we understand and process information, is a central function in our adaptation to our environment. A disturbance in cognition will lead to a disturbance in feeling and behavior. Correcting the disturbance in cognition will correct the disturbance in feeling and behavior. This emphasis on information processing is an obvious shift from the historical interest in affect, impulse, and conflict on the one hand and in behavior on the other.

In this chapter Dr. Beck discusses a variety of social phobias, performance anxiety, test anxiety, and anxiety in social situations. The treatment implications flow naturally from his conceptualization of these disorders. The term *evaluation anxieties* refers to a primary fear of being observed and evaluated and a primary cognitive distortion in which a critical evaluation is a catastrophe in terms of total failure, loss of love, loss of self-esteem, and so on. The anxiety may lead to an inhibition of functioning in social situations, which then itself becomes the problem.

It should be noted that besides cognitive therapy's very effective approach to social phobias, other popular approaches include group therapy, social-skills training, assertiveness training, psychodynamic exploration of factors such as inhibited exhibitionism, and medication.

Evaluation Anxieties

Aaron T. Beck

THE ESSENCE OF EVALUATION ANXIETIES

Before the Fall

A person entering a socially threatening situation is like someone walking a tightrope. He feels *vulnerable* to a serious mishap if his performance is not *adequate*. For *safety's* sake, he must conform to a rigid set of *rules* regarding appropriate actions and movements. The greater his *confidence* in his skill, the less likely he is to make a potentially fatal *misstep*. If he has a *failure* of nerve, his *performance* may be sabotaged by primitive reflex reactions—freezing, motor *inhibition*. Thus, this exercise is a test of his *ability* and *maturity*. Smooth performance reaffirms his *image* of himself and maintains his *status*. Failure would shatter this image. Finally, every action is *observed* by a crowd of *evaluators* and appraised as clumsy or skillful, and he is *judged* according to his confidence and competence. The italicized words here represent crucial aspects of the psychology of evaluative anxiety that will be described in this chapter.

The potential fall of the performer is paralleled by the "fall from grace" anticipated by an anxious person in the myriad of evaluative situations of everyday life. As in the case of the tightrope walker, *errors, missteps, inappropriate actions represent only a fraction of his overt behavior, but the damage is to the entire person*—or so he fears.

COMMON FEATURES OF EVALUATIVE THREATS

There are certain commonalities among the various situations in which an individual may experience "evaluation anxiety." The kinds of situation may be grouped as follows: (1) social situations—initiating or maintaining a person-to-person relationship; participating in a social gathering (for example, a party); (2) school or vocational situations—performance evaluation by teacher, supervisor, or peer group; taking a test or examination; confrontation with a superior over a conflict of interest; athletic competition; (3) transactions in the "outside world" while shopping or traveling, with salespersons, waiters or waitresses, taxi drivers, strangers.

A complex web of factors in these situations may aggravate or mitigate fears. These factors involve the question of evaluation and vulnerability and include the following: (1) the relative status of the individual and the evaluator in the area of power or social desirability; (2) the individual's skill in presenting an attractive or effective "front"; (3) his confidence in his ability to perform adequately in a given threat situation; (4) his appraisal of the degree of threat, the severity of potential damage, and the probability of its occurring; (5) the threshold of certain automatic "defenses" (verbal inhibition, blockage of recall, suppression of spontaneity) that can undermine individual performance; (6) the rigidity and attainability of the "rules" relevant to acceptable performance, behavior, and appearance; (7) the anticipated punitiveness of the evaluator for nonadherence to rules or substandard performance, and so on.

Vulnerability

The individual who is anxious on entering into an evaluative situation has a network of implicit questions.

1. "To what degree is this a *test* of my competence or acceptability? How much do I have to prove myself to me or others?"
2. "What is my status relative to that of my evaluators?" If the individual feels parity with or superior to the evaluator, then the rules are less narrow and more flexible and the prospective "punishment" for failure is less important.
3. "How important is it to establish a position of strength about relative power status (as in dealing with service personnel) or a position of acceptability in dealing with social evaluators (as in blind dates or speaking before an audience)?"
4. "What is the attitude of the evaluator? Is he accepting and empathetic or rejecting and aloof? Are his judgments likely to be objective or harsh and punitive?"
5. "To what degree can I count on my skills (such as verbal fluency) to carry me through the difficult evaluation?"
6. "What is the likelihood of my being undermined by distracting anxiety and inhibitions?"

Status and Ranking Order

A good part of the pressure to perform well is related to relative position on a vertical scale of power or social desirability. In a situation of confrontation with authority (teacher, supervisor, service personnel), the individual's perception of relative power determines his self-confidence and performance. If a person presents an appearance of self-confidence and competence, he reduces his "inferiority" on the power scale. If he perceives that he is lower, he is more likely to be less confident and less competent and thus will be vulnerable to being reduced in power even more. The dominance-submission dimension is generally also involved. The more dominant the individual perceives an evaluator to be, the more his own submissive tendencies are likely to be mobilized. Service personnel (physicians, cab drivers, receptionists, cashiers) are invested with authority and dominance by virtue of their position, which they can use to intimidate the individual.

In the case of a social confrontation in which a person wants to make a good impression, he is under pressure to maximize his social assets—attractiveness, dress, fluency, maturity, poise, grace. A high "score" on these assets may (depending on the values of the evaluator) make the person more desirable and thus ensure success in other encounters. A low "score" sets him up to be rejected.

A person may want to shun this type of confrontation because "failure" is painful. Moreover, avoidance leaves open the question of whether he is inferior, whereas a failure "confirms" his inferiority. Thus, social fearfulness is expressed in part by the experience of painful anxiety and the desire to reduce or avert the anxiety by avoiding or withdrawing from the aversive situation.

Self-Confidence

Confidence in one's ability to perform adequately in the confrontation is related to the perceived magnitude of one's expectations, their difficulty, and the anticipated punishment for inadequate performance.

A disparity in the individual's sense of his power or desirability in relation to that of the evaluator increases the magnitude of the task, because the criteria for acceptable performance are higher, and therefore the demands on him are greater. When he perceives himself in a "one-down" position, a person is less certain that he can fulfill these demands; and thus his global confidence in his competence is reduced. Moreover, if he anticipates a drastic "punishment" for inadequate performance (loss of job, suspension from school, termination of a relationship), his self-confidence may be further undermined. Other factors being constant, there is a reciprocal relationship between self-confidence and sense of vulnerability. As one goes up, the other goes down.

Rules and Formulas

In an obviously evaluative situation (for example, test taking, public speaking, making a date), there is a pressure to conform to arbitrary, rigid rules in order to avoid "punishment." The individual fears that he may not be sufficiently facile, fluent, and unflappable and thus experiences anxiety and other symptoms that militate against his attaining his goal. Deviations from these rules during performance raise negative evaluations and self-doubts, such as "I look timid, frightened," "What I say sounds stupid," "I'm so awkward," or "Will I foul it up?"

In public speaking, he believes he must adhere to stringent rules regarding the volume and tone of his voice, his articulateness and speed of speaking, his fluency and control of speech. The individual, thus, may fear that any departure from the rules may make him susceptible to disapproval and devaluation. In a social situation, deviation from the established canons may bring rejection.

In other types of interpersonal transaction (asking for information, requesting a raise), a breach of the rules may evoke hostility and overt devaluation. In such encounters, the individual is faced with such rules as "You shouldn't impose on people." Thus, if he makes a legitimate request or asserts his rights in a reasonable way, he may fear that "This seems like an imposition."

Automatic Protective Reactions

Automatic Inhibition

Reflex reactions in a dangerous situation have been discussed previously. Many people are susceptible to automatic inhibitory reactions that impede flow of speech, thinking, and recall. The "function" of these reactions under more primitive circumstances may have been to protect the individual from taking action that would provoke attack. Today this function is anachronistic and actually leads to dysfunction. Consequently, it is likely to evoke just the kind of attack that the individual would like to avoid. There does not appear to be any volitional component in this freezing reaction. It is mobilized completely contrary to a person's intentions and wishes.

Anxiety

Anxiety seems to be the product of a different system than is reflex inhibition. The function of anxiety seems to be to spur the person to take some action to reduce the danger. Then, he may be motivated to avoid going into a threatening situation or, if in the situation, to escape or minimize the danger by being inconspicuous (for example, not speaking up in class). It is obvious that, far from providing safety, the safety of protective patterns (inhibition blocking and anxiety-avoidance-escape) have a negative effect on performance. In fact, the anticipation of these reactions is in itself often sufficient to arouse anxiety and, then, to impair performance.

Faint

People in evaluative situations not infrequently feel faint and often fear that they will lose consciousness. This type of response is obviously highly inappropriate in an evaluative situation and may be a throwback to a primitive fear of being physically injured—as is the blood-injury phobia.

SOCIAL PHOBIAS AND SOCIAL ANXIETIES

Social phobias and social anxieties are concerned with one's exaggerated fear of being the focus of attention and devaluation by another person or persons. According to the third edition of the *Diagnostic and Statistical Manual of Mental Disorders* (DSM-III), the essential feature of social phobia is "a persistent irrational fear of, and compelling desire to avoid, a situation in which the individual is exposed to possible scrutiny by others" (American Psychiatric Association 1980, p. 228). This definition is probably too broad, in that it would encompass a huge proportion of the population as well as a significant number of patients now appropriately diagnosed as having a generalized anxiety disorder. In contrast to the definition of social phobia, the official definition of agoraphobia does specify that "normal activities are increasingly constricted as the fears or avoidance behavior dominate the individual's life" (p. 226). This restrictive criterion applied to the definition of social phobia would be more in keeping with the general concept of phobia. Moreover, DSM-III includes as examples of social phobias "fears of speaking or performing in public, using public lavatories, eating in public, and writing in the presence of others" (p. 227). Certainly the fear of speaking in public should not be included, since a very high proportion of the general population has this fear. If the more restrictive definition is used, a relatively small percentage of people with social anxiety would be considered social phobics.

PARADOXES OF SOCIAL ANXIETY

Unlike the phobias described in the previous chapters, a major feature of the social anxieties is that the actual fear (anticipation of being nervous and inhibited), prior to entering a situation, appears plausible and indeed seems to have a reasonable probability of being realized. Although a person with a phobia of heights, bridges, or elevators runs a minimal risk of falling or suffocating, an individual who is afraid that he will become tongue-tied when trying to carry on a conversation with a "blind date," or that his mind will go blank during an examination or interview, can reasonably expect these events to occur. The most interesting feature is that actually having the fear seems to bring on the undesirable consequence. A vicious cycle is created, whereby the anticipation of an absolute, extreme, irreversible outcome tends to make a person more fearful, defensive, and inhibited when entering the situation. On the other hand, the person who does not experience the fear of inept performance in a particular situation is substantially less likely to respond ineptly.

An important aspect of social anxiety, in which the fears are grossly inaccurate, is the individual's expectation that his inept performance in a social situation will be a fatal blow to his social aspirations. The expectation that one's life will be ruined by a specific rejection or failure is rarely borne out by experience. The content and the probability of such dire consequences are grossly exaggerated. Even when the extreme outcome does not occur after a particular unsettling experience, the individual, nonetheless, expects the bad thing to happen "next time."

The Fear of Being Evaluated

The central fear in the so-called social anxieties is that of negative evaluation by another person or persons—a fear that separates the social and the performance anxieties from agoraphobia. In the latter syndrome, a person may be afraid of wide-open spaces, fields, or beaches where there are no people, as well as closed-in groups or crowds of people. In agoraphobia, the fear of social disapproval appears to be secondary to the fear of losing control, fainting, going crazy, and so on. In contrast, in the social anxieties the central fear is of being the center of attention, of having one's "weaknesses" exposed, and consequently of being judged adversely by one or more people.

There is a symbolic confrontation in the social anxieties, whether the individual is calling a stranger on the telephone, trying to initiate a conversation in a social setting, or performing before a group. When the socially anxious person is engaged in a one-to-one encounter with another person or group of people, he believes that he is being scrutinized, tested, and judged.

Under observation are his performance, fluency of speech, self-assurance, and freedom from anxiety.

Unlike the agoraphobic, who is hypersensitive to internal signals suggestive of impending mental or physical collapse, the social phobic is hypersensitive to signals from other people regarding his acceptability. If he is receiving positive responses, he interprets them as a sign that he is making a good impression, and he feels less vulnerable and more self-confident. On the other hand, if he receives and integrates negative responses, he feels more vulnerable and less confident.

The physiological responses of the socially anxious individual may be similar to those of the agoraphobic person but are not as pronounced. As we shall discuss, he may feel the same type of sympathetic symptoms (rapid pulse rate, sweating) or parasympathetic symptoms (faintness, drop in blood pressure) as the agoraphobic; however, these evoke the fear that he will not perform adequately (which may be accurate), whereas the agoraphobic has the fear of an internal disaster (practically never accurate). It should be noted that some patients with public-speaking anxiety do, indeed, fear panic attacks, and some actually have a panic attack; but they are in the minority.

The Primal "Defenses"

The single factor that seems to be the most crippling to the socially anxious person is not the subjective experience of anxiety per se, although this indeed proves a handicap, but the various inhibitions, specifically those that interfere with his performance. Thus, the various types of inhibition—such as interference with verbal fluency, thinking, recall, and remote memory—are the most disabling factors in this disorder and, once they are involved in the vicious cycle, perpetuate the fear of going into the phobic situation.

These paradoxical responses to a threat, rather than priming the individual for more effective performance, actually impair his performance. The explanation seems to be, as we have said, that a primitive defensive system is mobilized as the individual goes into the social situation. This system, reminiscent of "freezing" and "atonic immobility" prepares the individual to cope with a *physical* assault but does not, of course, prepare him to perform effectively and maturely. Furthermore, the nature of this primitive innate response pattern is *designed* to produce immobility and muteness. Thus, paradoxically the defense against a challenge to speak up and actively participate in a particular situation triggers just the opposite of the demands.

DIFFERENTIATING SOCIAL PHOBIA FROM AGORAPHOBIA

In a landmark article, Amies and colleagues (1983) brought out in a systematic way a number of features that differentiate these two syndromes and consequently help to clarify the understanding of each. Eighty-seven people with symptoms of social phobia were compared with fifty-seven people with the symptoms of agoraphobia to determine whether the symptoms were part of distinct syndromes (the authors used the nonrestrictive diagnosis of social phobia according to DSM-III [1980]). The pattern of phobic situations was different in these two groups, as was the pattern of autonomic symptoms. Symptoms that could be observed by others were more frequent among the social phobics, whereas "fainting" was more frequent among the agoraphobics.

Situations that Provoke the Phobic Symptoms

The social phobics reported more severe anxiety in being introduced, in meeting people in authority, in using the telephone, whereas the agoraphobics reported more severe anxiety in being alone or in unfamiliar places, in crossing streets, and in public transport. The list of phobic situations is presented in Table 4-1.

TABLE 4-1 Comparison of Major Fears in Agoraphobia and Social Phobias

More severe when main complaint is social phobia	More severe when main complaint is agoraphobia
Being introduced	Being alone
Meeting people in authority	Unfamiliar places
Using the telephone	Crossing streets
Visitors to home	Public transport
Being watched doing something	Department stores
Being teased	Crowds
Eating at home with acquaintances	Open spaces
Eating at home with family	Small shops
Writing in front of others	Mice, rats, bats
Speaking in public	Snakes
	Flying insects
	Deep water
	Airplanes
	Blood, wounds

Source: Adapted from P. L. Amies, M. G. Gelder, and P. M. Shaw, "Social Phobia: A Comparative Clinical Study," *British Journal of Psychiatry* 142 (1983): 176.

In reviewing the situations that differentiate these two types of phobia, it becomes clear that the social phobic is concerned specifically about interpersonal situations, and that the center of the concern is being scrutinized by other people. The agoraphobic, in contrast, is concerned about being alone in unfamiliar or challenging places that present many kinds of stimulation and represent varying degrees of distancing or blocking from his home base (security). The social phobic, then, seems to encompass the notion of a *child being subjected to evaluation* by adults, whereas the agoraphobic seems to resemble the *child who has been placed in a strange place* for the first time. In the case of the social phobic, the other person or persons are involved in *paying attention* to the "child"; whereas in the case of the agoraphobic, the other people *ignore* him even to the point of not caring whether something disastrous happens to him.

In the study by Amies and colleagues (1983), the notion of being attacked is supported by the finding that the agoraphobic group is much more likely than the social phobic group to experience fears of small animals (mice, rats, bats), snakes, deep water, airplanes, injections, and so on. The typical agoraphobic's clustering of these fears suggests that this group is basically afraid of some kind of physical damage or attack.

Somatic Symptoms

Certain somatic symptoms tend to be far more pronounced in the agoraphobic than in the social phobic. As noted in Table 4-2, the agoraphobic is more likely to have typical "collapse" symptoms: weakness in the limbs, difficulty breathing, dizziness/faintness, and actual fainting episodes. This differentiation suggests that, in the agoraphobic, a different primal defensive response has been mobilized. This system—the parasympathetic—is generally associated with blood phobias but evidently also plays a role in agoraphobia.

TABLE 4-2 Comparison of Major Symptoms in Social Phobia and Agoraphobia

Item	Social phobia (%)	Agoraphobia (%)	P Less than
Blushing	51	21	0.001
Twitching of muscles	37	21	(0.07)
Weakness in limbs	41	77	0.001
Difficulty in breathing	30	60	0.001
Dizziness/faintness	39	68	0.01
Actual fainting episode	10	25	0.05
Buzzing/ringing in ears	13	30	0.05
Palpitations	79	77	NS*
Tense muscles	64	67	NS
Dry throat/mouth	61	65	NS
Sinking feeling in stomach	63	54	NS
Feeling sick	40	40	NS
Trembling	75	75	NS

Source: Adapted from P. L. Amies, M. G. Gelder, and P. M. Shaw, "Social Phobia: A Comparative Clinical Study," *British Journal of Psychiatry* 142 (1983): 176.
*NS = Nonsignificant.

THE PHENOMENA OF SOCIAL ANXIETY

In a clinical study, K. A. Nichols (1974) discusses the features of social anxiety in thirty-five cases observed over a 3-year period. The following clinical observations were drawn from different phases of therapy work, and each item was observed in at least 50 percent of cases.

1. The *perception* of disapproving or critical regard by others.
2. The *expectation* of disapproving or critical regard by others.
3. A strong tendency to perceive and respond to criticism from others that is nonexistent.
4. A feeling of being less capable and less powerful than others—low self-esteem.
5. Having rigid ideas of appropriate social behavior, and not being able to vary behavior in order to deal with difficulties.
6. Negative fantasy/imagination that produces anticipatory anxiety.
7. Heightened awareness and fear of being evaluated and judged by others.
8. A sense of being watched.
9. A discrimination and fear of situations from which sudden withdrawal would be unexpected and likely to attract attention.
10. A sense of being trapped/confined in such situations (that is, being socially closed).
11. An exaggerated interpretation of the sensory feedback related to tension or embarrassment.
12. Detection of bodily sensations within social situations.
13. A fear of being seen to be "ill" or losing control (that is, the physical signs of panic).
14. The experience of a progressive buildup of the discomfort.
15. The unpredictability of the anxiety response; the time available for prior fantasy and mood of the day seemed to be important determinants.

Nichols suggests that the incidence of social anxiety is related to some specific phase in development. He offers the late teens as a possible starting point. Finally, he adds that in the development of social anxiety, the role of personality traits and their associated cognitive aspects becomes important.

Shame and "Social Image"

The experience of shame is important in discussions of social anxiety because the socially anxious person is fearful of being shamed in many situations. Shame is an affect related to a person's conception of his public image at the time that he is being observed or believes he is being observed. His notion of his social image may be accurate or inaccurate; but if he *believes* that his image has been tainted, and he cares about the observer's opinion of him, then he is likely to feel shame. It should be noted that the possibility of being thought of as weak, inferior, or inept may be just as threatening as actually being talked about in these terms. In other words, what others think of him is the crucial ingredient of shame induction—irrespective of whether they communicate this opinion.

The key factor in the activation of shame is *exposure* to observation by one or more persons. This affect is triggered when a person realizes that he has been observed violating specific social norms, expectations, or demands, especially in relationship to appropriate appearance and behavior. His "deviant" appearance or behavior are judged (he assumes) to be reflections of his weakness, inferiority, ineptness, character flaw, or immaturity. The public sanctions for lack of conformity, by and large, take the form of making the individual feel inferior, depreciated, and immature. The actual social consequences may consist of covert depreciation or open expressions of disapproval, ranging from mild mimicking to overt ridicule. It should be noted that if a person manages to conceal his "substandard" behavior or engages in a shameful activity in private, then he does not feel shame.

A person who feels shame sees himself as relatively helpless in attempting to counteract his depreciated public image. He believes he is subject to painful group reprisals, such as public humiliation and ridicule, and is *powerless* to ward off these attacks. The social opinion is absolute, finalistic, irrevocable. It is futile for him to try to modify or appeal the group verdict, and he must accede to the right of the members of the group to amuse themselves at his expense. Any protestations only increase their enjoyment of his embarrassment. The individual acknowledges his "inept" behavior by statements such as "I made a public display of myself" and hangs his head or attempts to hide to avoid their gaze.

In his mind, the antidote for shame is to vanish from the shameful situation. A person will say, for example, "I should like to fade away," or, "I felt like merging into the woodwork." In contrast, anxiety is generally accompanied by the inclination to flee or by passive immobility.

Public relations deal in the currency of public appraisal, such as admiration or devaluation. A specific social group emphasizes surface values (peculiar to that group)—acceptable appearance, smooth performance, appropriate manners and dress, maturity—and gives public rewards (admiration, respect, special privileges). A person who deviates from the group norm may receive "punishment" through disdain, ridicule, isolation. We should emphasize that, if the opinion of members of the group is irrelevant or immaterial to him, he does not feel shame.

When we talk about the public image at a particular time, we do not imply that the "unacceptable" behavior is necessarily observed by a group. The interaction may be with another person with whom there is no personal relationship but who is a representative of the social group—that is, a stranger on the street, a telephone operator. Along the same lines, it appears that strangers can enforce shame more readily than can one's intimates. Thus, it may be practically impossible for parents to shame a child for his infractions of their domestic rules. Yet the child can be exquisitely sensitive to shame induced by strangers or by his own peer group for minimal deviation from group norms.

Shame is a form of *social influence*. Other people attempt to produce shame in us so as to control our behavior now and in the future. Typically, a person is exposed to a situation that produces shame. Although this may be the first experience in which he links this type of situation with this unpleasant affect, the memory is stored, and it influences the ways he approaches similar situations in the future. In a sense, a particular rule is set up by the individual: "If I behave in such a way, then I will be ridiculed and feel shame." It is the affect of shame that puts "teeth" into the rule. The individual thus is inclined to follow the rule and avoid the shame that would result from its violation.

Anxiety and shame differ in many ways. For one thing, anxiety generally occurs before one enters a stressful or threatening situation and may continue during the situation. But it is relieved when the situation is over. The feeling of shame starts during the "exposure" to the shameful experience and may continue for a time after the experience has ended.

Fear of Loss of Love or Abandonment

In intimate relationships, the demands are more "personal" than in "public relationships" and have to do with satisfying the specific needs and expectations of a particular person rather than with preserving an image. The expectations generally center on intangible qualities such as consideration, understanding, and caring. If a person does not meet those expectations of the significant other person, the sanctions take the form of withdrawal of affection or rejection. The affect derived from this sort of sanction is sadness. The qualities valued in intimate relations (kindness, empathy, warmth) are more often associated with "character traits," whereas those admired by the group are related to appearance and performance. In intimate relationships, a person is less likely to be concerned about group norms and, to a certain extent, can drop his façade. The concern in the intimate relationship is usually with unconditional and total acceptance without having to preserve appearances.

Fears of loss of love or abandonment may at times become entangled with the same concerns about performance as do the other evaluation anxieties. In these cases, the individual fears that he will not live up to the expectations or demands of a loved one. He may then slide into the same rut as the socially anxious person: (1) A sense of vulnerability because the other person has the power to terminate the relationship. He may come to fear that nothing he can do is good enough. (2) A sense of being continually judged and possibly disapproved of. (3) A defensive inhibition, so that his actual behavior becomes stilted and artificial. (4) "Catastrophizing" about the consequences of rejection. For example, a woman was in a continuous state of "high anxiety" over the possibility of being rejected by her lover. She believed that he was judging "everything" about her—how she dressed, spoke, prepared meals, arranged their social life. She worried that a single misstep would induce him to break the relationship. She sought continual reassurance that he was not displeased with her. Ultimately, he did leave her—not because of any deficiencies in her performance but because he could not tolerate her incessant requests for reassurance.

Public-Speaking Anxiety

The various disabilities and symptoms involved in severe public-speaking anxiety encapsulate the various facets of evaluation anxiety: vulnerability to being the center of scrutiny or to being judged harshly, negative predictions, reduced self-confidence, sense of incompetence, being handicapped by involuntary inhibition, impaired control of thoughts and speech, adherence to stringent rules, expectation of "punishment" for breaking the rules.

On Being Able to Function

The first hope of a person who attempts to speak in public is to be able to "function." The speaker must be able to maintain an upright position, keep his balance, open his mouth, and speak intelligibly. If he cannot do this, it means that "he has no control over the functioning of his mind and body"—a devastating blow to his self-confidence. Since control over "mind and body" is ultimately essential for survival, the undermining of his functioning by the primal mechanisms represents a symbolic threat. Specific symptoms such as swaying, a quavering voice, faint feelings, loss of fluency, rigid postural control, all mean to him, "I can't control myself—I can't perform adequately—anything can happen to me." The sense of being victimized by internal processes is similar to the experience of the agoraphobic, except that it does not imply the presence of a life-threatening or disintegrating disorder.

This demonstration of lack of control is perceived (or so the speaker believes) by the audience. The person then experiences not only the fear of being unable to function but also the greater fear that his lack of functioning will be judged by the audience as an indication of his "sickness, nervousness, immaturity, neurosis, inadequacy."

Role of Anxiety

Although the subjective aspects of anxiety are difficult to describe, they seem to be universally experienced in response to a sense of threat in the evaluative situation. The physiological symptoms are initially of the sympathetic type: increase in blood pressure, pulse, and perspiration. These symptoms, however are not infrequently followed by a faint, dizzy, or wobbly feeling (parasympathetic). The faint feeling is sometimes a result of the drop in blood pressure and may be related to the pooling of blood in the lower extremities. Similarly, dry mouth and/or sweating are autonomic reactions.

Anxiety itself serves as a "stimulus" to further negative conceptualization. First, the unpleasant experience itself serves to distract the person from the task at hand just as would a sudden sharp pain. Second, he interprets anxiety as a dramatic sign that he is not functioning well (and *will not* function well). The anxiety itself, rather than any focused systematic assessment of his capability, is taken as the index of dysfunction. He has a concept such as, "This is a sign that I'm not making it." Next, his global self-confidence is eroded. As the individual's attention is diverted to his anxiety, and as his cognitive-motor apparatus is diverted to danger, there is likely to be an increase in his overt "nervousness" as well as increased difficulty in performance.

Performance Feedback

The typical individual with public-speaking anxiety uses feedback from the audience to tell him whether he is effective. If the response is negative, then his functioning is likely to suffer. If he decides that the audience considers him inadequate, this judgment may activate his notions of inadequacy and trigger nonadaptive "protective" responses. He may become disabled, impaired, possibly even mute. In actuality, he could function if he *believed* that he was capable of functioning in these circumstances. The negative response from the audience makes him believe that he cannot function at a good level, and thus starts the vicious cycle.

The dysfunctional attitudes "interact," are often accentuated by a negative response from the audience, and lead to a barrage of negative thoughts. ("They can tell I'm nervous. They believe I'm weak. They're downgrading me.") As a result, the individual subjectively experiences a decrease in his sense of being able to influence the audience, and he feels his power draining out of him. As he becomes increasingly "weak and powerless," he senses great danger and feels vulnerable to attack or disapproval from the audience. The net effect is a catastrophic drop in his confidence in his functional capacities to see him through this crisis.

Cognitive Set during Speech

A person's cognitive set prior to presenting a speech includes a wide variety of negative attitudes and evokes unpleasant cognitions. The overall set is one of perceiving the audience itself as threatening, ready to pounce on any misstep. His view of their expectations is that he must speak clearly and articulately, that his content must be appropriate and interesting, that his manner must be free and confident, but not too casual or informal. He believes that any deviation from these rules will evoke a critical response. His self-perception is that he will be naked, exposed, and inadequate and that, furthermore, he will suffer crippling inhibitions and painful anxiety that will impair his performance and open him to criticism or ridicule. This set is manifested in automatic thoughts such as "I won't be able to do it," "They will be disappointed in me," or "I will make a fool of myself."

At the onset of the speech, the cognitive set consists of self-monitoring and evaluation of the audience response. This set is represented by negative evaluations and dire predictions: "I look silly"; "I'm not expressing myself well"; "I'll forget what I want to say"; "I sound childish"; "I won't be able to go on"; "I'll be forced to stop"; "I'll be disgraced." The interpretation of the audience response is based on selective focus and is expressed in such thoughts as "They're bored"; "They think I look pathetic"; "They wish this was over."

The cognitive set thus primes the person to meet a danger. The public speaker is prepared to deal with an adversary whom he perceives as more powerful than himself and who is poised to attack or to abandon him. The speaker feels vulnerable and exposed and does not perceive that he has effective weapons to ward off the anticipated attack. Hence a primitive defensive response is evoked—rigidity, inhibition of articulation. The problem is that the audience is not an enemy out to attack him, and that, consequently, the defensive protection does not protect him at all. In fact, it cripples his functioning and sets him up for what he wishes desperately to avoid: reduced control over his cognitive and physical functioning, and his appearing to the audience to be weak and incompetent.

Test Anxiety

Test anxiety can illustrate the processes involved in the anticipation of a specific confrontation with an evaluative situation—apprehension regarding available resources for dealing with the "danger"—and in the mobilization of primitive "defenses" against the threat. Let us take the case of a good student who is anxiety prone. Several months before the exam, he is confident that he will do well and is probably reasonably realistic in appraising his ability to be adequately prepared. He may even overestimate his chances for success ("self-serving bias").

At some point, as the date of the exam approaches, the possibility of not doing well enters into his thinking. As the exam assumes the character of a serious threat, his orientation to the test starts to point toward the consequences of failure—a blow to his self-esteem, an obstacle to future plans, a personal defeat, a disgrace in the eyes of his friends, disappointment to his family.

Focusing on the prospect of his performance's being evaluated, in addition to the possibility of failure and its consequences, affects his self-confidence. As the notion of threat takes hold, there is an automatic shift in his cognitive organization to a "vulnerability set." The student's attention is drawn to his various possible weaknesses—omissions in his coverage of the material, deficiencies in comprehension, difficulties in collating and expressing what he has learned. These flaws are given progressively greater salience and tend to overshadow his positive achievements and abilities. In fact, he may seriously question what he has learned and his ability to cover the additional material necessary for the test. Raising such questions casts doubt on how successfully he will perform on the test.

As the threat of doing poorly (by his standards) increases, his anxiety increases and may propel him to greater efforts to cover the material. As he studies, each difficulty, delay, or obstacle becomes a threat in itself and elicits a warning such as "You'll never be prepared in time."

Now let us suppose that the day of the exam has arrived. The vulnerability set is dominant. The student is concerned about his own weaknesses and the probability of examination questions or demands that may attack unknown gaps in his knowledge or comprehension. As the student looks at the exam, his cognitive set influences him to see the demands as enormous and his own resources as minimal. If the questions are realistically difficult, then the discrepancy between the demands and his own resources may be great. This discrepancy is translated into a threat: "I may not be able to handle this. I may blow it."

At this point one of the most disabling—and intriguing—phenomena associated with test anxiety may occur. His mind goes "blank," he has difficulty regaining access to material with which he is thoroughly familiar, and his reasoning ability seems to be paralyzed. The blocking is a component of test anxiety as well as of other evaluation anxieties that is difficult to explain. One possible explanation is that the individual perceives the task as overwhelming his available resources. For example, the questions may seem far beyond his comprehension or knowledge or ability. The perception (or misperception) that the test is overwhelming may have the same effect on him as when a task is indeed overwhelming. It can be postulated that, when confronted with a demand that overtaxes its capacity, the cognitive apparatus shuts down part of its capacity, just as an electric company under analogous circumstances automatically shuts down part of its capacity. Another possible explanation of the massive inhibition of recall, reasoning, and verbal expression may be that the primitive inhibitory reflexes are activated in this confrontation to serve the anachronistic function of diverting all attention to the danger.

The cognitive component is obvious in cases of progressive test anxiety. While the student continues to grapple with the questions or instructions, he tends to exaggerate flaws in his knowledge and understanding and in his responses. Each flaw takes on the form of a danger and increases the prospect of a failure.

Most students, of course, seem able to mobilize their resources when confronted with an actual test; and once they begin writing, their thoughts begin to flow, and the vulnerability set is damped down. The seriously test-anxious subject, however, is unable to turn down or turn off the vulnerability set. He continues to operate at two levels: One deals with actual questions on the exam; and the other, with continual warnings, predictions, and self-evaluations. Notions such as "You're stupid," "You'll never finish in time," "You can't understand," place a great tax on his cognitive capacity and thus reduce efficiency and performance (Sarason and Stoops 1978). Some students pass from the defensive phase (body rigid, fists clenched) to the helpless phase (feeling faint, limp, and so on)—a response that suggests a parasympathetic reaction. Others may respond with a panic attack—overwhelming anxiety and uncontrollable desire to escape—and, indeed, may abruptly leave and not return.

A SYNTHESIS

To the *sensitive subject*, being evaluated (for example, taking an examination, speaking in public, or going out on a date) is akin to being subjected to a painful probing. It may be likened to a dentist's probing teeth for an area of decay or a cavity. The evaluative situation is viewed as a confrontation or challenge that puts the subject on the defensive. He assumes that it is incumbent on him to prove himself to the evaluators and to *conceal* his presumed defects, ineptness, ignorance; whereas it is their role to *reveal* his ignorance, stupidity, and ineptness. Because he views the other persons (audience, graders of the test, dates) as looking for weaknesses, he assumes that they will pounce on every slip, flaw, or sign of nervousness and downgrade him for it. Thus, he stiffens after each misstep and imagines the immediate negative reaction of the evaluators and the long-range negative effects.

Since he regards himself as vulnerable, his reaction is self-protective: he automatically retracts into his shell so as to conceal any soft parts. In actuality, this retraction is expressed in the form of inhibition. Unfortunately for him, the inhibition not only conceals weaknesses (since it prevents him from saying or writing anything "stupid") but also interferes with effective presentation of the self. Consequently, the subject is undone by the very primal (reflex) mechanism designed to protect him.

The premonitory fears lead to stiffness *before* an encounter. The subject braces himself to absorb the impact of the aggressive scrutiny of the evaluators. This type of inhibition, however, interferes with spontaneous self-expression. Thus, at the onset of an encounter, his mind goes blank, he stutters, and he cannot focus on what he has to say or write. Moreover, he perceives the examination questions as being more difficult than they are, the audience as more unfriendly, and the date as more disdainful. He also underestimates his coping capacity. "Breaking the ice" consists of lifting the inhibition through action, by discovering that he does not need to retract and can allow free play of his personality or skill without reprisal.

REFERENCES

American Psychiatric Society (1980). *Diagnostic and Statistical Manual of Mental Disorders* (3rd ed.). Washington, DC: APA.

Amies, P. L., Gelder, M. G., and Shaw, P. M. (1983). Social phobia: a comparative clinical study. *British Journal of Psychiatry* 142:174–179.

Nichols, K. A. (1974). Severe social anxiety. *British Journal of Medical Psychology* 47:301–306.

Sarason, I. G., and Stoops, R. (1978). Test anxiety and the passage of time. *Journal of Consulting and Clinical Psychology* 46:102–109.

5 Generalized Anxiety Disorder

This chapter discusses both generalized anxiety disorder (GAD) and the use of cognitive therapy techniques in phobia therapy. GAD includes such concepts as free-floating anxiety, the chronic worrier, and the frequently seen generalized "neurotic" patterns that are marked by some hypochondriacal concerns, low self-esteem, chronic anxiety, and anxious preoccupations. This chapter delineates the current view of the syndrome, along with the emerging treatment implications.

GAD often presents one of the most difficult syndromes to treat, even for those experienced in the treatment of phobias. Patients may overcome their phobias but remain compromised by a syndrome of chronic anxiety. Some concrete techniques are given here for treating this pervasive problem, whether in the form of a residual symptom or of a primary disorder.

Dr. Coleman has worked with Aaron Beck at the Center for Cognitive Therapy and is a clear proponent of the use of cognitive restructuring in working with phobias. The chapter demonstrates how some of Dr. Beck's ideas are used in practice. While it specifically elaborates upon cognitive therapy techniques for treating GAD, the same techniques will be found to be broadly applicable to other phobias, as well as to patients with a variety of nonphobic problems, especially that of depression.

Generalized Anxiety Disorder

Ronald E. Coleman
Carol A. Gantman

A comprehensive treatment package for generalized anxiety disorder is presented below. Initially, current diagnostic conceptions regarding generalized anxiety disorder (GAD) are reviewed. Then, treatments are described for the somatic and cognitive aspects of GAD.

DIAGNOSIS: CURRENT STATUS OF GAD

The emphasis on GAD has increased in the most recent version of the *Diagnostic and Statistical Manual on Mental Disorders* (DSM-III-R) (American Psychiatric Association 1987). In DSM-II there were only two categories, anxiety neurosis and phobias. Generalized anxiety disorder was heavily emphasized as the major symptom picture of anxiety neurosis. In DSM-III, however, GAD was precluded as a diagnosis if an individual's anxiety was due to another physical or mental disorder, including another anxiety disorder such as panic disorder, agoraphobia, or obsessive-compulsive disorder. In DSM-III this resulted in the de-emphasis of GAD, despite the common-sense observation of many general-practice physicians as well as mental-health practitioners that GAD requires specific attention. This de-emphasis resulted in a relative lack of attention by clinicians regarding psychotherapeutics for GAD.

In DSM-III-R the diagnosis of GAD may be made despite the presence of another Axis I diagnosis, provided that the focus of the individual's anxiety and worry is unrelated to the other diagnosed disorder(s). That is, GAD may be diagnosed as long as the GAD symptoms are seen as separate from, for instance, the concern about the depression, or the worry and anticipation about having a panic attack, or the worry over social embarrassment in social phobia. Thus, in DSM-III-R, GAD is no longer excluded in favor of another diagnosis. As DSM-III-R notes, often an associated panic disorder or a depressive disorder is present. Likewise, according to the impression of physicians in general practice, GAD may be present when patients present with complaints about symptoms with a physical basis.

"The essential feature of this disorder is unrealistic anxiety and worry (apprehensive expectation) about two or more life circumstances, e.g., worry about possible misfortune to one's child (who is no longer in danger) and worry about finances (for no good reason), for six months or longer, during which the person has been bothered by these concerns more days than not" (APA 1987, p. 251). Symptoms of motor tension, autonomic hyperactivity, and vigilance and scanning need to be present and to be differentiated from anxiety symptoms present only during panic attacks. Specifically, at least six of the following 18 symptoms need be present in GAD:

Motor tension

1. Trembling, twitching, or feeling shaky
2. Muscle tension, aches, or soreness
3. Restlessness
4. Easy fatiguability

Autonomic hyperactivity

5. Shortness of breath or smothering sensations
6. Palpitations or accelerated heart rate (tachycardia)
7. Sweating or cold clammy hands
8. Dry mouth
9. Dizziness or lightheadedness
10. Nausea, diarrhea, or other abdominal distress
11. Flushes (hot flashes) or chills
12. Frequent urination
13. Trouble swallowing or "lump in throat"

Vigilance and scanning

14. Feeling keyed up or on edge
15. Exaggerated startle response
16. Difficulty concentrating or "mind going blank" because of anxiety
17. Trouble falling or staying asleep
18. Irritability

Prevalence of GAD

Data on the epidemiology of GAD differ, depending on the diagnostic criteria used (Schedule for Affective Disorders and Schizophrenia, SADS; Research Diagnostic Criteria, RDC; DSM-III), duration of psychopathology and diagnostic method (interviewed by clinician, nonclinician, questionnaire). Unfortunately, the excellent 1982 Epidemiologic Catchment Area (ECA) study did not survey GAD. This study found high rates for anxiety overall. For instance, it found rates for agoraphobia that ranged from 2.7 to 5.8 per 100.

Other studies found rates for GAD to be high, consistent with the ECA findings regarding other anxiety disorders (see Weissman and Merikangas 1986 for a review of this area). Rates of prevalence range from 2.5/100, looking at a 1-month period in a 1975 community survey in New Haven, using the SADS, to 5.2/100, over a 1-year period for a Zurich sample, using DSM-III, to 6.4/100 over a 1-year period in a 1979 National Survey of Psychotherapeutic Drug Use, which derived DSM-III diagnoses from responses on the SCL-90. These findings suggest that GAD is at least equally as prevalent or frequently occurring as agoraphobia, commonly thought of as the most frequent anxiety-disorder subtype.

Differentiation of GAD from Panic Disorder

It is helpful to review the differences between the two most similar anxiety disorders. Generalized anxiety disorder (GAD) and panic disorder (PD) involve similar physiologic responses. That is, physiologic symptoms in the PD list are the same as for GAD except for the following few PD symptoms: numbness or tingling sensation (paresthesias), chest pain or discomfort, fear of dying, and fear of going crazy or of doing something uncontrolled. However, in panic disorder, individuals experience discrete periods of intense fear or physical discomfort (panic attacks) that are unexpected. During some of these panic attacks the physiologic symptoms appear and accelerate in intensity within 10 minutes of the observation of physiologic symptoms. To diagnose PD at least four attacks must have occurred within a 4-week period, and one or more attacks need to be associated with at least a month of persistent fear of another attack. This is in contrast to GAD, which must be present on more days than not over at least a 6-month period.

There is a body of research findings that, taken together, support the notion that panic disorder and GAD differ. Among the biophysiological evidence is the following:

First, genetic-heritability studies tend to indicate that there is more concordance among panic-disorder cohorts than among GAD cohorts (Anderson et al. 1984, Hoehn-Saric and McLeod 1985). Second, pharmacological treatments of choice seem to differ for panic disorder and GAD. Benzodiazepines are the current treatment of choice for GAD. However, except for Xanax, the benzodiazepines do not seem effective for preventing panic attacks. Conversely, three classes of medication seem effective for treating panic disorder: Xanax, tricyclic antidepressants, and MAO inhibitors. The literature suggests that, except for Xanax, these latter pharmacologic interventions are not specific for GAD. Third, physical-challenge tests administered to individuals with panic disorder and with GAD tend to yield different effects (Breier et al. 1985, Dittrich et al. 1983). That is, when these individuals are administered a lactate infusion intravenously, the panic-disordered individuals tend to have physiologic arousal similar to that experienced during a panic attack. Individuals with GAD do not seem to become aroused. Lastly, the physiologic picture that patients describe seems different for the panic-disordered versus the GAD individual, when anxious. That is, the panic-disordered seem to have more cardiovascular (cardiac, vascular, and pulmonary) involvement than do GAD individuals (Hoehn-Saric 1982).

Clinically, the GAD individual experiences less intense somatic response (less panic) than someone with PD. Further for the GAD patient there is an earlier, more gradual onset, longer chronicity, more widely disturbed cognitive processes (irrational worry about a variety of situations), and grossly observed, mild or no avoidance of situations (Hoehn-Saric and McLeod 1985).

Nature of Symptoms: GAD

Symptoms of GAD may be divided conveniently into the following categories:

Somatic

Individuals with GAD vary in their concern over somatic symptoms. The GAD sufferer may experience the same concerns as the panic-disordered individual, over heart rate and felt intensity of beat as well as difficult breathing, shortness of breath, and fast shallow breathing. The range of the symptom picture extends along a dimension from individuals who may have few, vague somatic complaints to those who have frequent, specific somatic complaints.

The most typical somatic complaint found in the vast majority of cases as reported by Beck and Emery (1985) is the inability to relax.

Cognitive

Whereas the individual suffering from panic disorder is concerned most about his or her physical status, and ultimate fears of possibly dying, going crazy, or losing control, the GAD sufferer's central focus is the anticipation of difficulty in a few major or many situations. The GAD sufferer is a worrier, anticipates difficulty in a variety of situations, and is upset about aspects of psychosocial situations and about tasks needing to be accomplished. This is in sharp contrast to the individual experiencing panic disorder, who worries about vulnerability of body functions. The GAD sufferer has a heightened sense of vulnerability regarding his or her capability or adequacy in various situations. Unlike the social phobic, who anticipates and expects social embarrassment and ridicule and is concerned about his or her ability to perform, given this fear, the GAD individual is more concerned with the adequacy of ongoing performance.

A common cognitive impairment of GAD is difficulty in concentration, as reviewed by Beck and Emery (1985). Consequently, cognitive impairment is a frequent concern of GAD patients, as is the fear of losing control. This suggests that those experiencing GAD, similar to those with panic disorder, worry about the possibility of somatic symptoms becoming aroused and undermining them. An additional frequent complaint in GAD is the fear of rejection. This concern reflects the GAD individuals' major worry over the adequacy of their performance and their associated worry about the attitude of others toward them.

Anticipatory anxiety is most central to the individual with GAD. For instance, a teacher says: "I am worried whether I will be prepared for the first day of school. I don't know if I will be able to handle the questions these third-graders will throw at me." A manager in a large food store says: "The boss may find out that I am not able to do the job here. If I make any more mistakes I will be in trouble."

Cognitive Aspects of Avoidance in GAD

GAD in its past conceptions has been associated with free-floating anxiety. By definition, it was assumed that external causes of the individual's anxiety would rarely be ascertained. However, cognitive and behavioral therapists have long seen the value of detailed analysis to determine the source of the anxious and stressed individual's upset. That is, the GAD patient can identify specifically those situations in which he or she *anticipates* having difficulty (and worries about), those situations into which he or she enters and *worries* about adequacy of performance, and those situations that were troublesome in the past and are *worried about restrospectively*. Thus, anxiety for the GAD individual is not truly free-floating in nature.

By definition, the GAD diagnosis is not identified with avoidance as is the phobic, social phobic, or agoraphobic. In fact, individuals experiencing generalized anxiety seem to enter situations that they dread. In these situations, however, they will be cautious, timid, because of their worry about functioning adequately. Thus, though they may enter many situations in which they are anxious, they may avoid assertion or avoid becoming the focus of others' attention owing to fear about poor performance and subsequent negative consequences. Often the GAD individuals' anxieties are associated with situations that occur in their everyday life and cannot be avoided completely. Nevertheless, to the extent that they engage in self-protective, cautious behavior that helps them eschew performance evaluation, GAD individuals do avoid.

The case of Steve provides an example of the relative avoidance of the individual with generalized anxiety. Steve was afraid to confront his boss about the policy of using Steve's staff in other store departments during periods of high customer traffic. Steve was particularly anxious about his ability to manage his department and worried that he would make a mistake when deciding policy or when deciding how to use his employees. Although he was afraid he would be caught in a mistake and tended to avoid his boss, Steve spoke to the boss every day. He was, however, unable to discuss his concerns with his boss. Though he remained on the job, Steve's anxiety about his performance kept him in a passive, anxious position in relation to his boss.

A second case illustrates the difference in avoidance between types of anxiety disorders. Susan had applied for and been offered a job, yet decided to turn it down. In Susan's view the new job meant increased responsibility, because she would be teaching older children in the elementary school. When she turned down the job, she rationalized that she didn't want the additional pressure, but apparently she felt badly about it. Her husband and children made fun of her decision. Some time later, Susan sought therapy for help with her panic attacks. In addition to panic attacks, she had trouble going out of the house.

In treatment, Susan at first was forthright in her description of panic attacks and agoraphobia, but she was reticent to give a history consistent with GAD. Treatment for panic disorder was successful over the first few sessions. During these sessions she was given assignments to do things she avoided in order to confront the possibility that she might experience panic. One of these tasks was to go out of the house for walks. As a reason for not wishing to go on walks Susan gave an interesting diagnostic clue: she did not want to talk to neighbors that she encountered. Now, this aversion might have been a part of panic disorder as a result of not wishing to display anxiety to another, or as a result of wishing to avoid being trapped should a panic attack occur. Nevertheless, the therapist suggested that Susan, in fact, walk out of her house daily and stop to talk to neighbors whom she encountered. The therapist expected that Susan would do this with some difficulty if she were either agoraphobic or socially phobic. Susan reported, though, at the next session, that she was able to leave the house easily and she did speak with neighbors.

As a result she felt much relieved. She reported she had been afraid that those she spoke with would think she lacked brightness; she was afraid to reveal a lack of social intelligence. The basis of Susan's avoidance of neighbors was her fear of revealing how she privately felt about not having taken the new job.

The therapist began to see that a diagnosis concurrent with the panic disorder, and probably predating it, was GAD. Once the going-out-of-the-house situation was confronted, Susan had no difficulty speaking with neighbors, no concerns about being trapped, and was in touch with her sense of anxious concern in relation to impressing others. This was a case of GAD "avoidance" rather than that of an agoraphobic. In later sessions Susan reported the full extent of her worries over her abilities and her fear that others would learn of her "ineptness."

In general, a careful analysis of situations will reveal that the GAD individual has tendencies to avoid situations and may be tentative in other situations, owing to anxiety over performance.

TREATMENT OF GAD

The discussion of GAD treatment will be divided into three symptom areas: somatic, cognitive, and avoidance. The treatment program for GAD includes the following components:

Physiologic arousal management

Relaxation techniques

Cognitive therapy

Exposure therapy (behavioral experiments)

Somatic Treatments

As mentioned above, symptoms in GAD may differ in variety and intensity from those in PD. In the latter there is more cardiovascular involvement; in the former, more cognitive concern over chronic states of nervousness and aspects of muscular tension or other forms of bodily discomfort (e.g., stomach distress). However, as in PD, GAD somatic symptom distress may be improved with the treatments described below.

Physiologic Arousal Management

In GAD, when a patient is troubled by particular organ-system arousal, such as difficulty with breathing, dizziness, or worry over cardiac function, *physiologic arousal management* (PAM) techniques may be applied, as in the treatment of PD. In PD, individuals are frightened by the unexpected surge of somatic symptoms. These bodily reactions seem to lead to assumptions that physical harm is occurring, or will occur, through specific organ damage, or through loss of general control (e.g., fainting). Others interpret the experience of lack or loss of control of somatic response as "going crazy." Those who do not develop PD but have transient panic experiences may make accurate or benign attributions about the experience or may deny or minimize the importance of their physiological arousal.

Physiologic arousal management first focuses attention on specific organ systems involved in the panic attack. The purpose is to encourage "exposure" to the frightening central aspects of PD, the curious and unexplained intense physiologic arousal (Barlow et al. 1984, Clark 1986). Second, with exposure to specific frightening organ-system arousal, techniques may be applied for management of the arousal.

Relaxation Techniques

Purpose. In GAD, relaxation may serve several purposes. First, patients usually conceive of relaxation training as palliative when imagining themselves in stressful anxiety-producing situations. The relaxation response applied to anxious moments may reduce the anxiety somewhat and enhance the individual's functioning, but it will not, as some patients hope, do away with anxiety in those situations. The therapist must convey clearly that training in relaxation will help the patient remain in vivo but will not necessarily eliminate anxiety entirely.

A second use of relaxation training is the reduction of general anxiety and tension levels. GAD individuals may have a heightened level of anxiety outside of difficult situations, owing to their propensity to anticipate anxiety. Relaxation training may aid in the reduction of this aspect of anxiety.

Additional Concerns in Relaxation Training. A concern mentioned above is that the patient know what is reasonable to expect from relaxation training. Sometimes patients expect that a learned relaxation response will reduce anxiety in an anxiety-related situation to near zero. Of course, this is not always possible.

Another concern is that relaxation and meditation may produce relaxation-cued anxiety (Barlow et al. 1984). An individual while sitting quiescent may be exposed to somatic feedback (twitches, tingling, pains), anxiety-inducing thoughts, or both. Some individuals may be frightened during relaxation training by the opportunity to focus on their bodily functioning. This possibility calls for therapist vigilance and awareness during relaxation training. It is to be expected that among individuals prone to relaxation-cued anxiety will be some with a diagnosis of anxiety disorder. Individuals who fall in this diagnostic category are hypervigilant over their somatic activity and their anxiety-provoking ideation.

On the positive side, it may be that extensive relaxation responses are not necessary. It has been found that the extent of the biofeedback or relaxation response is not correlated with the outcome of anxiety reduction as measured at post-test (Barlow et al. 1984). Therefore, in spite of nonmaximal effect of relaxation, significant anxiety-reduction effects may be achieved. This suggests that the usefulness of relaxation training and the relaxation response may be due to its distracting as well as its relaxing properties. It may be effective as a coping device, which the patient may actively use, even though extensive relaxation was not achieved. This suggests that brief training in relaxation procedures is as effective as intensive long-term training in the relaxation response.

We employ very brief relaxation-induction procedures as described below.

Diaphragm Breathing. This procedure teaches relaxed, average deep breathing, which uses the diaphragm muscles, as contrasted with fast, shallow breathing, in which muscles of the chest, shoulders, rib cage, and tummy may be tense and tight. The procedure may be taught briefly and is simple to do. It entails instructing the patient to experience the feeling of slow, deep breathing. While experiencing this, the patient is instructed to notice the use of the diaphragm muscles and the associated relaxation of muscles in the torso. Patients are given homework to practice diaphragm breathing several times a day for several days, so that it becomes a habit. After this training, when the patient is anxious and experiences difficulty breathing, he or she is more likely to be able to apply this breathing procedure.

Scanning. This procedure combines a breathing exercise with a search through the body for muscle groups that have tension. The individual is instructed to scan through the muscle groups of the body, to look for areas of tension. Starting with the first muscle group, the individual is told to scan these muscles for tension while drawing a breath in, and to release any tension found during the next breath out. The next muscle or muscle group is reviewed at the next inhale, and, if tension is discovered, it is let go on the subsequent exhale.

This procedure is useful if repeated through the day. It achieves a variety of effects. It teaches people where in their body they react with tension. It gives them ongoing feedback about the situations that elicit anxiety. It cuts off anxiety arousal before it starts and in this manner may reduce the general level of anxiety.

To use this technique people need to use cues in their environment that remind them to scan, frequently and periodically, through the day.

Deep-Muscle Relaxation. Deep-muscle relaxation involves teaching tension-release cycles for groups of skeletal muscles (Bernstein and Borkovec 1973). The muscle group is tensed for 10 to 20 seconds; then the tension is released. The contrast between muscle tensing and muscle relaxation heightens the perceived response. Any muscle fatigue achieved may promote relaxation also.

After some training and practice it is important to shorten the time it takes to achieve induction of relaxation, and to develop ways to apply the relaxation response in vivo.

Conclusion. Somatic treatment for GAD may differ from that for PD. There are average differences between the two disorders in terms of amplitude and chronicity. GAD somatic symptoms tend to be less intense and more chronic; GAD patients more typically complain of tension and "nervousness" and vague bodily complaints. PD patients complain more typically of cardiovascular symptoms. Thus, for GAD patients we tend to rely more on relaxation training procedures, and for PD patients we rely more on PAM procedures. Note, again, however, that there is extensive overlap of symptoms between GAD and PD. Many GAD patients have focal organ-system problems involving worry about the heart, breathing, or dizziness, and they benefit from use of PAM approaches.

Cognitive Therapy

The treatment approach most consistent with the cognitive distortion in GAD is cognitive therapy. As mentioned above, GAD individuals have concerns about their ability to cope in a myriad of life's situations. They are worried about their adequacy and efficacy. Intervention is required at the cognitive dysfunctional level with regard to the patients' anticipation of these situations, their self-evaluations during them, and their concerns afterward. In worrying about their efficacy, ultimately they are concerned with their possible lack of success financially, vocationally, and—through the eyes of others—relationally.

Cognitive therapy aims to help the patients question, as a result of their re-evaluation of their cognitions, whether the danger of failure and/or rejection, according to objective evidence, exists. This task is accomplished collaboratively between patient and therapist. The patient's job is to provide the personal meanings (cognitions and emotions) that he or she attributes to upsetting events. The therapist's role is to socialize the patient into this approach and to provide the structure of how to challenge and evaluate the patient's anxiety-related cognitions. Cognitive treatment is an educational process in which the patient learns these procedures through practice in order to develop new habits of thinking that may eventually be applied in vivo. Thus, if it is to succeed, the process not only is an insight procedure that explores a new manner of thinking, but also it requires between-session homework assignments for practice in habit acquisition (Coleman and Beck 1981).

Steps in Cognitive Therapy.

1. Identify cognitions associated with anxiety.

The patient learns the tenets of the cognitive viewpoint and learns to "catch" cognitions.

2. Observe the effect of the cognitions on feelings and behavior.

Once the cognitions have been elicited, the relationships between thought and feeling and between thought and action are reviewed. "How would a person feel," says the therapist, restating the patient's cognition, "if he thought that each time he spoke to his boss, the boss was going to remind him about failing to get the Jones account? And how would that person behave toward his boss if he had that thought?" This approach is typical of the Beck (Beck et al. 1985) Socratic style, in which the therapist poses the issue and the patient is sometimes the provider or collector of marshaled evidence and the arbiter of decisions ("How would this make you feel or act?").

3. Evaluate the accuracy of the cognition.

This and the fourth step (rational responses) are the core of cognitive restructuring activity for the patient. There are many methods for helping the patient examine alternatives to his automatic viewpoint.

One need not leave the office to marshal evidence regarding automatic thoughts and their accuracy. People need only examine their own experience and their ability to use logic to evaluate their thoughts.

Review of Logic. Often patients may be assisted in examining their thinking for evidence of faulty logic. Often patients *catastrophize* in their anxiety-related thinking; in anticipating danger, they jump to the worst conclusions. A typical example is the A student who tells his classmates after an exam, "I definitely flunked the test!"

In *overgeneralizing*, anxious individuals take one negative experience and translate it into the benchmark standard of their potential success, imagining this prototypical outcome to occur in all similar situations in the future ("I can't seem to be successful").

Similarly, patients *maximize* or exaggerate a critical remark. A wife reports, "Harvey said we should go on diets. He thinks I'm too fat." An anxiety-prone woman may view Harvey's remark as the definitive statement about the negative quality of their relationship, while *minimizing* her positive attributes, the positive qualities of the relationship, and her husband's positive comments and behaviors.

Review Evidence. In these procedures the patient brings into play his or her life experience to evaluate the accuracy of anxiety-related cognitions.

The most general procedure is a review of the evidence related to the thought in question. For example, a man just promoted to a new job was nervous about his ability to do it. His cognition was that he would never be able to succeed adequately at the new job. The therapist provided a series of questions that reviewed the evidence about this patient's proven ability.

Therapist: How similar is your new job to your old one?
Patient: Pretty much the same. Really I was given the responsibility and the authority to do what I actually did

before. Now I have the power to try and make sure it gets done. But I'll have to provide more reports and check on people.
Therapist: How do you feel about the reports and checking on people?
Patient: I think I can do it.
Therapist: Then, what do you think about doing the new job?
Patient: I guess I already do most of the job now. I guess I confused the added responsibility with thinking that there was a lot new I had to learn.

After additional discussion about the patient's ability to get along with workers he would now be supervising, he felt relieved and more positive about the promotion.

The method of *alternative conclusions* asks the patient to look at the situation another way. Often the therapist can use a two-column technique, asking the patient to list on the left column what he or she was thinking and on the right what possible alternative cognitions there might be. Obviously, the patient habitually takes the short, negative view and would benefit from achieving a broader perspective. Looking at alternatives encourages the patient to see that observations of situations may be attitudes or beliefs about them. These may be viewed as opinions, often having no particular accuracy. This is illustrated in the case of the man who was afraid to speak to his boss for fear the boss would ask about the Jones account. The patient had failed to close the deal after several presentations to the Jones Company. The patient felt at fault and inadequate about not having closed the sale.

Therapist: What do you think your boss would say to you?
Patient: That he is angry with me.
Therapist: Why would he be angry?
Patient: Because he will think I wasn't good enough to make the sale.

Therapist: Has Jones turned you down yet?
Patient: No.
Therapist: Then this seems like catastrophizing without much evidence as basis. What do you think?
Patient: Perhaps you are right.
Therapist: What other ways can you look at your boss's potential behavior when you approach him?
Patient: Well, although the Jones account is a big one, the boss may not even be thinking of it.
Therapist: Any other ways to look at it?
Patient: Well, I really still am negotiating with the Jones people; maybe they haven't come to a decision yet. Maybe the boss will encourage me to keep trying with Jones.

As a result of the discussion it became clear that the patient had not yet been turned down on the Jones account. But he felt he should have closed the deal by this point. Actually, the patient was not attending to how long it would take the Jones Company to reach a decision on the sale. Several departments in the Jones Company needed to make their input to reach a decision about the purchase of the patient's product. After this, the patient paid attention to estimating more accurately the amount of effort and length of time a sale required, and he put more effort into understanding the political and power climate in firms to which he made presentations.

The *reattribution technique* is applied when the patient takes on more of the responsibility or blame for a situation than seems necessary. Often individuals believe that they are responsible for the responses of those they are with as well as their own behavior. For instance, a psychology intern was complaining about the behavior of several of a small group of medical students to whom she was lecturing. She was concerned that they looked less than interested, with one seeming to fall asleep. The intern was asked whether any of the medical students indicated interest. She answered in the affirmative. It was pointed out that the intern was taking responsibility for preparation, presentation, and the behavior of her audience. She was encouraged to reassign less than 100% of the responsibility for the situation to herself. Review of information about on-rotation, hard-working, possibly moonlighting medical students was also helpful in the reattribution process.

This example brings us to the use of *information*. It is often helpful to impart information to patients to reduce cognitive distortions. Anxious patients frequently ask whether they are going crazy. While caution requires hesitation to give a guarantee, the therapist may review definitions of "crazy"—that is, review aspects of psychotic behavior, such as delusions and hallucinations. Contrast between such definitions and the patient's experience of anxiety is reassuring. As well, imparting information about the extant list of anxiety symptoms may help some patients, who are struggling to distinguish between physiological arousal that is emotional and their arousal that they fearfully interpret as due to a physical disorder.

Behavioral Experiment. Generally, patients may evaluate their cognitions by actually collecting objective data. Thus, review of evidence need not rely solely on the patient's range of experience. The patient may go out and observe additional experience, take a poll, or do library research.

Evaluation of the accuracy of automatic anxiety-related thoughts may best be done prospectively rather than retrospectively. This is particularly true of GAD patients, who are constantly predicting large and small negative outcomes related to their functioning. These patients benefit from writing down their predictions of doom and gloom and comparing them with actual outcomes. Thus, they may begin to see their anticipations in terms of hypothesis testing. They learn to hold their final decision on the value of their negative thought until they live through the experience. In a similar vein, these anticipatory anxious thoughts may be labeled predictions and likened to weather predictions. We know that the probability of weather predictions' being accurate is far from even 80% correct. The patients may begin to see the probability of accuracy of their own predictions. They learn the value of empiricism, of waiting until they get to the situation to evaluate their performance.

Behavioral experiments may be devised to test an individual's cognition. The patient who was reluctant to go out because she was hesitant to see neighbors was avoiding the possibility that she would be viewed by them negatively. A mutually agreed-upon task to go out to say hello and talk to neighbors was able to provide evidence that supported a more positive self-attribute. The patient realized that her neighbors were friendly and enjoyed speaking to her.

Patients with anxiety disorder frequently have cognitions about their somatic arousal, believing that something is wrong physically. This may occur with some frequency in the GAD patient. As part of exposure techniques, behavioral experiments are important to evaluate cognitions regarding physical vulnerability. Anxiety patients who have these concerns are similar to "cardiac cripples," whose concern about anticipated physiological stress results in avoidance of safe physical activity. Thus, prescribing physical activity for someone who is anxious about possible tachycardia would enable him to confront the potential danger of this activity (physical activity is prescribed taking into account the patient's age, physical health, and physical conditioning).

Rational Responses. The last step in cognitive therapy is to replace the automatic thought with a rational response consistent with the new evaluation of the automatic thought. Often this may be accomplished with the use of a five-column technique. On a five-column paper, patients describe (1) the problematic situation, (2) their emotion in that situation, (3) their automatic thought associated with the emotion, (4) their evaluation of the automatic response, and (5) a more rational response (see below). The page may be used in stages that follow cognitive therapy's steps in training.

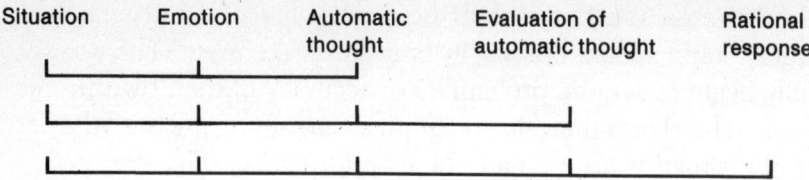

The patient uses first the first three columns, to collect automatic thoughts; then the first four columns, to evaluate the accuracy of the automatic thoughts; then all five columns.

The above steps occur over several to many sessions. Over sessions, once patients become adept at evaluating the accuracy of their cognitions, they are encouraged to begin to apply their re-evaluations on the spot.

Avoidance

Although by definition GAD patients seem not to actively avoid, we have seen that their vulnerability to worry over efficacy leads them to avoid risk-taking in many situations. The therapist's task is to encourage exposure that confronts the patient's tendency to avoid risk-taking. The avoidance topography is not geographical as in many phobias; it is defined by the situational dangers as elicited from patients' anxiety-related cognitions. Thus, eliciting the cognitive meaning that the patient attributes to events aids in revealing the situational niches he or she avoids.

Exposure (Behavioral Experiments). It is the job of the therapist, in collaboration with the patient, to encourage exposure to situations the patient avoids (Coleman 1981). Sometimes with GAD patients the situation that needs to be confronted is obvious—for example, when the activity in question involves a dramatic change, such as the need to apply for a job. There is nothing to be done, finally, but for the patient to confront the situation to see what will happen. He may utilize aids, advice, training in coping skills, and, where possible, successive approximation toward the goal. More often, with the GAD patient, what is to be approached is an aspect of the situation that the individual finds difficult. This may involve an intervention calling for the patient to be more assertive with another, or an intervention calling for him to master more complex tasks or consider goals that engender greater risks and greater rewards.

Cognitive therapy. *Treatment—Initial Session(s)* In the initial session, after the diagnosis of GAD is made, the precipitating complaint and the cognitive, somatic, and avoidance symptoms need to be reviewed. The precipitating complaint(s) and worst symptoms then need to be ascertained and a treatment plan developed. It is best to attack the most handicapping symptoms first.

Often the patient presents with an additional diagnosis, such as panic disorder or depression with a background history or substrate of GAD. As soon as the panic, depression, or initial difficulty in life is resolved, the need for treatment of GAD emerges more clearly. This was illustrated above in the case of the woman who did not take a teaching job offered to her, because she anticipated difficulty. After her husband ridiculed her, panic attacks developed. Some breathing exercises, cognitive therapy about her worst fears, and exposure to avoided situations soon resolved the panic attacks. The diagnosis of GAD then was easier to make. The patient communicated her pervasive doubts about her abilities and how these had undermined her, overwhelmed her, and led her to avoid a new job.

CASE STUDIES

The Case of Steve

> Steve, a 35-year-old supermarket manager, came into therapy owing to pressure over work. A refurbishment of the store 6 months earlier had enlarged his department along with the rest of the store, while making his storage/preparation area smaller. Worried about his adequacy in his job, Steve worried what others would think of him should he fail. As a result, over time, as the

difficulty at the store continued, he became increasingly insecure among friends and family. Also he reported difficulties breathing and nervous tension. In his initial session he informed the therapist he had taken the week off from his job, and it became increasingly clear that he was afraid to return to work.

In the first two sessions, as information was gathered, the therapist also described a treatment plan to Steve. The plan was to provide relaxation training for his nervousness and tension, PAM for his concerns over breathing, and cognitive interventions for job issues, in order to assist Steve in his return to work. He was given a rationale for cognitive therapy, and the procedure was explained to him. He was given brief relaxation training in the form of diaphragm breathing exercises.

During his week off, Steve was consumed by worries about the difficulties of the job. He personalized these difficulties ("Can I do the job?") while giving himself a hard time about his troubles ("I shouldn't be going through this"). He was given homework: to read about cognitive therapy, to practice breathing exercises, and to collect automatic thoughts.

During the week he continued to have negative cognitions and generalized anxiety. He thought, "I can't go back to work," and "Why can't I cope?"

Several serendipitous, positive things happened during the week between the second and third sessions. In retrospect the therapist saw these behavioral experiments that supported Steve's more rational responding. First, Steve talked on the phone to his boss and mentioned some of his concerns. The boss was reassuring, and Steve was surprised and relieved. Second, Steve revealed to his parents that he was troubled. They were understanding, and again he was surprised and relieved. Third, he spent some time with friends. They were friendly; Steve was relieved.

Steve felt that these responses were confirmation that people did not view him as such a failure. He returned to work the next week, not expecting to get through the day, a difficult Monday. At work Steve continued to have extreme doubts about his ability and somatic arousal. Throughout the week, however, he was able to challenge his dysfunctional thoughts, using the column technique, and he was able to calm down his somatic arousal with relaxation techniques.

Table 5-1 is an illustration of Steve's column work and the rational responses he produced after reviewing the available evidence.

Steve dealt well with the problems of catastrophizing and accompanying physiological arousal. He was able to reduce his catastrophic thinking. When he did this, his sense of being overwhelmed was reduced sufficiently to allow him to focus on one job or problem at a time. He was also able to arrive at alternative ways to look at the situation. As he gained the ability to focus on the work situation with less upset and anxiety, he was better able to apply appropriate coping skills.

In the next session Steve reported making a mistake that led to self-doubt about his decision-making ability. He had bought some tomatoes from a farmer who came directly to the store, a purchase of a type he occasionally made. The bottom boxes of tomatoes

TABLE 5-1 Dysfunctional Thought Record

Situation	Feeling	Automatic thought	Rational response
Monday morning. Work. Store a wreck. Shelves empty.	Anxiety Tension	I don't think I can find the time to get done all that I want to.	Don't panic! Do one thing at a time. It will all get done in due time.
Monday at work. Afternoon. Under extreme stress.	Tension	Don't know what to do first. Trying to do too much.	[*Written that night*] By the end of the day it all worked out. Must find a way to cope with the tension during the day.
6 A.M. Tuesday. Woke early.	Worried Scared	Still nervous about work. Monday was no picnic. At times it almost seems unreal.	Monday is a very difficult day. And maybe I can schedule my people better. It would make it easier. It was also the first day back. I did OK.

were rotten. Steve ruminated over the wasted dollars, worrying whether he was capable of being back at work. He and the therapist worked out rational responses in the subsequent session, as shown in Table 5-2.

Over the subsequent weeks Steve came up with other rational responses of his own, regarding a variety of situations. It appeared that the cognitions related to anxiety typical for Steve were:

Overwhelmed with problems
Catastrophizing
Perfectionistic
Concerned about opinion of others

Steve and the therapist continued to work on decatastrophizing, on focusing on one thing at a time, on coping rather than trying to be perfect, and on trusting that others would like him regardless of his performance. Steve worked with the therapist in this way, using the dysfunctional thought record to analyze his cognitions, and using relaxation procedures, over a ten-session period. At the end of that time he had much lower anxiety and was low in measures of depression. He seemed to be coping and was more assertive and more flexible in work. His improvement was maintained at 9-month follow-up.

TABLE 5-2 Dysfunctional Thought Record

Situation	Feeling	Automatic thought	Rational response
Sitting in meeting, worrying about mistake.	Panicky Tense Light-headed	Feel what I did was a big mistake. Maybe I shouldn't be the boss.	People make mistakes. It does not mean I cannot do my job. I will correct it, or I will live and learn from this.
Still worrying.	Tense Anxious Weak	Very worried about what I did being a big mistake.	I can't change it now. Less thought and more action! I should have done this before so I would not put myself through this.

Case of Susan

This case illustrates the co-occurrence of GAD with another anxiety disorder—in this example, PD.

Susan's initial complaints were about panic attacks that included difficulty in breathing, face flushed, hands sweaty, and the feeling that she wanted to scream out and run. She experienced panic attacks approximately once a week, over a period of several months, from the time she turned down an offer to move from substitute to permanent status as teacher of a third grade. She had rationalized the decision to others, knowing herself that she was afraid she could not handle the job.

Accompanying the panic attacks were avoidance of stores, of church, and of others ("People bore me"), together with obsessive thinking about stabbing and killing. Before the advent of panic attacks, Susan had been a worrier with low self-esteem.

Susan was treated with breathing exercises, both to help with her difficulties in breathing and as a relaxation response for her anxiety. The supplying of didactic information and reframing of her experience of anxiety attacks also proved helpful. Avoidance behavior in situations such as church and stores was treated with a program of exposure to these situations. As mentioned earlier in the chapter, Susan was encouraged to talk to neighbors. She was asked, while doing so, to collect her dysfunctional thoughts about her sense of inadequacy during social encounters. The social avoidance was quickly overcome, revealing a GAD-like pattern of worry over social contact rather than one of phobic or socially anxious avoidance.

The cognitive therapy and PAM for panic symptoms reduced the intensity of Susan's panic attacks to the point where she was increasingly successful in entering previously avoided situations. Over a period of several weeks her distress was markedly reduced, her thoughts of killing and stabbing disappeared, and her avoidance behavior was gone, though she had some anxiety in the previously avoided situations. After five sessions she insisted she was improved to the point where she did not need to come again. As her therapist felt that treatment was not yet complete and told her this, he kept an open door.

A month later Susan called her therapist, saying she was troubled by problems she had not acknowledged previously. She was able to admit she never had intended to get a permanent teaching job, owing to self-doubt about her performance. As a result, she was furious at herself for being weak. Throughout the period when she was deciding whether to accept the teaching job her husband had encouraged her to take it. When she refused it, he ridiculed her. This, according to Susan, was "objective evidence" of her weakness.

It was apparent that the patient in prior sessions had minimized evidence of premorbid GAD in order to present herself in a good light. Now, freed of the pain of anticipating panic attacks, she was able to focus on the nature of her life's compromises due to GAD. The therapist and Susan began a new round of therapy to address the GAD symptoms.

Treatment included continued attention to somatic arousal, focus on cognitive therapy for situations that were anxiety provoking, and, a bit later, emphasis on assertion. Collection of dysfunctional thoughts with the dysfunctional thought record revealed a number of themes. The twin themes of "fear of doing" and perfectionism were present. Susan revealed in detail her concerns about moving out into the work world. She and the therapist worked on these issues. An additional major theme was that Susan was "worried about what people would think." After several sessions it was evident that her lack of self-confidence currently expressed itself with her children and husband as lack of assertiveness. During one session, Susan discussed a difference of opinion with her husband over discipline of one of her children. She had not been able to express herself to her husband, though she was upset by how he had handled the situation. Susan recognized this as a pattern. Though she was reluctant to confront her husband, this crisis became her opportunity to do so. The subsequent talks she had with her husband made a dramatic difference in her feelings about herself and led to her taking risks in other situations.

On follow-up, six months after therapy was completed, Susan reported that she had taken a teaching job in grade school. Her anxiety was minimal, her relationship with her husband was improved, and she continued practice on assertion.

This case illustrates the importance of noting the presence of GAD as a co-occurring diagnosis that may have preceded and precipitated another Axis I diagnosis.

Case of Leonard

Leonard's case illustrates briefly the co-occurrence of GAD with depression. It is unclear whether GAD was in the premorbid history of the depression. In this case, after the successful treatment of depression, symptoms of GAD remained.

Leonard was a young television program director who had experienced a meteoric rise in his field. Depression began after a job promotion. He felt that he had more responsibilities than he could handle and that he did not have the pertinent experience he needed. Also he felt unsupported by his boss. Throughout this period his marriage was strained.

Cognitive-behavioral therapy for depression, a brief hospitalization, and treatment with tricyclic antidepressants were helpful in alleviating the depression. He was referred at the end of his hospitalization to continue cognitive-behavioral treatment to facilitate his return to work. At this time Leonard had no symptoms of depression, though he doubted his ability to do his job. He had somatic symptoms of GAD, and he wondered whether he had the ability to accomplish much.

The therapist concentrated on Leonard's many worries over functioning effectively at work. Cognitive therapy, as in the case of Steve above, focused on comparing Leonard's negative thoughts about how he would perform at work with his actual experience of the situation. Gradually, Leonard began to regain confidence in his ability to work. Issues involving relationship and personal self-concept were addressed toward the end of therapy.

CONCLUSION

Examination of the clinical syndrome of GAD suggests that it is amenable to cognitive-behavioral treatments. The treatment package described resembles in some ways, and in some ways differs from, the treatment for PD. The treatment package for GAD includes—for somatic arousal—physiologic arousal management (PAM) and relaxation training. For cognitive aspects it includes cognitive therapy for the widespread anticipation of ability to perform adequately. For the aspects of avoidance in GAD it includes cognitive therapy and exposure for the situational niches avoided.

GAD has received renewed diagnostic importance. That is, DSM-III-R gives GAD renewed emphasis, regardless of the presence of other Axis I diagnoses. This, plus the evidence for its high incidence, suggests that GAD is an anxiety disorder to which psychosocial treatments need give attention. Despite the availability of psychosocial tools, however, there is a paucity of discussion about or research on psychosocial treatments for GAD (Lindsay et al. 1987). Perhaps this is why clinicians pay scant attention to a problem that most general- and family-practice physicians probably see daily.

The treatment package described here has been found effective clinically in the treatment of GAD. It is comprised of tools that, separately, have been effective cognitive and behavioral interventions for other anxiety disorders. Especially given the widespread use but questionable effectiveness of benzodiazepines, it is time to examine cognitive-behavioral packages such as described here for the treatment of GAD.

REFERENCES

American Psychiatric Association (1987). *Diagnostic and statistical manual of mental disorders* (3rd ed. rev.). Washington, DC: APA.

Anderson, J. A., Noyes, R., and Crow, R. R. (1984). A comparison of panic disorder and generalized anxiety disorder. *American Journal of Psychiatry* 141:572-575.

Barlow, D. H., Cohen, A. S., Waddell, M. T., et al. (1984). Panic and generalized anxiety disorders: Nature and treatment. *Behavior Therapy* 15:431-449.

Beck, A. T., Emery, G., and Greenberg, R. L. (1985). *Anxiety Disorders and Phobias: A Cognitive Perspective*. New York: Basic Books.

Bernstein, D. A., and Borkovec, T. D. (1973). *Progressive Relaxation Training*. Champaign, IL: Research Press.

Breier, A., Charney, D. S., and Heninger, G. R. (1985). The diagnostic validity of anxiety disorders and their relationship to depressive illness. *American Journal of Psychiatry* 142:787-797.

Clark, D. M. (1986). A cognitive approach to panic. *Behaviour Research and Therapy* 24:461-470.

Coleman, R. E. (1981). Cognitive-behavioral treatment of agoraphobia. In *New Directions in Cognitive Therapy*, ed. G. Emery, S. D. Hollon, and R. C. Bedrosian, pp. 109-119. New York: Guilford Press.

Coleman, R. E., and Beck, A. T. (1981). Cognitive therapy for depression. In *Depression: Behavioral and Directive Intervention Strategies*, ed. J. F. Clarkin and H. I. Glazer, pp. 111-130. New York: Garland STPM Press.

Dittrich, J., Houts, A. C., and Lichstein, K. L. (1983). Panic disorder: Assessment and treatment. *Clinical Psychology Review* 3:215-225.

Hoehn-Saric, R. (1982). Comparison of generalized anxiety disorder with panic disorder patients. *Psychopharmacology Bulletin* 18:104-108.

Hoehn-Saric, R., and McLeod, D. R. (1985). Generalized anxiety disorder. *Psychiatric Clinics of North America* 8:73-87.

Lindsay, W. R., Gamsu, C. V., McLaughlin, E., et al. (1987). A controlled trial of treatments for generalized anxiety. *British Journal of Clinical Psychology* 26:3-15.

Weissman, M. A., and Merikangas, K. R. (1986). The epidemiology of anxiety and panic disorders: An update. *Journal of Clinical Psychiatry* 47(supp.):11-17.

6 Childhood Phobias

The understanding of anxiety in childhood and adolescence has undergone the same radical changes as those described in the introductory chapter with regard to adults, both in diagnosis and in treatment. There seems to be an easier acceptance of symptomatic treatment for childhood phobias than for those of adulthood. For example, a parent with a child who refuses to attend school will be likely to seek therapy that promises short-term symptom relief. For the parent's own phobia, however, there may be no effort to seek therapy, or a traditional exploratory psychotherapy may be attempted. The effectiveness of the treatment now available for anxiety in childhood might perhaps have a salutary effect on the mental health of the future adult, in that a rapid remission encourages a more normal and age-appropriate developmental progression. But, as Dr. Koplewicz points out, diagnostic accuracy in anxiety disorder in childhood is of especial importance to avoid missing the diagnosis of a more insidious and serious pathological process.

Childhood Phobias

Harold S. Koplewicz

ANXIETY DISORDERS

Anxiety disorders of childhood and adolescence, according to the DSM-III-R, are avoidant disorder, separation anxiety disorder, simple phobia, overanxious disorder, and obsessive-compulsive disorder. These disorders are pathologic states of normal anxiety conditions. Several hypotheses have been postulated for their etiology:

1. Normal developmental maturation does not occur in a group of anxious children.
2. The parents, usually the mother, condition these children to be anxious. This hypothesis is hard to prove, since most parents of anxious children are nonsymptomatic, and they are the ones requesting help for their child.
3. A group of children is predisposed to anxiety disorders in the same way certain children are predisposed to chronic ear infections, seizures, or any other physical illness.

Even though the etiology of the anxiety disorders is still unknown, effective treatment approaches including psychotherapy and pharmacotherapy have been developed. The possibility that more than one hypothesis is true often indicates an individualized treatment approach, utilizing psychotherapy, parent counseling, and medication. This chapter will review the current state of the art in the treatment of the anxiety disorders of childhood and adolescence.

Avoidant Disorder of Childhood and Adolescence

Anxiety normally occurs at certain developmental stages throughout childhood. Its absence may be a pathological sign. Alternatively, anxiety is termed a disorder when the anxiety reaction continues past the normal developmental stage and causes the child discomfort and dysfunction. Normal stranger anxiety occurs in infants between the ages of 7 and 11 months. For example, while being examined by a physician, the baby may look up at the doctor's face and begin to cry. One hypothesis for the baby's anxiety reaction is that his brain has developed to the stage that he can distinguish his mother and father from strangers, and he becomes "distressed" at the difference. The absence of stranger anxiety may be a symptom of certain pathological conditions. The differential diagnosis would include hearing or visual impairment or possibly neglect or abuse.

A nonpathological absence of stranger anxiety would result from the effects of multiple caretakers on normal children. A child from a large extended family being examined by his pediatrician would look up at the doctor and think, "This isn't my mother, this isn't my father, this isn't my Uncle Pete, this isn't Cousin Rose," and by the time he had compared the doctor to all the images in his mind of his relatives, he would be back in his mother's arms. Therefore, no anxiety or distress would be expressed. Similarly, children of working parents may also have multiple caretakers and may not experience stranger anxiety.

Stranger anxiety that persists past the age of 2½ years is a pathologic condition. For example, a child may have a warm, satisfying relationship with his parents and immediate family but become electively mute, socially uncomfortable, and isolated when a stranger or friend of the family enters the house. As the child enters adolescence, these symptoms cause greater dysfunction. This condition is known as *avoidant disorder of childhood and adolescence*. It is common, and frequently these children and adolescents suffer "quietly" and do not present for treatment.

Case Example

> Elizabeth is a 16-year-old who presented to a children's anxiety clinic at her parents' request. She had always been a shy child. In elementary school, although she was a good student, she often refused to read out loud or answer questions in class. She had one close friend and spent most of her free time with her parents. During adolescence Elizabeth's social awkwardness became more obvious and problematic. Her avoidant behavior interfered with the psychosocial developmental tasks of adolescence. Her behavior in social settings included posturing and elective mutism. She was socially isolated and withdrawn from her classmates.
>
> At the recommendation of her guidance counselor, Elizabeth's parents took her to a therapist. The doctor utilized an analytic approach, which resulted in nonsignificant gains. Essentially, Elizabeth spent the sessions in silence. After several months the parents took her to an anxiety clinic at a university-affiliated hospital. The differential diagnosis included avoidant disorder and schizoid disorder. The prognosis for a child with avoidant disorder is possibly a continuation of her symptoms in the form of a social phobia. The child with schizoid disorder presents with peculiar social skills but is not anxious about his social deficits. The prognosis for this child may include schizophrenia.

Most individuals have experienced social phobic reactions at a large cocktail reception. One has the sensation of being scrutinized. Eating in restaurants and using public bathrooms may become problematic. It is easier to treat a child with avoidant disorder than an adult with social phobia. The adult has a lifelong pattern, while the child's symptoms may be of only a few years' duration.

In the adult population, patients who have social phobia have been treated with group therapy and with either Nardil or placebo (Liebowitz et al. 1986). Both groups received social-skills training. The group that also received Nardil had a significant decrease in symptoms over the placebo group. Nardil is effective in the treatment of atypical depression. Rejection sensitivity is commonly seen in atypical depression and is probably a key feature of social phobia, therefore providing a possible rationale for efficacy of an MAOI antidepressant in this anxiety disorder.

Treatment

The treatment of choice for avoidant disorder is group therapy. A social-skills training group is the most effective route (Cartledge and Milburn 1986), most often optimally composed of eight to ten patients, all of whom have social-skills deficits. The group may include both sexes with an age range of approximately three years (e.g., 12-15 years, 15-18 years). The treatment is short-term, consisting of 12-18 sessions. Each session is goal specific—teaching how to conduct phone conversations, speaking in front of a group, dealing with parents. The group therapy includes relaxation techniques. The patients are encouraged to have contact with their group members outside of sessions.

Consideration of pharmacotherapy is indicated in patients with severe anxiety or rejection sensitivity that limits the effectiveness of psychotherapy. In these cases, a short-term trial of a minor tranquilizer should be made an adjunct to the psychotherapy. In adolescent patients who will comply with the necessary dietary restrictions, a trial of an MAO inhibitor can be considered.

Separation-Anxiety Disorder

The normal child between 18 months and 2½ years old experiences separation anxiety. We expect that a child will be anxious when his mother leaves the room. Sometimes, a child playing comfortably in his own room will suddenly need to see his mother. The first day of nursery school or even kindergarten, children may become very upset, clingy, and experience separation anxiety. After a few days, this anxiety decreases and eventually disappears. The child becomes comfortable in the school setting. This is a normal sequence. When separation anxiety behavior persists past the age of four, and causes distress and dysfunction, it is separation anxiety disorder (SAD). In SAD, children experience, (1) illogical worry that something is going to happen to threaten the integrity of the family, (2) distress upon separation, and (3) homesickness (American Psychiatric Association 1987). The illogical worries can be present in nightmares in which separation themes are prominent. Fears about kidnapers coming into the home and taking the child or killing the parents are common. The threat to the integrity of the family is a key feature to these worries. Distress upon separation presents most acutely on Monday and other school day mornings. These children will state that "Sunday nights and Mondays are the worst days of the week." Homesickness can present with school refusal or termination of sleep-over dates. Sleep-away camps will represent a great difficulty. Homesickness may affect a child so that he is terribly uncomfortable and often experiences physical symptoms at school. Younger children experience more gastrointestinal complaints while the adolescents more frequently complain of cardiovascular symptomatology (Gittelman-Klein and Klein 1980).

Case Example

> Adam, a first-grader at a new school, was an attractive 6-year-old with curly blond hair. He was homesick and weepy and complained daily of stomachaches at school. Physical examination disclosed no organic etiology. Adam admitted to the pediatrician that the stomachaches occurred only on weekdays. He also realized that they disappeared with his mother's presence.

Treatment

The treatment approach should include the parents and school as well as the child. The first goal will be to get the child to attend school. The longer the child has been out of school, the more difficult the treatment (Gittelman-Klein 1975). If the child does not respond within a month to a vigorous behavioral child-therapy approach, medication should be added to the treatment regimen. In the adult population with panic disorder and agoraphobia, 50% had childhood SAD (Klein 1964). Tofranil (imipramine) is effective in the treatment of panic disorder and has efficacy in children and adolescents with SAD (Gittelman-Klein et al. 1971).

The relationship between panic disorder with agoraphobia and SAD is very close, and they occur together frequently. In one study comparing adult patients with panic disorder with agoraphobia versus simple phobia, 47% of those with panic disorder with agoraphobia also had SAD, while only 22% of those with simple phobia reported a current diagnosis of SAD. In adults with a diagnosis of panic disorder with agoraphobia, 50% report a history of childhood separation anxiety versus the adult simple-phobic population, which reports a history of 27% (Klein et al. 1980). In another study, parents of children with SAD were compared to parents of children with attention-deficit disorder with hyperactivity (ADDH). The parents of the separation-anxiety-disordered children reported histories of separation anxiety in 19% of the group versus 2% in the ADDH group (Gittelman-Klein and Klein 1980). In a survey done in the general population, adults with a diagnosis of depression with agoraphobia reported that 24% of their children had separation anxiety versus no incidence in the children of adults with depression without an anxiety disorder (Weissman et al. 1982). Xanax (alprazolam), which has proven efficacy in the treatment of anxiety disorders in the adult population, has been used in an open clinical trial with children and adolescents with SAD with positive results (Sheehan et al. 1984, Koplewicz and Gittelman-Klein 1986).

Simple Phobia

A normal child will experience fear of many common things, such as the dark, dogs, at 3 to 5 years of age. When the fear causes dysfunction and severe distress, it is considered a simple phobia—an illogical fear of a harmless object. Some common objects of simple phobias are snakes, elevators, bugs, and planes. Many children, adolescents, and adults experience simple-phobic symptoms but never require treatment, because they are able to avoid the feared object, and therefore do not experience distress or dysfunction. With support and reassurance, a simple-phobic reaction in childhood may remit.

Case Example

> Sam, a 3-year-old, had developed a fear of pigs. The onset of this phobic reaction occurred while he was visiting relatives who lived on a farm. Sam repeatedly asked to see the pig. When he was taken to the pen, however, a piglet ran at him and nipped his ankle. Although he suffered no physical harm, the entire day Sam spoke of nothing else but his fear of the pig's eating him. For several weeks Sam had nightmares about the pig and was fearful of visiting his relatives, going for a drive in the country, or visiting the zoo.

Treatment

Children may develop phobias of many different types of animals or objects (such as snakes, elevators, bugs). If the condition persists and the child's functioning is impaired, a treatment that includes desensitization should be started. No medication has efficacy in the treatment of simple phobias.

Overanxious Disorder

Children may experience anxiety before tests, recitals, or plays. This is known as performance anxiety. However, a child who experiences excessive worries about performance before, during, and after the test may have an overanxious disorder. Such children often have "pseudoprecarious worries." They are overly concerned about the future and what others think of them. The overanxious child frequently presents to the pediatrician with physical complaints that prove to have no organic etiology.

Case Example

> Jennifer, a 7-year-old, is described by her parents as a "nervous wreck." She has headaches and stomachaches all the time. Jennifer admits to worrying about everything: "I worry about money, I worry about the future, I worry where I will go to school when I am older." Jennifer refused to go to the rooftop playground at her school. She was fearful that a gust of wind would blow down the fence and possibly she would fall or get hurt. Her teachers state that she "tries her hardest" all the time. She requires their constant reassurance that she is doing her school work correctly. Her dinner conversation centers around test and school performance.

Treatment

The treatment for a child with overanxious disorder requires the participation of the school, the parents, and the child. The parents often are overachievers and may be anxious about their performance and the child's, but usually not to the child's pathologic extent. Behavioral-therapy approaches can be effective with these children (Ollendick and Gruen 1972). The parents require counseling on how to focus on other issues beside the child's performance. The initiation of low doses of minor tranquilizers may be necessary because of the increased anxiety these children experience when performance discussions and teacher checkups are eliminated. To date, a systematic study of the efficacy of minor tranquilizers in the childhood population has not been done.

Obsessive-Compulsive Disorder

In school-age children, rituals and superstitions are not uncommon. Fear of "stepping on a crack, breaking your mother's back" is an example. Obsessive-compulsive disorder (OCD) usually presents in school age or early adolescence. Its range of severity is wide. Obsessions are illogical ideas or thoughts that one has to keep repeating in one's head. The compulsion is a purposeless behavior or ritual. The most common obsessions and compulsions are related to germ contamination (American Psychiatric Association 1987). A feeling of dread is common and necessitates the compulsive behavior. Quite often, children with OCD are secondarily depressed.

Case Example

> David, a 16-year-old, presented with a 4-year history of OCD. At age 12 he became intensely worried about his height. He began measuring himself repeatedly and comparing his height to that of everyone he met. His concentration and then his school functioning decreased. He described the symptoms as ego dystonic. David was demoralized and at times said he wished he could die so his symptoms would end.

Treatment

Treatment for children and adolescents with OCD should include cognitive-behavioral therapy. Clomipramine (Anafranil), a tricyclic antidepressant, has been studied in this population and has efficacy in the treatment of OCD (Flament et al. 1985). Currently, clomipramine has not been approved by the Food and Drug Administration.

Fluoxetine (Prozac) has been studied in adults with OCD with positive results (Turner 1985). In single-case studies in the childhood and adolescent population Prozac looks promising as a pharmacologic approach.

CONCLUSION

The anxiety disorders of childhood and adolescence are common. The treatment approach often requires the active involvement of the parents and school as well as the child.

The treatment of avoidant disorder of childhood and adolescence is social-skills training. This treatment consists of a short-term group therapy. Further research following adult models is needed to test the efficacy of MAO inhibitors in this childhood disorder.

The treatment of separation-anxiety disorder (SAD) consists of psychotherapy and pharmacotherapy. The utilization of behaviorally oriented psychotherapy is effective in 40% of children with school phobia (Gittelman-Klein and Klein 1971). Based on a double-blind placebo-control study, Tofranil is the medication of choice for this disorder. Open clinical trials of alprazolam (Xanax) with children and adolescents with SAD have been promising. Further research is needed before this medication can be used in the treatment of this population.

Simple phobia is the most common anxiety disorder of childhood. Treatment is required only when the child experiences distress and dysfunction as a result of the phobia. The treatment of choice is desensitization. At present no drug treatments are available.

Children and adolescents with overanxious disorder infrequently present to a mental-health professional. Worries about performance and the future are symptoms that can be useful for academic success. Frequently, a child will experience physical symptoms secondary to the overanxious disorder before a psychiatric consultation is eventually obtained. The most efficacious treatment involves the parents and school as well as the child. In some cases, a short-term trial of a minor tranquilizer can be instituted along with psychotherapy. To date, there are no double-blind placebo-control studies of medication for this disorder.

The treatment of children and adolescents with obsessive-compulsive disorder includes cognitive behavioral therapy and pharmacotherapy. Clomipramine (Anafranil) has proven efficacy for children and adolescents with OCD. Fluoxedine (Prozac) is a promising alternative to clomipramine; however, further research is required in the childhood and adolescent population.

The treatment of anxiety disorders in children and adolescents is very promising. Treatment models utilized in adults, which include psychotherapy and pharmacotherapy, are proving effective in the childhood and adolescent population.

REFERENCES

American Psychiatric Association (1987). *Diagnostic and Statistical Manual of Mental Disorders* (3rd ed. rev.). Washington, DC: APA.

Cartledge, G., and Milburn, J. F., eds. (1986). *Teaching social skills to Children: Innovative Approaches*, 2nd ed. New York: Pergamon Press, Inc.

Flament, M. F., Rapoport, J. L., Berg, C. J., et al. (1985). Clomipramine treatment of childhood obsessive compulsive disorder: A double blind control study. *Archives of General Psychiatry* 42:977-983.

Gittelman-Klein, R. (1975). Pharmacotherapy and management of pathological separation anxiety. *International Journal of Mental Health* 4:255-271.

Gittelman-Klein, R., and Klein, D. F. (1971). Controlled imipramine treatment of school phobia. *Archives of General Psychiatry* 25:204-207.

Gittleman-Klein, R., and Klein, D. F. (1980). Separation anxiety in school refusal and its treatment with drugs. In *Out of School*, ed. L. Hersov, pp. 321-341. London: Wiley.

Klein, D. F. (1964). Delineation of two drug-responsive anxiety syndromes. *Psychopharmacologia* 5:397-408.

Klein, D. F., Gittleman, R., Quitkin, F., et al. (1980). *Diagnosis and Drug Treatment of Psychiatric Disorders: Adults and Children*, 2nd ed. Baltimore: William and Wilkins.

Koplewicz, H. S., and Gittelman-Klein, R. (1986). *Short-term psychotherapies of children and adolescents*. Paper presented at the Meeting of American Academy of Child and Adolescent Psychiatry, Washington, DC.

Liebowitz, M., et al. (1986). Phenelzine and social phobia. *Journal of Clinical Psychopharmacology* 6:93-98.

Ollendick, T. H., and Gruen, G. E. (1972). Treatment of a bodily injury phobia with implosive therapy. *Journal of Consulting and Clinical Psychology* 38:389-393.

Sheehan, D. V., et al. (1984). Some biochemical correlates of panic attacks with agoraphobia and their response to a new treatment. *Journal of Clinical Psychopharmacology* 4:66-75.

Turner, S. (1985). Fluoxetine treatment of obsessive-compulsive disorder. *Journal of Clinical Psychopharmacology* 5:207.

Weissman, M. M., Kidd, K. K., and Prusoff, B. A. (1982). Variability in rates of affective disorders in relatives of depressed and normal probands. *Archives of General Psychiatry* 39:1397-1403.

7 Flying Phobia

Captain "Slim" Cummings enters the field of phobia therapy from a different perspective: His background is as a pilot rather than as a mental-health professional. In the early days of the field, nonprofessionals who had a personal involvement in helping phobics often made substantial contributions. Captain Cummings perceived a need to help those in the grip of this seemingly mysterious, incapacitating illness. A tradition began within this field, comparable to that of Alcoholics Anonymous, for paraprofessionals, who are often former phobics themselves, to be of assistance to those who are currently afflicted. Slim began his program in 1974, and it is clear that he intuitively incorporated, through a commonsense, "seat of the pants" approach, techniques not very different from those developed by the professionals. One difference, perhaps, is that he emphasizes educational material concerning accident rates, troublesome airplane noises, and the like to a greater extent than other therapists might. He is also obviously adept at using group process and group therapy for maximizing therapeutic gains. For those interested in treating fear of flying in individual therapy, it should be noted that this program can also be conducted with considerable success on an individual basis, in the therapist's office, with "homework" flights structured for practice.

Flying Phobia

T. W. Cummings

How common is the problem of fear of flying? Several surveys, including an extensive one prepared for the Boeing Airplane Company, indicate that 25 million adults in the United States are fearful about flying: one out of ten. A 1984 Gallup Poll for *Newsweek* magazine asked over a thousand people, "When you fly, how often are you frightened?" Sixty-five percent answered "never." But a full 35% admitted they were afraid: 21% sometimes, 11% always, and 3% percent most of the time.

The fear of flying seems to be the most common phobia of all. Furthermore, it encompasses several other phobia groups. Acrophobics and claustrophobics avoid flying for obvious reasons; agoraphobics, who resist venturing out, do not even consider venturing up.

Admittedly, many of the 25 million people who avoid flying have what might be called a simple, or novelty, fear, which subsides as soon as someone takes their arm and guides them on board. We have all heard about a grandparent who reluctantly boarded a plane for the first time and within a few minutes after takeoff became a carefree, enthusiastic flyer. But there are still millions who need the guidance of a phobia specialist. They are skeptical that anyone can help them, because their feelings are so intense and so threatening.

Those who seek to control their feelings only become more frustrated and helpless. When asked why he did not fly, the well-known sports commentator, John Madden (who shuttles across the country on trains or in his private bus), responded curtly, "I'm claustrophobic, and that's it." His remarks reflect the feelings of millions: hopelessness.

If the fear of flying is the most common phobia, it is also the most treatable. Therapists and counselors who work with fearful flyers must actively seek out this population, make them aware that help is available, and teach them how to release themselves from their bonds of fear to participate in the miracle of flight.

In this chapter I will summarize the methods we have found to be effective in working with some 2,000 people who have attended our seminars over the past 14 years. I hope to provide the reader with the essence of the four three-hour sessions that comprise the seminars and to explain the procedures we use to allay terrifying feelings on our "graduation flights."

THE FIRST EXPERIMENTAL SEMINAR

It was not until I joined Pan Am, after World War II, that I began to realize that fear was keeping many people grounded and many others disturbed while aloft. Help, if any, was scarcely available to them at that time. I had an educational background and interest in psychology. With Pan Am's encouragement, I organized an experimental seminar for fearful flyers in Miami in 1974.

Three hundred people responded to a story in the *Miami Herald* announcing the seminar. After the first fifty were accepted as participants, a psychologist friend of mine agreed to attend the seminar to observe and to advise me. We held ten two-hour meetings spread over a two-month period, culminating in a round-trip Pan Am flight to Key West. Halfway through the course a minor airliner accident occurred, and several participants dropped out. I was discouraged. I was also apprehensive. Some of the participants were predicting panic attacks on the graduation flight. A few thought that if one panicked, all would panic, resulting in a stampede. A midair bedlam!

Although in twenty-eight years of airline flying, I had never had anyone panic on a flight, I wondered if these people were somehow—and unpredictably—different. Since then, extensive psychological research has shown that phobic anxiety is categorically different from the personality disorganization of psychosis: phobics never erupt in the raving episodes they imagine will occur in flight. I wish I had known that at the time. As it was, I consulted many therapists about in-flight panic, and the consensus seemed to be that it was highly unlikely because of two prime factors: (1) the sharing and caring that was developing within the group and (2) their confidence in my guidance and leadership, which was probably affected by my airline affiliation and credentials as a pilot.

The seminar attracted continual press coverage, and the presence of television cameras added to the pervasive tension on the day of the graduation flight. Three of the participants did not board. One of them was overweight and "overpale." I was glad he chose not to join us. On boarding, a well-dressed woman hesitated in the galley alcove, not moving back to a seat. She had taken off her shoes and held them under her arm. I asked her what was going on, and she tearfully told me that it had suddenly occurred to her that—as a little girl—she had reacted to being threatened by "tucking my shoes under my arm and running as fast as I could go." She somehow resisted that impulse and joined the others.

With an empathetic cockpit and cabin crew, I knew we could handle whatever problems arose. But the probing television cameras still worried me. If the evening news carried the picture of even one person coming unhinged, my hopes for Pan Am's continuing interest in the program would be over. There was much at stake.

What happened was unpredictable indeed. Yes, there were

fear, anxiety, wringing hands, tears, and wild-eyed vigilance. But no one panicked, became hysterical, fainted, or screamed. Shortly after takeoff, a contagious elation, joy, and triumph spread through the cabin. It seemed that everyone was engulfed in the celebration of each other's courage. Each person had created a unique miracle; I had served only as their guide. But I knew I had discovered an exciting endeavor, which I could pursue as a fulfilling second career.

Since then (I retired from Pan Am in 1977 at age 60, the compulsory retirement age for airline pilots), we have conducted close to 150 seminars throughout the United States and in London. The seminars—and our cassette tapes, books, and individual counseling—have enabled thousands of people grounded or restricted by fear to become comfortably, even joyously, airborne. During the past six years my wife, Carmen Cummings— who holds a master's degree in counseling psychology—has worked with me.

PRESEMINAR PROCEDURE AND FIRST SESSION

Our seminars actually begin several weeks before the first scheduled meeting. We send each participant two sixty-minute cassette tapes, which provide an understanding of how a phobia develops and ways to cope with it, and a booklet that answers questions about flight and fear. We urge our participants to become as familiar and comfortable with these materials as possible.

The tapes present a simple relaxation procedure (parts of which are summarized below) and then sequentially lead the listener through the details of a typical airline flight, from the arrival at the airport through taxiing, takeoff, cruise, descent, and landing. Through the tapes, I, as narrator, am able to "sit beside" the listener on this flight, discussing feelings and explaining the aircraft's sounds and movements.

The seminars include a maximum of twenty participants and

consist of four evening sessions, usually from 7:00 to 10:00. A hotel meeting room is used for the first two sessions.

Many of the people who contact us express an urgent need to overcome their fear. Jobs, travel obligations, even family relationships may be impaired. The need is well identified, but most people who are fearful about flying are also fearful about doing anything about it. The fear is too immense, too intimidating. Therefore, in the first minutes of the seminar, participants are heartily congratulated as the few who decide to challenge the problem. Despite their abiding skepticism about being helped, their courage is commendable. We ask that everyone stand and applaud those similarly courageous around them. And then, with louder applause, we ask that they clap for themselves.

Motivation has brought these people to the seminar. Its components are loved ones, jobs, travel, and self-esteem. No matter how long or how severely they have been fearful, it is this desire to change that gets them moving.

People who have never flown and who avoid it because they feel threatened by the very thought of it comprise only 10% of the attendees. The remainder of the group is quite evenly divided between those who have stopped flying because of the relentless stress of the experience and those who continue to fly but do it miserably. The futile aim of this latter group is to try to avoid the experience of flight through liquor, sedatives, the white-knuckled grip, closed eyes, or sitting rigidly, resisting all aircraft movement. Some even try to defy gravity by sitting "lightly" in their seats. These devices of avoidance are counterproductive, serving only to reinforce the problem. Each flight becomes just another practice session in being fearful.

A mild drink might relieve a mild anxiety. But the seriously fearful people who seek our help have found that booze doesn't release them from the grip of their fear. One man told me that even after "a dozen martinis" he was still both sober and scared during an entire flight. After landing, liquor took its effect, and he suddenly was so drunk that two attendants had to help him disembark.

A few recovering alcoholics attend our seminars. They quickly perceive that, like Alcoholics Anonymous, our program embodies the strength of a group drawn together by a common problem. What emerges from both groups is a common desire to change, a common caring, and a common courage. As in A.A., our participants refer to themselves by their first names only. Recovering alcoholics also know that trying to find out why one drinks, or why one is phobic about flying, will not solve the problem. What will help them is doing something about it. Insight may come later.

We get down to the business of helping participants understand the nature of their phobia by helping them to admit its source in themselves and acknowledging their own responsibilities in combating it. We conduct a symptomatic survey. One of our questions is: "Do you believe your fear to be rational, irrational, or both?" The people who admit that their fear is irrational recognize that it is not the airplane that causes the problem but rather their own emotional, phobic response to flight or the contemplation of flight. Two-thirds of the participants, however, respond that their fear is either rational or a mixture of rational and irrational concerns. To cope with the exaggerated, distorted stories and assertions of this latter group, we must present the truth: the facts about the safety of air transportation. We distribute current facts and statistics about air safety, and then present this information along the following lines:

> The media seldom mention anything about air *safety*. Most of the stories on film and in print are about accidents, overcrowded skies, overworked controllers, poorly trained pilots, and inadequate maintenance. Fearful flyers, looking for ways to justify their resistance to flying, will grab at these stories, dwell on them, and repeat them with convictions of real danger. These stories can be refuted only by presenting the facts and statistics about how safe air travel really is.
>
> The Airline Deregulation Act of 1978 established open price competition among all airlines, bringing air fares down and allowing millions more to fly. Only 270 million people flew in 1977. In 1987 that number had increased 66% to 450 million. The resulting crowded terminals and

flight delays brought frustration, anger, and fear. But has deregulation compromised *safety*? Table 7-1 confirms the only reasonable answer.

The facts are, simply, the facts: *despite a 50% increase in passengers over the ten years since deregulation, there has been a 25% decrease in the number of fatalities and a 40% decrease in the number of fatal accidents.*

The first-century philosopher Epictetus put it well when he wrote: "People are disturbed, not by things, but by the views which they take of them."

The years 1983, 1984, and 1986 were fatality-free years for airline flying. During 1986 and until the August 1987 crash during takeoff in Detroit, the U.S. Scheduled Airlines transported 700 million people an average distance of 800 miles, through 10 million takeoffs and landings in all kinds of weather *without a single passenger fatality*. After the Detroit tragedy, syndicated columnist George Will wrote: "When a crash crystallizes anxiety about air safety, journalism should stress the news—yes, news—that flying is astonishingly safe. Travel on U. S. commercial airlines is the safest form of transportation ever devised."

What about more specific concerns—midair collisions, for example? For all the talk about near-misses, there has been only one midair accident involving a commercial airliner within the last decade: the collision of a B-727 with a private plane over San Diego in 1978. United States carriers have since logged 50 million takeoffs and landings without a single midair fatality.

Compare air travel with highway travel. Forty-eight thousand people lose their lives on our nation's highways every year—a daily average of 130 deaths, not to mention the thousands incapacitated by injuries. This carnage rarely hits the evening news, since it is not news at all, but simply the commonplace, predictable toll that happened yesterday, is happening today, and will happen tomorrow. The plain truth is that the average *daily highway* fatality figure of 130 exceeds the *yearly air* average of 120. According to a 1986 article in *Time* magazine, "On a mile

TABLE 7-1 Air Safety before and after Deregulation

Time frame	Total passengers	Total fatal accidents	Yearly average	Total passenger fatalities	Yearly average
1967–1977	2 billion	50	5	1600	160
1978–1988	3 billion	30	3	1200	120

to mile basis, Americans are nearly 100 times as likely to die in car accidents as in plane crashes."

Living, day to day, involves some element of risk. Walking, the oldest form of locomotion, takes a yearly toll of 7,000 lives. More people die of bee stings than airline flying. Many fearful flyers nervously suck on cigarettes as they charge that air travel is too risky. Government figures blame smoking for killing 350,000 each year.

We go on to brief descriptions of the extensive training and continual review of pilots, the preparedness of flight attendants in safety procedures, the strength of modern jetliners, and the basics of radar and traffic control. In one sense, my own credentials as a former pilot can become countertherapeutic at this early stage, since they tempt participants to keep the discussion in the abstract, impersonal realms of engineering and statistics. "Aren't the skies too crowded?" "Isn't maintenance dangerously lax?" Each of these hypothetical "I gotcha" questions can give birth to hours of increasingly picayune discussion, none of it applicable to the problem at hand.

We try, therefore, to cover the facts without dwelling on them. The bottom line is that flying is 99.99998% safe—a figure, notes the author Robert Serling, that "compares most favorably with virtually any form of human activity, including taking a bath." Our point, and we make it emphatically clear, is that our participants' problems have nothing to do with airplanes or the reality of flight. Their problems are their own feelings, which are what they are here to address.

"But why," they often ask, "if it is so safe to fly, am I so scared?" This excellent question signals a willingness to begin to address themselves to their feelings and demands an encouraging response. "First," I say, "it has nothing to do with intelligence. People who seek our help are above average in education and achievement. You are well able to reason. But in contemplation of a flight your intellectual, reasoning mind is bypassed by the strong emotional impact of fear. As Einstein said, 'Imagination is more powerful than knowledge.'"

We then present them with the antidote to fear, which we call AAA/BM or "Triple-A/BM." The acronym stands for the following coping tools that diffuse the phobic response:

Awareness

As a fearful flyer, you have no power to change the manner of flight, the plane, the pilot, or the weather. You can only change your emotional response. Concentrating on your fear can be terrifying. From fearful thoughts come fearful feelings: an inevitable sequence. Without *awareness* of why this dreaded experience occurs and what can be done about it, the problem is reinforced with each flight. But your response can be changed, once you become aware that the problem and its solution lie within yourself.

Acceptance

Many fearful flyers, confused and frustrated by their feelings, will try to shut them off, ignore them, or deny them. Trying to suppress those feelings only increases them. Progress in treatment will not begin until you acknowledge and accept your feelings. As scary as the feelings are, they need not be embarrassing or demeaning. It's okay to be afraid. Admitting it and accepting how it has affected you marks the beginning of its demise.

Action

Fearful flyers *re*-act. As anxiety moves on to fear, adrenalin enters the bloodstream, the heart rate increases, the chest and abdominal muscles tighten, the throat dries, and the palms may become cool and sweaty. The reactions to danger, real or imagined, are physiologically the same. This body response is automatic, seemingly uncontrollable. When confronted by real dangers, our aboriginal ancestors in caves would either fight or flee in response to these neurological imperatives. As a phobic flyer, you are in no danger, but neither can you fight or flee. It is a lonely experience, but it need not be one of helplessness. *Re-action* is the problem. The solution is in *action*.

Breathing

Breathing is the first action we prescribe. You can interrupt and moderate the automatic fear response by consciously taking control of your breathing and movement. Three slow, deep breaths can be a powerful tool in coping with flight fright. Hold each inhalation for the count of three ("one thousand, two thousand, three thousand"), exhaling slowly and fully after each.

A participant in my first Miami seminar came to the third meeting with a story. He had received an emergency call that his mother was gravely ill in Chicago. Worried enough to visit her, but "paralyzed" at the thought of flying, he managed to obtain a seat right next to the aircraft door, so that if he panicked he could run out before the door closed. As the last passenger was boarding—and as he got ready to bolt—he suddenly remembered the breathing exercises. He did them, with difficulty and disbelief, but he told us that it was the breathing exercise that had enabled him to stay on that plane. It shifted his focus.

Today, even the most skeptical fearful flyers swear by this simple procedure. We know that one doesn't have to believe in these exercises to benefit from them. But you must do them. You must act.

Many professional entertainers and athletes use deep breathing and movement to dissipate performance anxiety. Some seminar participants report previous attacks of hyperventilation; these attacks do not recur after they take charge of their breathing.

Movement

As fear progresses, all the muscles of the body, including those related to digestion and respiration, tighten. As breathing and movement become restricted, the symptoms intensify. You can arrest, even reverse, this response by moving the arms, legs, and torso. Several years ago, a participant on a flight out of Dallas stood up to show me that his hands were trembling and that he couldn't stop them. I suggested that he "go with the problem" by shaking them faster. He did that easily, and after half a minute or so I told him that he could stop any time he chose to. Much to his surprise, and mine, the trembling stopped. His deliberate action changed his involuntary reaction.

We now call this exercise the "shakeoff." With forearms extended, vigorously snap your wrists, letting your hands flap. This movement seems to elicit considerable enthusiasm—and laughter—among our groups when we suggest that they are "shaking off the crap," which is their fear.

Combine hand snapping with stomping, marching heavily in place. Stretching your arms gently upward often relieves shoulder muscle tension. Slowly rotating the upper torso also helps.

Effect of the Exercises

The breathing/movement exercises help to unite everybody in the group. After practicing them together, the participants are better able to verbalize and share their doubts and encouragements with each other. If somebody falters, other understanding and sensitive members of the group will move in to pick up the spirit of the hesitant one. This sincere demonstration of caring adds immeasurably to the strength of the receiver. And caregivers, in the act of comforting others, get their minds off their own worries.

We teach these exercises whether our group numbers two or twenty. We first practice them in the classroom, where the odd behavior is more easily accepted because of the strong empathy among participants. Although conspicuous behavior is something fearful flyers most wish to avoid, they will risk embarrassment standing in a circle with the group. In doing so, they gain strength by finding out that nothing embarrassing happens. Over the course of the seminar we rehearse these exercises at the terminal, in the waiting lounge, and on a parked airplane.

Effect of Sharing Experiences

We take some time at the end of the first session to have everyone sit in a circle and share why they came to the seminar. Their tales are both frightening and funny. Some remember movies about flying, vivid media pictures and stories of crashes, or dreams of crashing, falling, dying. Some say that the fear started when they separated from home to attend college, go to work, or get married. Others feel that they may somehow jeopardize the good fortune of a promotion or parenthood by flying; being on an airplane becomes, in their minds, an act of unacceptable irresponsibility. To one woman, who had made repeated flights accompanying her fatally ill husband to a clinic in a distant city, the airplane became associated with sadness and death.

Some say they have experienced a "bad flight," a hard landing, or a flight through rough weather. Other people admit that their flights have been smooth, but that they held on tightly, expecting bumps at any minute. Oddly enough, the very few participants who have actually been in aircraft accidents, even when fatalities have occurred, seem more receptive to treatment than those who entertain fantasies about plummeting earthward in a ball of fire.

A sense of caring begins to emerge in the group. Whereas at first many exchanged horror stories about flying, now their attention has shifted to sharing feelings and hopes.

PREPARING FOR THE GRADUATION FLIGHT

For the better part of the last two meetings, we use the passenger cabin of a parked jet transport as our classroom. To prepare fearful flyers for the graduation flight, they must have the opportunity to board, sit in, and move about a stationary aircraft. This can be arranged with an airline that serves the city where the seminar is held. The bigger the airline, the more likely it is to have an aircraft parked at a gate for an hour or longer. The most accessible are those that arrive in the evening and remain at the airport overnight.

Therapists should arrange these visits through the airline's passenger service manager, or somebody with a similar title. Because an airline employee must accompany the group onto the plane, a request for a full hour's time on board might be refused. However, a request for fifteen to thirty minutes will most likely be granted. Once the group has boarded, that time limit may expand without difficulty, or the group may be able to board a second aircraft.

These practice sessions are so important because, without the threat of takeoff, the participants can learn new ways of responding to the phobic environment. For example, the oversensitive reaction of some people to the sound of the closing of the cabin doors can be substantially reduced as they watch us open and close the door several times.

We urge those who object to a window seat to sit in one for ten seconds, or thirty, or to shake and stomp in one for a full minute. The experience may elicit a lot of stress, but it provides a great opportunity to prove to themselves that the exercises work. It gives them a sense of being in control in a time of real stress. As one person in the group begins confronting situations he or she has been avoiding, others will begin to take risks also.

We also introduce and practice a procedure called *terrible turbulence training*, which will serve them well on the graduation flight and later. The seat-belt sign is turned on. With everyone seated together and with seat belts fastened, we ask them to simulate mild turbulence by bouncing up and down. As they join in the spirit, we suggest they increase the intensity. Soon everyone is bouncing and laughing. The seat-belt sign is then turned off. The movement and laughter have brought relaxation, and the point of the exercise is made clear. Although turbulence has been a dreaded experience for many group members, the next time they encounter it in flight they will vividly recall sharing this "crazy" exercise. We even suggest that when the "fasten seat belt" sign comes on in flight, they start jostling before the plane encounters any bumps. Practicing for it helps.

We are progressing slowly toward a face-to-face encounter with flight—the object of their phobia. Bertrand Russell pointed out that "a fear which we are unwilling to face grows worse by not being looked at." The only certain remedy for a phobia is confrontation. More knowledge about air transportation is not enough. Determination and courage are not enough. The understanding gained through psychological counseling is not enough. The fear of flying can be vanquished only by confronting flight. This can be accomplished via supportive, permissive, knowledgeable exposure to it.

As the day of the flight approaches, the participants inevitably begin to anticipate the big event. Dr. Robert L. DuPont has designated the phobic anxiety syndrome as "a malignant disease of 'what-ifs.'" Such obsessive, future-oriented speculations nurture all phobias. The fearful flyer's initial feeling of uneasiness doesn't become a problem until it is ignited by "what if." "What if I cry? Shake? Scream? Faint? Panic? Have a heart attack?" This anticipation of embarrassing or disabling behavior seems to be the biggest barrier in reaching the essential goal of all phobics' confrontation.

The fearful flyer must become aware of how obsessive and destructive the "what if" pattern is, and—more important—what can be done to interrupt the pattern that will either keep him or her from boarding the plane or make the flight a miserable experience. The phobic person, sinking in a quagmire of "what-ifs," can be rescued by the reality of "what *is*." "What ifs" refer to the future, and no one can live—feel joy or fear—in the future. "What is" refers to this moment, this reality, the NOW.

One way to interrupt the "what if" process is to ask the sufferer to measure his anxiety state on a scale of one to ten (one being tranquil and ten being the worst level imaginable). Evaluating the threat in this way automatically shifts the focus away from the anxiety. If people say they are at five or above, we urge their participation in the breathing/movement exercises, assuring them that the anguish will subsequently subside to a more manageable level.

The fourth, and last, meeting before the flight is an emotional and powerful one, as more fears and hopes begin to surface. We list several of the "what ifs" on a blackboard. Many have to do with the fear of embarrassing behavior. We urge everyone to give themselves permission to be embarrassed. Putting a big "so" in front of the "what if" will diminish the threat. "*So what* if I cry? *So what* if I faint?" (It must be noted that the fears of falling, crashing, and dying are common "what if" fears of the fearful flyer. Nightmares about falling are not uncommon among the general population. In my opinion, the fear of crashing relates more to "crashing" emotionally rather than physically. And many who express thoughts about crashing still come on the graduation flight with us.)

The meeting concludes with everybody sitting in a circle and sharing reasons for being on the next day's flight. The testimonies are very moving and affirming. Warm handshakes and embraces follow. Their faces are brighter and their voices firmer than the first night. We remind them that only in the experience itself will they realize that 95% of their anxiety has been anticipation. For those who are still unsure whether they will fly, we tell them to come to the airport to see the others off.

THE GRADUATION FLIGHT

We prefer graduation flights of about an hour's duration. Those that depart around noon will be less crowded than those leaving at 8:00 or 9:00 A.M. Remaining at the flight's destination for a couple of hours before returning will allow time for refreshment and to process the flight experience. Wide-bodied jets are somewhat roomier and therefore preferable, though by no means essential, for these "maiden voyages." In any case, seating in the forward area of economy class affords a smoother and quieter ride. Ticketing and seating arrangements for the flight can often be handled more easily and cheaply through a travel agent than through the airline's busy phones or the long lines at the airport.

The participants who assemble in the boarding area for the graduation flight represent a variety of emotions. A few are excited about the prospect of how much this flight can mean to them. Some seem to turn aside as they glumly fix their attention on a series of discomforting "what ifs." A participant in Boston showed up for the flight carrying a large cardboard box. She had printed a bold message on it, and as we boarded she held it up for her fellow passengers to heed: BEFORE BOARDING PLEASE DEPOSIT ALL "WHAT IFS" AND "YES, BUTS" IN HERE.

It is not unusual for a participant to come to me on graduation day with a frown and say, in all seriousness, something like, "I'm confused because I slept quite well last night and even ate some breakfast this morning. That worries me because it just isn't like me to do that before a flight." Evidence of improvement is often difficult to accept, after the burden of fear has persisted for so long.

We gather together for at least an hour before the flight. As we move into a circle and join hands, I remind everyone that feelings of anxiety, worry, anticipation, and excitement are indeed appropriate for this big event, this opportunity. Other big events, like getting married or giving a speech, have carried similarly mixed reactions.

We arrange to board before the other passengers, so that we can meet the cockpit and cabin crew and get settled into our seats. The time after boarding and before the entrance door closes is critical. The urge to escape from all the stress is often a very powerful one. Just by stepping into the plane, the person has successfully handled a present reality, but the anticipations are threatening. "I recognize that some of you may feel miserable right now," I tell them. "But I know from experience that you will be okay if you stay with us. I also know that you will be very disappointed if you get off. Don't let fear make the decision for you. *Choose* to stay, knowing what this achievement will mean to you."

There seems to be a very thin line between the decision to stay on or to disembark. Once, many years ago, after we had begun to taxi toward the runway, and as I was walking through the cabin attending to each participant, a woman looked up at me and pleaded, "I wanna get off! I wanna get off!" There was a whine in her voice, as if she were a little child. It seemed to me that she was waiting for a "father figure" to tell her what to do. Knowing how important the flight was to her, I said firmly, "I want you to stay right there in that seat, and that's it!" That proved to be what she needed to be told.

We all sit together in the same section of the plane. Soon after boarding and during taxiing and awaiting clearance for takeoff we go through our relaxation exercises. We applaud all evidences of courage. We stomp our feet. We also encourage crying as a way of letting go, flowing. The caring touch of others in the group is helpful also.

We watch particularly for the loners, those who do not communicate and share their feelings. Besides the "Triple-A/BM," we ask these people to locate some particular part of their body where the fear or pain seems to be centered. Then we suggest that they intensify it. They rarely succeed in this effort, but in trying to they gain a sense of control instead.

Takeoff is usually regarded as the most disturbing aspect of flight, perhaps because it symbolizes departure from familiarity, home, and terra firma. As we taxi onto the runway for the takeoff, everyone joins hands, takes two deep breaths, and leans back in their seats. We remind them not to close their eyes. As the takeoff roll begins, I ask everybody to "wiggle their toes, wiggle them faster and faster as we accelerate." This distraction works wonders.

The transition from fear to courage starts soon after takeoff, even as the landing gear is still retracting. Applause is spontaneous. Joy and enthusiasm spread rapidly through the group. Some are entranced by the view out the window. Others take reluctant peeks. A few who have never left their seats on previous flights now cautiously stand. Particularly noteworthy is the apparent lack of concern about heights or being closed in. A few may ask worried questions about sounds and movement, but this monitoring gradually decreases as "what ifs" give way to "what is."

Actually, the problems are few and quite easily addressed. To the 10% who have never flown, it is a flight of wonder. To all, the flight is a celebration of courage, and many regard the accomplishment as the happiest, most important event of their lives. Many, consequently, will stop smoking, lose weight, or improve their lives in other ways. This is sometimes referred to as the umbrella effect.

An expression we often hear is "I can't believe how well I did on that flight." These people, and everyone else, are urged to make this experience believable by repeating it soon again, preferably in two weeks. Everyone is cautioned that, without a reaffirming flight, the old specter of fear may stealthily creep back. Participants who have grown close through so much sharing often make arrangements to fly together.

In a survey of more than 200 seminar participants, almost half graded themselves as high on perfectionism. The perfectionist seeks to have everything carefully arranged and predictable. This is an impossible goal, which always creates frustration and tension. After the graduation flight, the perfectionists, even though they may have been grounded for twenty years, minimize their achievement in statements such as "I didn't do as well as I hoped I would." The pursuit of perfection has been called "a dangerous form of madness." We are all imperfect, and it is that imperfection that makes us likable, laughable, and kindred spirits.

Usually, about 10% of those who attend the seminar do not come with us on the graduation flight. Some will write that they flew a few days later. I distinctly remember one woman, a travel agent, who didn't join us on the flight but lingered at the airport to observe the others when they returned. When she saw how happy the others were, she promptly bought a ticket for a similar flight leaving in thirty minutes.

Nearly 40% of our participants indicate that they have had psychological therapy. Although the seminar is a giant step, we recognize that some of those attending are having difficulty with problems unrelated to the fear of flying. We recommend that they seek professional counsel. Occasionally we will introduce a local psychologist to the group, who may also assist us in the seminar.

CONCLUSION

People have always been intrigued by the wonder of flight. Ancient civilization left flying to the gods. The Roman messenger of the gods was Mercury, with wings on his helmet. The Greeks found their god symbol in Pegasus, the winged horse. Early Christians deified those who were selected to ascend into heaven by giving them wings and calling them angels.

Now, here in the United States, more than a million people speed comfortably through the skies every day. Although millions are still intimidated by the thunder of takeoffs, the sheer audacity of flight, it is these very wonders that have established today's jet aircraft as the ultrasafe method of transportation.

For the past fourteen years it has been my privilege to see how much the quality of people's lives is enhanced by the decision to confront their fear of flying. It has been an inspiration to me to play a part in this growth experience. I hope the ideas presented in this chapter will encourage others to offer their help in this needed area.

> Nothing in life is to be feared. It is only to be understood.
>
> —Marie Curie

REFERENCES

Cummings, T. W., and White, R. (1987). *Freedom from Fear of Flying.* New York: Pocket Books (Simon and Schuster).

8 Obsessive-Compulsive Disorder

Edna Foa and her colleagues at Temple University Medical Center have developed one of the best known and most effective programs in the treatment of obsessive-compulsive disorders. She has taken ideas, such as Stampfl's "implosion therapy" and other behavioral techniques, which on the basis of a small number of cases had been suggested as effective for obsessive-compulsive disorders, and systematically tested them in a series of research studies over the past 20 years. This chapter concisely reviews the main points of the treatment program that has been developed in accordance with these research findings.

Although obsessive-compulsive disorder (OCD) is relatively rare, it has served as the model for an important step in treatment of mental disorders. Previously, it was held that obsessions were thoughts and compulsions were acts. Experience with psychotherapy has favored a functional definition, that obsessions are what increase the anxiety and compulsions are what decrease it. For example, in the childhood rhyme, "Step on a crack, break your mother's back," not stepping on a crack is a compulsive avoidance that reduces the anxiety of the obsessive thought of doing harm to mother.

Although phobias and obsessive-compulsive disorders are similar in many respects, the treatment of OCD is frequently more difficult, and success seems to be less complete and slightly less stable than with phobic disorders. Before the development of the new techniques, however, OCD was generally found to be quite refractory to psychotherapeutic intervention. As in the treatment of phobias, the primary mode of today's OCD therapy is through some form of desensitization. In vivo exposure is even more important with OCD, however. At some point, either in the therapist's office or on his own, the patient must directly confront the contaminant or perform the anxiety-provoking act. Furthermore, he must do so without also performing a compulsive behavior or having a thought presumed to undo the anxiety-provoking contact. For example, the person must leave the house after checking the locks only once, or touch something on the floor without afterward washing hands, or think of the word "death" without then performing the ritual of counting to four a specified number of times. This treatment regimen is known as "exposure with response prevention." The anxiety engendered by contact with the contaminant gradually diminishes with exposure over time, if the undoing response is prevented. In the program described here, this goal is achieved in conjunction with supportive psychotherapy. Marital therapy is a frequent adjunct, because ritualizers so often involve family members—as, for example, in the case of a housewife who makes all family members partially disrobe before entering the house.

Obsessive-Compulsive Disorder

Edna Foa
Gail Steketee

The concept of obsessive-compulsive neurosis has been discussed for over 100 years. Esquirol (1838) provided the first written account, but it was not until the beginning of this century that attempts were made to arrive at a formal definition (e.g., Lewis 1936, Schneider 1925). It is generally agreed that obsessive-compulsive disorder is characterized by recurrent or persistent thoughts, images, impulses, or actions, accompanied by a sense of subjective compulsion and a desire to resist it. Some patients, identified as obsessionals, suffer from obsessional thoughts, images, or impulses without manifesting overt repetitious actions. However, the majority of obsessive-compulsives complain of both intrusive disturbing thoughts and repetitious, stereotyped actions. Here we will describe a treatment plan designed for the latter patient population.

It is customary to refer to thoughts and images as "obsessions" and to repetitious actions as "compulsions." We find this classification unsatisfactory, since it is based on the modality of the symptoms rather than on their function. We suggest instead a distinction that rests on the relationship between anxiety or discomfort and symptoms. Accordingly, thoughts, images, and actions that elicit anxiety or discomfort will be denoted as obsessions. On the other hand, overt behaviors and, more rarely, conditions that are anxiety reducing are termed compulsions.

Compulsions take a variety of forms, of which the two most common are washing and checking. *Washers* are patients who feel contaminated when exposed to certain objects or thoughts; their compulsive behavior consists mostly of excessive ritualistic washing and cleaning. *Checkers* are patients whose compulsions consist of repetitious checking and/or ritualistic stereotyped actions performed to avoid future "disasters" or punishment. Sometimes rituals are related to anxiety-evoking obsessions in a direct, rational way (e.g., checking to see if the stove is off in order to avoid possible fire); other rituals are not rationally related to the obsessions (e.g., dressing and undressing to prevent one's husband from having an accident).

Both washing and checking can be found in the same patient. For the purposes of outlining a treatment plan, however, they will be considered separately. The following case descriptions are illustrative of each type.

> *Case 1.* Jane is a 30-year-old married woman with two children. She felt contaminated (a nonspecific feeling of being dirty, accompanied by extreme anxiety and discomfort) when in contact with her home town. Her symptoms began at age 16, when Jane felt contaminated by Christmas ornaments stored in her parents' attic. At first, only these ornaments were disturbing, but within a short period of time, everything that had been in direct or indirect contact with them led to anxiety and a concomitant urge to wash. In addition to feelings of contamination, the ornaments also produced strong feelings of sadness and depression. At the time she applied for treatment, Jane avoided anything associated with her home town, including family members. These elaborate avoidance efforts, however, proved inadequate to protect her. Jane continuously found herself confronted with items from her home town, such as chocolates manufactured there and sold in food stores, where they contaminated other groceries.

Such encounters made it necessary for her to engage in extensive washing and cleaning rituals to restore a state of noncontamination. Jane was motivated to seek treatment when her grandmother, whom she loved and had not seen for 7 years, became seriously ill. The fear of contamination prevented Jane from visiting her.

Case 2. Mike, a 32-year-old patient, engaged in checking rituals that were triggered by a fear of harming others. When driving he felt compelled to stop the car often to check whether he had run over people, particularly babies. Before flushing the toilet, Mike inspected the commode to be sure that a live insect had not fallen into the toilet—he did not want to be responsible for killing any live creature. In addition, he repeatedly checked the doors, stoves, lights, and windows, making sure that all were shut or turned off so that no harm, such as fire or burglary, would befall his family as a result of his "irresponsible" behavior. In particular he worried about the safety of his 15-month-old daughter, repeatedly checking the gate to the basement to be sure that it was locked. He did not carry his daughter while walking on concrete floors in order to avoid killing her by accidentally dropping her. Mike performed these and many other checking rituals for an average of four hours a day. Checking behavior started several months after his marriage, 6 years before treatment. It increased 2 years later, when Mike's wife was pregnant with their first child, and continued to worsen over the years.

REVIEW OF TREATMENTS

Obsessive-compulsive disorders have long been considered among the most intractable of the neurotic disorders. As recently as 1961, Breitner (1960) noted that "most of us are agreed that the treatment of obsessional states is one of the most difficult tasks confronting the psychiatrist and many of us consider it hopeless" (p. 32). Traditional psychotherapy has not proven effective in ameliorating obsessive-compulsive symptomatology (Black 1974). In a sample of 90 inpatients, Kringlen (1965) found that only 20% had improved at a 13- to 20-year follow-up. Somewhat more favorable results were reported by Grimshaw (1965): 40% of an outpatient sample were improved at a 1- to 14-year follow-up.

Early Forms of Behavioral Treatments

Some improvement in the prognostic picture emerged with the application of treatments derived from learning theories. These methods can be divided into two classes: (1) exposure procedures aimed at reducing the anxiety/discomfort associated with obsessions, and (2) blocking or punishing techniques directed at decreasing the frequency of either obsessive thoughts or ritualistic behaviors.

The most commonly employed exposure treatment was systematic desensitization. Despite initial claims for its efficacy with obsessive-compulsive disorders, a review of the literature indicated that systematic desensitization effected improvement in only 30% to 40% of the cases reported (Beech and Vaughan 1978, Cooper et al. 1965). Treatment procedures utilizing prolonged exposure to feared cues (e.g., paradoxical intention, imaginal flooding, satiation, and aversion relief) have also been employed with this population. Improvement with these procedures, which have been examined largely through case reports, has not exceeded 60%, with the exception of aversion relief, which proved effective to varying degrees for each of five patients.

The second set of treatment methods, blocking or punishing procedures, includes thought stopping, aversion therapy, and covert sensitization. Thought stopping has proven largely ineffective in several case studies. Aversion therapy using electrical shock, the snapping of a rubber band on the wrist, or covert sensitization has fared somewhat better. As with the exposure procedures discussed above, our knowledge of the efficacy of blocking techniques is based largely on case reports, which tend to be biased toward positive outcomes.

If, as suggested previously, obsessive-compulsive symptomology is composed of obsessions that evoke anxiety and compulsions that reduce it, then treatment should consist of techniques that decrease anxiety and procedures that suppress compulsions. It follows that the simultaneous use of interventions directed at both obsessions and compulsions would be expected to yield superior results to treatment directed at only one set of symptoms. In the foregoing reports, investigators rarely attempted to match the treatment procedure to the target symptoms. An exception was the use of aversion relief (Marks et al. 1969, Rubin and Merbaum 1971), where compulsive behavior was followed by the administration of electrical shock (blocking), and shock was terminated upon contact with the feared situations (obsessions). Treatment was successful in the two patients who underwent this procedure. Another treatment program that addressed both obsessions and compulsions was exposure and response prevention. This program has proven highly effective and has become the treatment of choice for this disorder. A summary of the research on this procedure follows.

Exposure and Response Prevention

In 1966, Victor Meyer developed a therapeutic program, later labeled *apotrepic therapy* (Meyer et al. 1974), which consisted of two basic components: (1) in vivo exposure to discomfort-evoking stimuli, i.e., placing the patient in the real-life feared situation, and (2) response prevention, i.e., blocking the compulsive behaviors. The results were impressive; of the 15 patients treated with this program, 10 were rated as much improved or symptom free, and five were rated as improved. Only two patients relapsed during the follow-up period. At the same time, Stampfl and Levis (1967) formulated a therapeutic procedure consisting of prolonged imaginal exposure to fear-evoking scenes. Called "implosive" therapy, this method was applied primarily to phobics. A few reports with single patients suggested that this therapy might reduce obsessive-compulsive symptoms.

Variants of in vivo exposure and response prevention have been investigated in numerous studies. In contrast to the relatively poor prognosis for obsessive-compulsives with traditional psychotherapy, the overall success rates with these two behavioral procedures were quite high—about 75% of patients improved markedly with these treatments (e.g., Marks et al. 1975, Emmelkamp and Kraanen 1977). Slightly better results have been noted with a combination of imaginal and in vivo exposure (Foa and Goldstein 1978). (Extensive reviews have been done by Foa et al. [1985] and Rachman and Hodgson [1980].) At present, exposure in vivo and response prevention, sometimes with the addition of imaginal exposure, have been adopted as the treatment of choice for obsessive-compulsive ritualizers. Is it necessary, however, to apply all three procedures? To answer this question, a series of studies examining the role of each of the three treatment components was conducted.

Differential Effects of Exposure in Vivo and Response Prevention

Since obsessions evoke anxiety, therapy of obsessive-compulsives should include procedures that reduce the obsessional anxiety. To this end, prolonged exposure to an obsessional stimulus has been found to decrease anxiety (Foa and Chambless 1978, Grayson et al. 1982, Nunes and Marks 1975). If rituals are maintained only because of their ability to reduce obsessional anxiety, then—as suggested by Marks (personal communication)—prolonged exposure alone should effectively ameliorate them and response prevention should be unnecessary. Negating this proposition are observations that in some cases prolonged exposure eliminated anxiety, yet compulsive behavior persisted (Marks et al. 1969, Walton and Mather 1963). Perhaps, then, exposure and response prevention operate through separate mechanisms, both of which are required to reduce obsessive-compulsive symptoms successfully.

In a series of five single-case studies, Mills et al. (1973) found that response prevention alone virtually eliminated ritualistic behavior, whereas exposure alone produced either no change or an increase in compulsions and subjective urges to ritualize. (Anxiety was not measured in this study.) However, contact with the discomfort-evoking stimuli was brief, therefore the failure of exposure to reduce compulsions may have been due to inadequate exposure. In two additional series of single-case experiments (Turner et al. 1979, 1980), response prevention decreased ritualistic behaviors but affected anxiety only minimally. Exposure ameliorated anxiety but did not enhance the efficacy of response prevention in reducing ritualistic behavior.

In a series of studies, we extended these case reports to investigate the short- and long-term effects of both exposure and response prevention (Foa et al. 1984). In one experiment 32 obsessive-compulsives with washing rituals were treated with 15 sessions (over three weeks) of in vivo exposure only, response prevention only, or the combination of these two procedures. The results indicated that immediately after treatment deliberate exposure decreased anxiety to contaminants more than did response prevention. Ritualistic behavior, in turn, was ameliorated more by response prevention than by exposure. The group who received both treatments benefited most on measures of anxiety associated with contaminants and time spent washing (Figures 8-1 and 8-2). At a 9-month follow-up the superiority of the combined group was retained on measures of obsessive anxiety. With regard to compulsions, at follow-up the three groups did not differ on time spent washing; however, on other measures of compulsions—urges to ritualize and severity of main ritual—the combined group improved the most.

Exposure in Vivo versus Exposure in Imagination

As stated earlier, imaginal exposure has been employed in the treatment of obsessive-compulsives. Some authors reported success with this procedure (Frankl 1960, Stampfl 1967); others

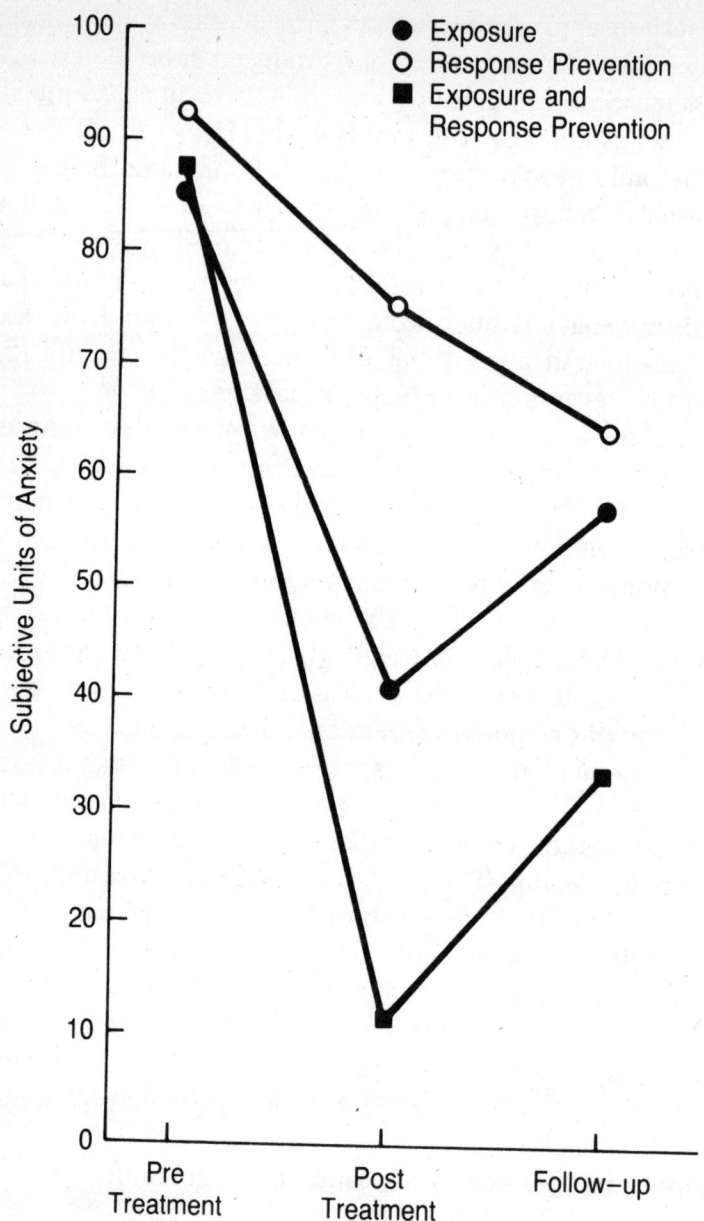

FIGURE 8-1 Mean highest subjective anxiety levels during exposure test for the three treatment groups before and after treatment and at follow-up

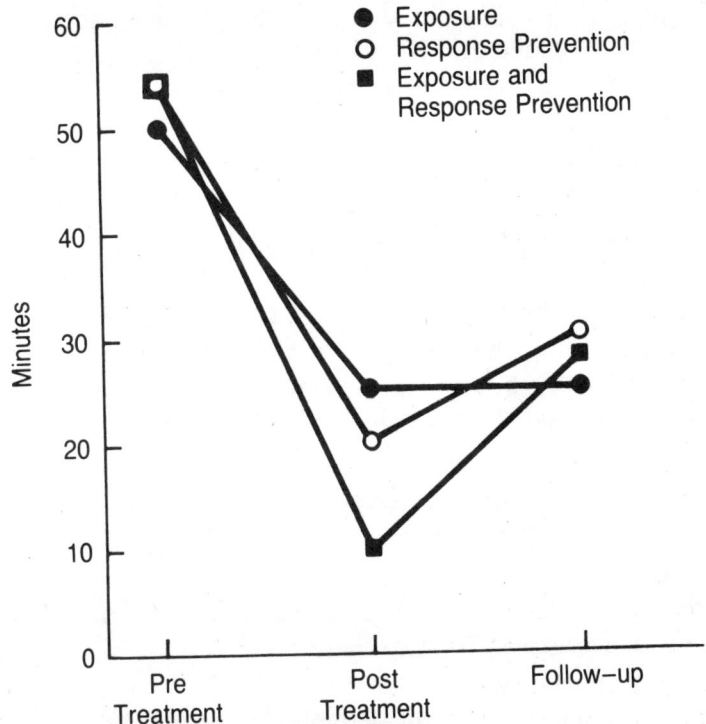

FIGURE 8-2 Self-monitored washing time for the three treatment groups before and after treatment and at follow-up

have found it ineffective (Wolpe 1964, Marks et al. 1969, Rachman et al. 1970). The literature suggests that actual confrontation with feared situations is superior to exposure in fantasy with simple phobics (e.g., Emmelkamp and Wessels 1975, Marks 1978, Mathews 1978). It stands to reason, therefore, that when obsessive fear is evoked primarily by tangible cues (e.g., urine, dirt), exposure in vivo will fare better than imaginal exposure.

For many patients, however, anxiety is generated both by tangible cues from their environment and by anticipation of harm that might ensue from confrontation with these cues; the latter (e.g., death, disease, house burning down) can be presented only in fantasy. For example, the patient who is afraid of running over someone and therefore constantly rechecks his path, can be exposed in vivo to his fears by requiring him to drive without checking. Obviously, the exposure session will not include the actual hitting of a pedestrian and leaving him behind to die because of failure to check carefully. Exposure to such a "disaster" can be accomplished only in imagination.

If it is important to match the content of the exposure situation to a patient's internal fear model (Lang 1977), then those who fear disastrous consequences (which cannot be produced in reality) should improve more with the addition of imaginal exposure. To study this issue, data from 49 obsessive-compulsives were analyzed (Steketee et al. 1982). Twenty-six patients (9 checkers and 17 washers) received 10 to 15 daily two-hour sessions of exposure in vivo. Twenty-three patients (7 checkers and 16 washers) received 90 minutes of imaginal exposure followed by 30 minutes of in vivo exposure.

On the basis of percent change scores of assessor-rated obsessions and compulsions, patients were divided into three groups: (1) "much improved" were those who showed treatment gains of 70% or more; (2) "improved" were those who evidenced treatment gains of 31% to 69%; and (3) "failures" were those who improved 30% or less. The results for post-treatment and for follow-up (mean, 11 months) are given in Tables 8-1 and 8-2, respectively.

These results suggest that the addition of imaginal exposure to in vivo exposure does not affect short-term treatment gains but does increase on the maintenance of such gains. When data at

TABLE 8-1 Exposure in Vivo Versus Combined Imaginal and In Vivo Exposure at Post-treatment

	Outcome			
	Much improved	Improved	Failures	Total
Imaginal and in vivo exposure	14	7	2	23
In vivo exposure	14	12	0	26
Total	28	19	2	49

TABLE 8-2 Exposure in Vivo Versus Combined Imaginal and in Vivo Exposure at Follow-up

	Outcome			
	Much improved	Improved	Failures	Total
Imaginal and in vivo exposure	15	1	5	21
In vivo exposure	12	7	6	25
Total	27	8	11	46

post-treatment and at follow-up were cross-tabulated, only 19% of patients who received imaginal exposure lost gains over time, in contrast to the 40% relapse rate among those who received exposure in vivo only. (The χ^2 value was significant at the .08 level). It appears, then, that when feared disasters are not directly addressed, the reduction of discomfort to environmental (concrete) situations tends to be temporary, perhaps because the core of the fear—that is, concern with future catastrophes—has not changed. It is important to note that not all patients who did not receive imaginal exposure lost gains at follow-up. Perhaps patients who can generate their entire internal fear model (including fears of disasters) when presented with concrete cues do not require the addition of imaginal exposure.

In summary, the results of the studies discussed argue for the use of deliberate in vivo exposure in combination with response prevention in the treatment of obsessive-compulsives. They also suggest that imaginal exposure be added for those who manifest fears of future catastrophes.

CLINICAL IMPLEMENTATION OF TREATMENT

The treatment program consists of three stages: an information-gathering period, an intensive exposure/response-prevention phase, and a follow-up maintenance period. These are summarized below.

Information-Gathering Period

The goals of the first interviews with the patient are twofold: establishing a diagnosis and collecting information pertinent to treatment planning. First the nature of the obsessions must be explored. The vast majority of obsessive-compulsives describe external cues that evoke anxiety. The therapist should solicit highly specific information about these cues in an attempt to identify the sources of concern. Such identification is important but often quite difficult, because contamination "travels" and neutral objects become contaminants through contact (which may be quite remote) with the source of contamination. It is impossible, for example, to understand the patient who fears touching leather items, animals, and men without the knowledge that all of these are contaminated only because they are associated with "maleness" (i.e., leather from male animals). Ascertaining the source of fear is important not only for comprehending the patient's conceptual structure but also for determining the situations to which patients must be exposed. If treatment omits direct confrontation with the source of fear, a relapse often occurs.

Anxiety/discomfort may be generated by internal cues, including thoughts, images, or impulses that are disturbing, shameful, disgusting, or horrifying. Examples of these cues are number sequences, impulses to stab one's child (triggered, in turn, by external cues such as knives or scissors), thoughts that one's spouse may have an auto accident on the way home, and images of having sex with Christ. Some patients are reluctant to disclose their obsessions, but they can usually be encouraged by direct questions, a matter-of-fact attitude, and reassurance that most normal individuals also have unwanted thoughts.

Often, the external and internal obsessional cues are associated with anticipated harm, which for some patients may constitute the primary cause for discomfort. Although the specific content of the feared disasters varies from patient to patient, most washers fear that contamination will result in disease, physical debilitation, or death to themselves or others. Most checkers fear being responsible for an error that will lead to physical harm (e.g., leaving the stove on and thereby burning the house down) or to psychological harm (e.g., setting the table incorrectly and being criticized by a significant other; writing "I am a homosexual" on a check and thereby losing others' respect). Those with repeating rituals are typically concerned that their upsetting thoughts will come to pass (e.g., an accident happening, losing control and stabbing someone, punishment from God). The information about the external fear cues determines the exposure in vivo program; knowledge about the internal cues and feared disasters constitutes the basis for imaginal exposure.

Both active and passive forms of avoidance behavior are exhibited by obsessive-compulsives. Whenever possible they, like phobics, seek to circumvent passively situations that provoke discomfort. Most avoidance patterns are clear-cut (e.g., refraining from using public toilets, shaking hands, touching garbage, using the stove, or taking out the trash). Sometimes, however, they can be quite subtle. Examples include sidestepping brown spots on the sidewalk (possible dog feces), touching doorknobs at their less-used base with fingers only (to be washed later), sitting forward on chairs to avoid the spot that others usually contact, wearing only slip-on shoes to avoid having to touch laces or buckles. It is important to identify avoidance behaviors and to prohibit them during treatment since even minor avoidances prevent full exposure to the fear cues and therefore may serve to maintain that fear. Additionally, retention of avoidance patterns may reinforce the patient's belief that they protect him from the "danger" inherent in exposure.

Active forms of avoidance, i.e., ritualistic behavior, have already been described. They consist of washing, cleaning (including wiping with alcohol or spraying with Lysol), checking, repeating actions, placing objects in a precise order, and repeatedly requesting reassurance. They also include cognitive rituals, such as praying, thinking "good" thoughts, and listing events mentally. The function of rituals is to reduce anxiety associated with the obsessions. The relationship of each ritual to fear and to passive avoidance behaviors should be ascertained. When such a relationship is lacking, one should question the diagnosis of obsessive-compulsive disorder and consider the possibility of a psychotic disorder.

On the basis of information about the internal and external fear cues, the feared harm and the active and passive avoidance behaviors, a treatment program can be designed.

THE TREATMENT PROGRAM

Exposure

For external fears in vivo exposure is recommended over imaginal techniques (Emmelkamp and Wessels 1975, Rabavilas et al. 1976). Research has determined that for most patients the speed with which the most anxiety-provoking object is confronted matters little (Hodgson et al. 1972). But since patients prefer gradual exposure, we usually employ a five- or six-step hierarchy. For example, a patient who feared contamination from feces, urine, sweat, and other body secretions was first asked to hold doorknobs continuously, especially those to public restrooms. In the second session, discarded newspapers were added to the doorknobs. In later sessions, he was introduced to sweat and toilet seats. By the sixth session, the patient was exposed to fecal material, which he feared most. The remaining nine treatment sessions were devoted to all of the above contaminants, with particular focus on the most disturbing ones. Although modeling (the therapist demonstrating contact with feared items) was not found to enhance the effectiveness of exposure (Rachman et al. 1973), some patients find it helpful.

Longer periods of exposure are superior to brief interrupted ones (Rabavilas et al. 1976), but no information about the optimal exposure time is available. Nor do we know the best point at which to terminate an exposure session. For obsessive-compulsives, discomfort begins to dissipate after anywhere from 30 to 60 minutes; this reduction continues for up to 90 minutes (Foa and Chambless 1978, Rachman et al. 1976). Since the amount of habituation of discomfort during an exposure session was found to be related to treatment outcome (Foa et al. 1983a), one- to two-hour sessions are recommended.

The anxiety associated with internal cues and anticipated future disasters is best treated by imaginal exposure (i.e., "flooding"). The following is an example of an imaginal exposure scene for a patient with fears of contamination by "leukemia germs":

> Imagine that you are sitting in the waiting room at Mercy Hospital waiting to see your brother who had surgery. As you are looking around you, you notice a sign to the Oncology Department. You read it and start to feel the familiar sense of contamination. You know that leukemic patients have probably sat on the very chair you are sitting in now. You feel the contamination on your back and under your legs, spreading to your entire body. You wonder who sat on your chair in the past. You can visualize a man, balding and thin from chemotherapy. Just as you're sitting there you see a very thin woman, her hair with patches of baldness, who comes and sits next to you in the waiting room. . . .

Response Prevention

As for phobics, the passive avoidance of obsessive-compulsives is blocked by definition when deliberate exposure is instituted. However, nonavoidance does not automatically eliminate overt compulsions. As noted earlier, to achieve maximal reduction of compulsions, response prevention needs to be implemented. The degree of strictness of the response prevention program has varied across studies, ranging from normal handwashing to total abstinence from washing for days. How strict response prevention should be is unknown. In our treatment program, washers are requested to refrain from all washing and cleaning except for one 10-minute shower every fifth day. Dishwashing and other activities that normally necessitate contact with water are carried out with gloves or are assigned to someone else during treatment. Checkers are permitted a single check of items that are normally checked after use, such as stoves and door locks. Other objects judged not to require routine checking (e.g., unused electrical appliances, discarded envelopes) may not be checked.

In some treatment programs, patients are supervised for 24 hours. In others no supervision is employed. The amount of supervision seems to affect outcome minimally, perhaps because motivated patients will comply with treatment instructions without supervision and unmotivated ones will circumvent them. We typically request that patients have a designated supervisor whose task is to provide support and encouragement to resist urges to ritualize. We do not use physical force to prevent ritualistic behavior.

Cognitive rituals are more difficult to treat, possibly because they are less under the patient's control than overt rituals. Blocking techniques such as thought stopping, aversion treatment, and distraction may be of help, but information about the efficacy of these methods for covert symptoms is not yet available. In using blocking procedures with cognitive rituals, it is important to distinguish between obsessions and cognitive compulsions, since the former calls for exposure rather than for blocking.

We will now illustrate the application of the treatment procedures in the clinical setting using two case illustrations, a checker and a washer.

TREATMENT OF A WASHER: THE CASE OF JANE

The treatment of Jane (described earlier), who feared contamination from her home town, is described below to illustrate the application of exposure and response-prevention treatment for a patient with washing rituals. The preliminary interviews with Jane revealed that her obsessions were focused primarily on external objects. Because of the absence of anticipated harm, the treatment program did not include imaginal exposure. In preparation for treatment, we wrote to Jane's mother, who lived in the contaminated home town, and requested that she mail us objects from home, including clothing, books, and ornaments from the attic. These were kept away from Jane until the beginning of treatment.

In the first session, Jane and the therapist went into the supermarket to purchase groceries located near the counter where the chocolate from her home town was situated. She touched these items to her face, hair, and clothing; anxiety increased to 50 SUDs (subjective units of disturbance, ranging from zero to 100) and declined to 20 SUDs after 90 minutes. Jane continued the exposure at home after the session, contaminating her entire house, including her bed, closets, drawers, etc. On the second day she brought into the session books, kitchen utensils, and some clothes that she had been avoiding because of their indirect contact with contaminants. On the third day, Jane handled and ate chocolates from her home town. In this session her high level of anxiety necessitated some coaxing from the therapist, starting with brief contact by one finger and gradually increasing it until she was able to touch the chocolate with her entire hand. In the next session, Jane was required to wear the clothes sent from home. In subsequent sessions, she wore her mother's clothes and touched the ornaments. Anxiety to the latter contaminant increased to 90 SUDs and required 3 hours to habituate to a level of 40 SUDs. The remainder of treatment concentrated on contact with various items from home. In the last (fifteenth) session the therapist accompanied Jane to her home town, where they went to her attic to handle all of the objects that still provoked some discomfort. She brought some of them back with her so that exposure to the source of contamination could continue.

Throughout this intensive 3-week program, Jane was instructed to refrain from washing her hands entirely and to limit her showering to 10 minutes every fifth day. To reinforce maintenance of her gains she was advised to return to her home town every 2 weeks over a period of 3 months. A follow-up 8 years later indicated that Jane's improvement had been maintained.

TREATMENT OF A CHECKER: THE CASE OF MIKE

Mike, the patient with the checking rituals described earlier, feared both external situations and the disasters that might ensue if he failed to ritualize. Treatment, therefore, included both imaginal and in vivo exposure, with the addition of response prevention. The first scene that Mike was asked to imagine was as follows: Mike was at school where he teaches. He failed to check the toilet bowl before flushing it. A school child came looking for his gerbil in the bathroom where the cage was kept. The cage was empty and the child cried, worrying that the gerbil fell into the toilet. Mike feared that he indeed flushed the gerbil down the toilet, since he failed to check. During the image, his reported anxiety climbed to 80 SUDs, gradually diminishing to 30 SUDs. In vivo exposure during the first session involved flushing toilets in public restrooms with eyes closed. The homework assignment was not to check the toilet at home before flushing it.

In the second scene Mike imagined that he had forgotten to check the windows and doors; a burglar entered and stole his wife's jewelry. She blamed him for the theft. In vivo, Mike was required to close doors and windows, checking briefly only once. Next, Mike was asked to imagine that he dropped his baby daughter on a concrete floor because he did not hold her properly. She was hospitalized for injuries and both his wife and parents accused him of carelessness. In vivo exposure consisted of walking with his daughter on a concrete floor until his anxiety reduced. In subsequent scenes Mike fantasized driving over a bump on the expressway and then worrying that he had run over someone. A police car pulled him over and charged him with a hit-and-run accident. His homework required city driving among pedestrians and potholes without stopping and without checking his rearview mirror or retracing his path.

At a 3-year follow-up, Mike reported 10 minutes of checking per day in contrast to 4 hours before treatment. Most of the excessive checking was done in the classroom in an attempt to prevent papers from being mixed up; some brief unnecessary checking of doors and windows at home also persisted.

TREATMENT COMPLICATIONS

Noncompliance

When confronted with a description of the exposure/response prevention program, about 25% of obsessive-compulsives who approach behavioral treatment decline to participate. This attrition process leaves in treatment only the motivated patients. Nevertheless, a few of them fail to abide by the agreed-upon rules, and a larger number try to bend them. Failure to resist rituals and persistence in avoidance patterns lead inevitably to a poor outcome.

It is unusual for an obsessive-compulsive patient to conceal ritualistic activity from the therapist. When this happens, the patient should be confronted with the implications of the failure to comply for treatment outcome. If noncompliance persists, therapy should be discontinued with the understanding that the patient may return when he or she is prepared to follow the treatment regimen. Continuance under conditions in which failure is likely to occur will leave the patient hopeless about future prospects for improvement.

Another motivational problem is posed by individuals who carry out exposure exercises without ritualizing but continue to engage in passive avoidance patterns. The persistence of such behaviors hinders habituation of anxiety to feared situations and may leave the patient with the erroneous belief that this avoidance protects him from harm. Failure to give up avoidance patterns also calls for a re-evaluation of continuation in treatment.

Familial Patterns

Family members have typically experienced intense frustration due to the patient's symptoms. It is not surprising that some are impatient, expecting treatment to result in rapid and complete symptom remission. Conversely, family members may continue to "protect" the patient from previously upsetting situations, thus reinforcing avoidance behaviors. Years of accommodation to the patient's peculiar requests have established communication patterns that are difficult to break. The above familial patterns may hinder progress in treatment and interfere with maintenance of gains, thus requiring therapeutic intervention.

Functioning without Symptoms

Many obsessive-compulsives have become socially and occupationally nonfunctional as their symptoms occupied an increasing proportion of their life. Successful treatment leaves them with a considerable void in their daily routine. Assistance in acquiring new skills and in planning both social and occupational activities should be the focus of follow-up therapy in such cases.

FAILURES AND RELAPSES

The interference of depression with treatment outcome has been widely noted (e.g., Rachman and Hodgson 1980, Foa et al. 1983b). Patients who exhibited severely depressed moods prior to treatment tended not to benefit from treatment and were particularly prone to relapse at follow-up. The alleviation of depression by pharmacological and psychological means should be considered for these patients before beginning behavioral treatment.

An anxious mood at the outset of therapy was also found related to patients' response to treatment but in a somewhat different manner than depression. Those with mild anxiety were more likely to succeed; those with high anxiety, unlike high depression, were equally likely to succeed or to fail.

A further stumbling block in treatment may be the patient's belief system regarding the likelihood that the feared consequences will in fact materialize. Foa (1979) observed that those who firmly believed that their worst fears would come to pass if they failed to protect themselves by ritualizing did not habituate to feared contaminants, either within an exposure session or across sessions. Unfortunately, reliable or valid measures of the degree of conviction have not yet been developed and thus the validity of these observations has not been tested in a controlled manner.

CONCLUSION

Innovations in behavioral treatment, particularly exposure and response prevention, have profoundly improved the prognostic picture for obsessive-compulsives. However, patients rarely find themselves entirely symptom free at the completion of this regimen. Maintenance of gains is problematic for about 20% of patients (Foa et al. 1983b). Relapse is most common among those patients who are only partially improved at the end of treatment. The implementation of drugs, specifically antidepressants, in combination with behavioral treatment may prove useful for those who manifest severely depressed moods at the beginning of treatment. More importantly, we need to develop maintenance programs that focus on the patient's interpersonal and occupational adjustment and provide support in the struggle to progress from a nonfunctional to a healthy lifestyle.

REFERENCES

Beech H. R., and Vaughan M. (1978). *Behavioral Treatment of Obsessional States*. New York: John Wiley.

Black, A. (1974). The natural history of obsessional neurosis, in *Obsessional States*, ed. H. R. Beech. London: Methuen.

Breitner, C. (1960). Drug therapy in obsessional states and other psychiatric problems. *Diseases of the Nervous System (Supplement)* 21:31–35.

Cooper, J. E., Gelder M. G., and Marks I. M. (1965). Results of behavior therapy in 77 psychiatric patients. *British Medical Journal* 1:1222–1225.

Emmelkamp, P. M. G., and Kraanen, J. (1977). Therapist-controlled exposure in vivo: A comparison with obsessive-compulsive patients. *Behaviour Research and Therapy* 15:491-495.

Emmelkamp, P. M. G., and Wessels, H. (1975). Flooding in imagination and flooding in vivo: A comparison with agoraphobics. *Behaviour Research and Therapy* 13:7-15.

Esquirol, J. E. D. (1838). *Des Maladies Mentales.* Vol. 2. Paris: Bailliere.

Foa, E. B. (1979). Failure in treating obsessive-compulsives. *Behaviour Research and Therapy* 17:169-176.

Foa, E. B., and Chambless, D. L. (1978). Habituation of subjective anxiety during flooding in imagery. *Behaviour Research and Therapy* 16:392-399.

Foa, E. B., and Godstein A. (1978). Continuous exposure and complete response prevention in the treatment of obsessive-compulsive neurosis. *Behaviour Therapy* 9:821-829.

Foa, E. B., Grayson, J., Steketee, G. S., et al. (1983a). Success and failure in the behavioral treatment of obsessive-compulsives. *Journal of Consulting and Clinical Psychology* 51:287-297.

Foa, E. B., Steketee, G., Grayson, J. B., et al. (1983b). Treatment of obsessive-compulsives: When do we fail? In *Failures in Behavior Therapy*, ed. E. B. Foa and P. M. G. Emmelkamp, pp. 10-34. New York: Wiley.

Foa, E. B., Steketee, G., Grayson, J. B., et al. (1984). Deliberate exposure and blocking of obsessive-compulsive rituals: Immediate and long-term effects. *Behavior Therapy* 15:450-472.

Foa, E. B., Steketee, G. S., and Ozarow, B. J. (1985). Behavior therapy with obsessive-compulsives: From theory to treatment. In *Obsessive-Compulsive Disorders: Psychological and Pharmacological Treatments*, ed. M. Mavissakalian, pp. 49-129. New York: Plenum Press.

Frankl, V. E. (1960). Paradoxical intention: a logotherapeutic technique. *American Journal of Psychotherapy* 14:520-525.

Grayson J. B., Foa, E. B., and Steketee, G. (1982). Habituation during exposure treatment: Distraction versus attention-focusing. *Behaviour Research and Therapy* 20:323-328.

Grimshaw, L. (1965). The outcome of obsessional disorder, a follow-up study of 100 cases. *British Journal of Psychiatry* 111:1051-1056.

Hodgson, R. J., Rachman, S., and Marks, I. M. (1972). The treatment of chronic obsessive-compulsive neurosis: Follow-up and further findings. *Behaviour Research and Therapy* 10:181-189.

Kringlen, E. (1965). Obsessional neurotics, a long-term follow-up. *British Journal of Psychiatry* 111:709-722.

Lang, P. J. (1977). Imagery in therapy: An information processing analysis of fear. *Behavior Therapy* 8:862-886.

Lewis, A. J. (1936). Problems of obsessional illness. *Proceedings of the Royal Society of Medicine* 29:325-336.

Marks, I. M., Crowe, E., Drewe, E., et al. (1969). Obsessive-compulsive neurosis in identical twins. *British Journal of Psychiatry* 15:991-998.

Marks, I. M., Hodgson, R., and Rachman S. (1975). Treatment of chronic obsessive-compulsive neurosis by in vivo exposure, a 2-year follow-up and issues in treatment. *British Journal of Psychiatry* 127:349-364.

Meyer, V., Levy, R., and Schnurer, A. (1974). A behavioral treatment of obsessive-compulsive disorders. In *Obsessional States*, ed. H. R. Beech. London: Methuen.

Mills, H. L., Agras, W. S., Barlow, D. H., et al. (1973). Compulsive rituals treated by response prevention. *Archives of General Psychiatry* 28:524-529.

Nunes, J. S., and Marks, I. M. (1975). Feedback of true heart rate during exposure in vivo. *Archives of General Psychiatry* 32:933-936.

Rabavilas, A. D., Boulougouris, J. C., and Stefanis, C. (1976). Duration of flooding sessions in the treatment of obsessive-compulsive patients. *Behaviour Research and Therapy* 14:349-355.

Rachman S., DeSilva P., and Roper, G. (1976). The spontaneous decay of compulsive urges. *Behaviour Research and Therapy* 14:445-453.

Rachman, S., and Hodgson, R. (1980). *Obsessions and Compulsions*. Englewood Cliffs, NJ: Prentice Hall.

Rachman, S., Hodgson, R., and Marzillier, J. (1976). Treatment of an obsessional-compulsive disorder by modelling. *Behaviour Research and Therapy* 8:383-392.

Rachman, S., Marks, I. M., and Hodgson, R. (1973). The treatment of obsessive-compulsive neurotics by modelling and flooding in vivo. *Behaviour Research and Therapy* 11:463-471.

Rubin, R. D., and Merbaum, M. (1971). Self-imposed punishment versus desensitization. In *Advances in Behavior Therapy 1969*, ed. R. D. Rubin, H. Fensterheim, A. A. Lazarus, et al., pp. 85-91. New York: Academic Press.

Schneider, K. (1925). Schwangs zus Tande un Schizophrenie. *Archiv für Psychiatrie und Nervenkrankheiten* 74:93–107.

Stampfl, T. (1967). Implosive therapy: The theory, the subhuman analogue, the strategy and the technique. Part 1. The theory. In *Behavior Modification Techniques in the Treatment of Emotional Disorders*, ed. S. G. Armitage. Battle Creek, MI: V.A. Publications.

Stampfl, T. G., and Levis, D.J. (1967). Essential of implosive therapy: A learning-theory-based psychodynamic behavioral therapy. *Journal of Abnormal Psychology* 72:496–503.

Steketee, G. S., Foa, E. B., and Grayson, J. B. (1982). Recent advances in the behavioral treatment of obsessive-compulsives. *Archives of General Psychiatry* 39:1365–1371.

Turner, S. M., Hersen, M., Bellack, A. S., et al. (1979). Behavioral treatment of obsessive-compulsive neurosis. *Behaviour Research and Therapy* 17:95–106.

Turner, S. M., Hersen, M., Bellack, A. S., et al. (1980). Behavioral and pharmacological treatment of obsessive-compulsive disorders. *Journal of Nervous and Mental Diseases* 168:651–657.

Walton, D., and Mather, M.D. (1963). The application of learning principles to the treatment of obsessive-compulsive states in the acute and chronic phases of illness. *Behaviour Research and Therapy* 1:163–174.

PART II

Techniques

9 Cognitive-Behavioral Therapy

Dr. Barlow and his colleagues at the Phobia and Anxiety Disorders Clinic of SUNY at Albany have made their notable contributions through years of research on a variety of issues that have direct clinical applicability to treatment of anxiety disorders. These issues include, among others, cognitive-behavioral therapy, marital therapy, relaxation training, and hyperventilation and breath control in panic disorders. This chapter emphasizes interoceptive conditioning, which is defined as the anxiety response that panic disorder patients experience in response to bodily experiences. That is, these patients respond to internal somatic cues, rather than to external circumstances such as heights or enclosed places. The bodily sensations in the early stages of a panic attack become conditioned as cues to impending panicky feelings and can thus themselves come to induce phobic anxiety. For example, someone who experiences rapid heartbeat during an anxiety attack might begin to feel anxious, or even panicky, if rapid heartbeat occurred while exercising. Reports of such experiences are quite common in phobics encountered in clinical practice.

The cognitive-behavioral approach currently is gaining credibility as an approach to treating the panic attack itself. There are reports that, although in vivo desensitization may result in significant improvement in functioning, many phobics continue to experience panic attacks. That is, they have learned to cope with the panic attacks in the phobic situation and will no longer avoid those situations, but the treatment has not had a direct impact on the panic disorder itself. The cognitive-behavioral approach promises to be effective treatment of the panic disorder, rather than addressing itself only to the phobic avoidance, as earlier treatments had done. The programmatic strategy includes modules. The cognitive element, of course, refers to Dr. Beck's cognitive therapy described above. The behavioral elements include relaxation training, breath control, psychoeducation, and desensitization of the interoceptive cues of the panic attack.

For more information on this treatment program, please write to Dr. David H. Barlow, Center for Stress and Anxiety Disorders, 1535 Western Avenue, Albany, New York, 12203.

Cognitive-Behavioral Therapy

Janet S. Klosko
David H. Barlow

At the Phobia and Anxiety Disorders Clinic, our treatment of panic attacks grew from experience with treatment of the phobic aspects of agoraphobia. In our clinic and elsewhere, studies showed consistently that treatment that focused upon exposure to feared situations significantly decreased avoidance behavior in most agoraphobic patients (Barlow 1985). Moreover, when we measured panic attacks directly, we found that exposure treatment, still focused upon avoidance of feared situations, also decreased panic attacks. For example, a clinical replication series of sixteen agoraphobic patients at our clinic showed that almost half the patients who reported panic attacks pretreatment were panic-free posttreatment (Klosko and Barlow 1986).

Concurrent with our research on treatment of agoraphobia we began a treatment project on treatment of panic disorder. At that time, like DSM-III, we viewed panic disorder in the same class as generalized anxiety disorder—both being disorders of anxiety states—rather than in the same class as agoraphobia. We began treatment of panic attacks with the application of self-control procedures, such as biofeedback and relaxation, and cognitive therapy. In a controlled-outcome study, we demonstrated some success (Barlow et al. 1984).

As our work continued, gradually our treatments of phobia and panic grew closer together. This occurred partly because it was so rare to find patients with panic attacks who did not exhibit phobic avoidance. Most often we found that, even in patients diagnosed with panic disorder rather than agoraphobia, most exhibited avoidance responding, though their avoidance might be subtle. For example, it was not unusual to find patients with panic disorder avoiding exercise, or heat, or the drinking of alcohol—or any other activity that might elicit panic-like sensations. They feared and avoided symptoms of panic attacks. We came to see similarities in agoraphobic avoidance of external anxiety cues and avoidance of internal anxiety cues. Our view emerged that internal events can serve as phobic stimuli and that individuals, through a process of interoceptive conditioning, starting usually from the first panic attack, can develop phobic avoidance of internal events. Consequently, for us the distinction blurred between agoraphobia and panic disorder. We began to view patients with these diagnoses on a continuum, with fear of panic as the key feature.

We thus began to experiment with exposure treatments of anxiety states. Particularly, we designed treatments in which, in addition to learning self-control and cognitive strategies, patients underwent exposure to panic symptoms and cues. Our evidence suggests this is an effective treatment of panic attacks (Klosko and Barlow 1986).

ASSESSMENT

Initial Assessment

All patients who present to the Anxiety Disorders Clinic undergo initial assessment by administration of the Anxiety Disorders Interview Schedule (ADIS) (Di Nardo et al. 1983), recently revised (Di Nardo et al. 1985). The ADIS is a structured interview designed to provide DSM-III and DSM-III-R diagnoses of anxiety and affective disorders and to rule out psychosis, substance abuse, and somatoform disorders. It provides detailed symptom ratings and includes the Hamilton Anxiety Scale (Hamilton 1959) and the Hamilton Depression Scale (Hamilton 1960). In addition, the ADIS assesses psychiatric and psychological history, situational and cognitive factors that influence anxiety, and comorbidity of anxiety disorders with one another and with other mental disorders. Reliability tests of the ADIS for 125 subjects, using Kappa coefficients, indicate good reliability for all anxiety disorders (Barlow 1985). Patients who participate in panic-disorder treatment projects at the clinic have been given a primary diagnosis of panic disorder, with a clinician's severity rating of at least 4 on a 0-to-8 scale.

Patients generally respond positively to the ADIS. It presents them aspects of their experience structured in a way they find educational. Often patients feel understood. After administration of the ADIS, the interviewer meets with the patient, explains the diagnosis, and describes treatment. Most patients who are offered treatment at the clinic agree to participate.

Pre- and Posttreatment Assessment Measures

In addition to the ADIS, psychophysiological and self-report assessment measures are administered to all patients pre- and posttreatment.

Psychophysiological Measures

Psychophysiological assessment lasts about an hour. A polygraph measures physiological responses of patients (forehead muscle tension, heart rate, skin resistance, and finger temperature) to relaxation and stressor tasks. This procedure has been described in detail by Andrasik and co-authors (1982).

Self-Report Measures

Self-report measures include both standardized questionnaires and self-monitoring. Questionnaires measure such factors as panic and generalized anxiety symptoms, fear and avoidance, somatic symptoms associated with anxiety, interference with functioning, depression, personality, and life events.

Patients engage in daily self-monitoring for two weeks pre- and posttreatment, and throughout treatment. Self-monitoring is a crucial part of treatment. Patients use a diary called the Weekly Record that provides information about levels of anxiety and related variables. This record was constructed by staff at the clinic over the course of several years. We have also developed a set of procedures to maximize compliance with recording, including instruction, review, and feedback. Patients record on the diary current levels of anxiety, depression, and pleasant feelings on 0-to-8 scales, four times each day. Such data serve as measures of background levels of these variables. In addition, patients record the following information about each discrete episode of anxiety they experience that they rate 4 or higher on the 0-to-8 scale: date and time of onset and offset of the anxiety episode; maximum level of anxiety during the episode; whether or not the patient considers this episode of anxiety a panic attack (according to DSM-III criteria); whether the patient considers the context of the episode stressful or nonstressful; and the symptoms the patient experiences. Data serve as measures of anxiety episodes and panic attacks, both spontaneous and situational. In addition, there is space on the diary for patients to describe the situation in which the episode occurred, relevant behavior and cognitions, and any comments they may have.

Recently, the clinic has begun to experiment with psychological induction of panic symptoms as an assessment measure.

Treatment

Generally patients receive 15 sessions of cognitive-behavioral treatment in weekly meetings. Treatment is administered individually, although recently we have treated small groups of panic-disorder patients. Treatment begins with presentation of the rationale. Patients are told they will learn skills to control panic-disorder symptoms in three response systems: physiological, cognitive, and behavioral. They are given education about the disorder. Individual symptoms are explained, with emphasis on the notion that symptoms are not dangerous. Active treatment phases are composed of one or more of the following components: progressive muscle-relaxation training; cognitive therapy; exposure to external anxiety cues; and exposure to internal anxiety cues and panic symptoms.

Progressive Muscle-Relaxation Training

This treatment component is based upon the model for training described by Bernstein and Borkovec (1973). It begins with a tension-relaxation phase, in which patients are taught to tense and relax muscle groups and to discriminate muscle tension levels. Exercises are gradually reduced from sixteen to four muscle groups. Then patients are taught relaxation by recall, in which they recall sensations of muscle release in muscle groups. Finally, patients are taught cue-controlled relaxation, in which they learn to associate the subvocalized word "relax" with muscle relaxation. Patients are instructed to practice relaxation at home twice per day and to maintain records of such practice. They are encouraged to use cognitive and relaxation skills learned in treatment in their daily lives and to carry out homework assignments for practice in use of the skill.

Cognitive Therapy

This treatment component was based upon the model for therapy described by Beck and Emery (1979). It includes presentation of didactic material, self-monitoring of automatic thoughts and self-statements, hypothesis testing, and behavioral experiments in the form of graduated homework assignments, from low to high anxiety.

Exposure to External Anxiety Cues

This treatment component consists of graduated in vivo exposure to phobic or otherwise stressful situations. Patients and therapists together construct hierarchies of feared situations, from low- to high-anxiety items. Patients expose themselves systematically to the situations through structured homework assignments.

Exposure to Internal Anxiety Cues and Panic Symptoms

This treatment component was developed by clinic staff through experience in treatment of panic disorders. It consists of exposure to internal cognitive and physiological cues of anxiety and panic using procedures such as imagery training of both stimulus and response propositions of images (Lang et al. 1983); induction of symptoms through imagery of anxiety-provoking situations and sensations; voluntary hyperventilation (Clark et al. 1985); physical exertion (such as running in place, spinning one's head); or other idiosyncratic methods for eliciting frightening physical symptoms, accompanied by deliberate catastrophic interpretations. Exposures proceed up a hierarchy of feared cognitions and somatic sensations, both in sessions with the therapist and in homework assignments the client carries out between sessions. A detailed description of the treatment protocol can be found in Barlow and Cerny (1988).

Patients are followed up at 3 months, 6 months, 1 year, and 2 years. Our research indicates that patients maintain positive treatment changes (Barlow et al. 1984). Many continue to improve after treatment ends. Treatment is designed to work against establishment of dependency relationships between patient and therapist. The emphasis on self-control strategies, graduated mastery experiences, generalization practices, and homework assignments between sessions increases the likelihood of maintenance of treatment gains.

CASE EXAMPLE

When she presented for treatment, M. was a 26-year-old married woman with a 4-month-old infant. She barely could discuss her first panic attack, which had occurred in the hospital after the birth of her baby, under the influence of Demerol. She thought she had been given too much Demerol and was dying. Two weeks later, at home, following an argument with her husband, she had an attack out of the blue. Her husband rushed her to the emergency room. Doctors there told her there was nothing wrong and sent her home. A week later she was back in the emergency room with another attack, and doctors there gave her Xanax (alprazolam). Despite her continuation on Xanax, the attacks persisted. Before she started treatment at the anxiety clinic, she withdrew from Xanax, a requirement of the particular research project in which she participated.

Interview and self-monitoring revealed that M.'s most severe panic symptoms were tachycardia, difficulty breathing, and shaking. She avoided hospitals; all drugs, including alcohol, and situations in which others took drugs (i.e., bars); arguments; and exercise. She avoided thinking and talking about anxiety and panic. For reasons she did not understand, late every afternoon she experienced panic symptoms. The most disturbing seemed to be feelings of unreality, which she connected with going crazy. She reported intense fear of panic, and preoccupation with death and dying. The last she related to a "bad trip" she had experienced on LSD as a teenager, during which she had the sense that she had died. (Interestingly, questioning revealed M. actually had had her first panic attack during this "bad trip." She attributed the experience to the drug, however, and did not consider it a panic attack.)

The early course of M.'s treatment illustrated a pattern that seems common to many cases of panic disorder. In the first few weeks she stopped panicking completely. At that time she felt elated; she felt she would never panic again. She was told that in all likelihood she would panic again and that, moreover, treatment would not be effective without her continued experiences of anxiety. By the fifth week of treatment she reported panic attacks again. In the early weeks she was taught relaxation and rebreathing skills to control the physiological components of anxiety. Through use of her self-monitoring records, she identified carefully the thoughts she associated with anxiety. In her case, such thoughts tended to be interpretations of physical sensations as dangerous, either because they signaled a panic attack, or because she thought they meant something was physically wrong. She was told as she learned to control anxiety symptoms, she would fear her sensations less.

For the exposure component of treatment, we developed a hierarchy of fear situations, activities, and sensations, from low to high anxiety. Her hierarchy was as shown in Table 9-1.

M. was encouraged to adopt a stance of approach to, rather than avoidance of, anxiety symptoms, in order to practice controlling them. We started with low-anxiety hierarchy items. Between sessions in homework assignments, she was instructed to enter feared situations, or engage in feared activities, until she reached a criterion of anxiety she felt able to control. Gradually we increased the criterion. For example, one of her first assignments was to swim until her anxiety reached a "3," to stop and control the anxiety until it was a "1," then to repeat the exercise several times. Toward the end of treatment she visited the hospital unit in

TABLE 9-1 Patient-M.'s Anxiety Hierarchy

Anxiety	Rating	Feared situation/activity/sensation
2	(low)	Swimming until her heart rate increased
2		Arguing with her husband when she disagreed with him
3		Numbness in her hands and legs
4		A sense of pressure in her head
4		Feeling unsure of herself at a staff meeting
4		Getting a floating feeling out of the blue
5		Getting shaky out of the blue
7		In a room with friends who were smoking marijuana, feeling the sensations of the drug
7		Visiting the hospital maternity ward where she had her baby
8	(high)	Taking Demerol at the hospital

which she had suffered her first attack, and she relived in imagination her Demerol experience.

In sessions, M. used such techniques as visualization, voluntary hyperventilation, and physical exercise to induce symptoms and practice controlling them. For example, early in treatment she induced lightheadedness, a low-anxiety item, by holding her breath and breathing shallowly. At other times she induced chest pain by tensing her chest muscles, and she induced trembling by tensing her arms and legs. Through visualization she re-experienced episodes of anxiety and panic she had experienced in the past week, and she rehearsed episodes she anticipated in the week to come. Toward the end of treatment, M. became willing in sessions and at home to visualize her first panic attack. At the end of treatment she still had panic attacks, but they were less frequent, less intense, and less severe; she feared and avoided panic symptoms significantly less; and she was no longer judged to have a clinical disorder. At 3-month follow-up, she had continued to improve.

FUTURE DIRECTIONS

We plan to pursue the development of treatment of panic attacks in a number of directions. Clinical experience continues to suggest ways to improve treatment, which we may study experimentally at a later time. Presently, with a group-comparison design, we are conducting a component-analysis study of our panic treatment. We are also conducting a placebo-controlled study that compares psychological treatment of panic to medication treatment with alprazolam. A next step would be to look at the combination of psychological and medication treatments. We do not expect the effect of combining psychological and medical treatments of panic to be simply additive. Clinical experience indicates medication at times interferes with psychological treatment. Patients tend to attribute decreases in symptoms to medication, and therefore they tend not to develop an adequate sense of mastery and self-control. Further, effective exposure treatment requires the patient to experience anxiety symptoms, and masking of symptoms by medication may make this difficult. We also are conducting single-case and group studies that evaluate the effectiveness of adding the component of exposure to interoceptive cues to treatments of agoraphobia.

REFERENCES

Andrasik, F., Blanchard, E. B., Arena, J., Saunders, N., and Barron, K. D. (1982). Psychophysiology of recurrent headache: Methodological issues and new empirical findings. *Behavior Therapy* 13:407-429.

Barlow, D. H. (1985). The dimensions of anxiety disorders. In *Anxiety and Anxiety Disorders*, ed. A. H. Tuma and J. D. Maser. Hillsdale, NJ: Lawrence Erlbaum Associates.

Barlow, D. H., and Cerny, J. A. (1988). *Psychological Treatment of Panic*. New York: The Guilford Press.

Barlow, D. H., and Craske, M. (1988). The phenomenology of panic. In *Panic: Psychological Perspectives*, ed. S. Rachman and J. D. Maser. Hillsdale, NJ: Lawrence Erlbaum Associates.

Barlow, D. H., Cohen, A. S., and Waddell, M. T. (1984). Panic and generalized anxiety disorders: Nature and treatment. *Behavior Therapy* 15:431-449.

Barlow, D. H., O'Brien, G. T., and Last, C. G. (1984). Couples treatment of agoraphobia. *Behavior Therapy* 15:41-58.

Beck, A. T., and Emery, G. (1979). *Cognitive Therapy of Anxiety and Phobic Disorders*. Philadelphia: Center for Cognitive Therapy.

Bernstein, D. A., and Borkovec, T. D. (1973). *Progressive Relaxation Training*. Champaign, IL: Research Press.

Clark, D. M., Salkovskis, P. M., and Chalkley, A. J. (1985). Respiratory control as a treatment for panic attacks. *Journal of Behaviour Therapy and Experimental Psychiatry* 16:22-30.

DiNardo, P. A., O'Brien, G. T., Barlow, D. H., Waddell, M. T., and Blanchard, E. B. (1983). Reliability of DSM-III anxiety disorder categories using a new structured interview. *Archives of General Psychiatry* 40:1070-1078.

DiNardo, P. A., Barlow, D. H., Cerny, J., Vermilyea, J., Vermilyea, B. B., Himadi, W., and Waddell, M. (1985). *The Anxiety Disorders Inter-*

view Schedule—Revised. Albany, NY: Center for Stress and Anxiety Disorders.

Hamilton, M. (1959). The assessment of anxiety states by rating. *British Journal of Medical Psychology* 32:50–55.

Hamilton, M. (1960). A rating scale for depression. *Journal of Neurology, Neurosurgery, and Psychiatry* 23:56–62.

Klosko, S. S., and Barlow, D. H. (1986). Cognitive-behavioral treatment of panic attacks. Poster presented at Association for the Advancement of Behavior Therapy, Chicago, IL.

Lang, P. J., Levin, D. N., Miller, G. A., Kozak, M. J. (1983). Fear behavior, fear imagery, and the psychophysiology of emotion: The problem of affective response integration. *Journal of Abnormal Psychology* 92:276–306.

10 Psychoeducation

This chapter is part of the psychoeducational material distributed to those attending Dr. Barlow's clinic. Most experts recommend the use of some body of educational material in the beginning stages of treatment, and this convention has considerable research support. This chapter addresses the questions frequently asked and provides an excellent manner of conveying this body of information.

Those who approach this book from a psychodynamic background may find the idea of "teaching" the patient objectionable. Notice, however, that all the authors in this section of the book emphasize the need to provide educational information. The reason is found in the nature of the panic attack, which is so overwhelming that it is experienced as a profoundly disturbing loss of psychological control. The anxiety-stricken patients often present with fears that they are "going crazy" or having a "nervous breakdown." Information about panic disorder relieves the patient's fear of loss of sanity. Further, because intense anxiety is so disorganizing in its effects on rational and purposeful thought, the information performs an additional service in the beginning stage of treatment as an understandable and supportive communication.

This chapter is an excerpt from the manual *Mastery of Your Anxiety and Panic*, describing the latest treatment program for panic attacks and panic disorder developed at the Center for Stress and Anxiety Disorders of the State University of New York at Albany. Information on obtaining this manual is available from Dr. David H. Barlow, Center for Stress and Anxiety Disorders, 1535 Western Avenue, Albany, NY 12203.

Psychoeducation

Ronald M. Rapee
Michelle Craske
David H. Barlow

PHYSIOLOGY OF ANXIETY

Anxiety is probably the most basic of all emotions. Not only is it experienced by all humans, but anxiety responses have been found in all species of animals right down to the sea slug. Anxiety experiences vary in severity from mild uneasiness to terror and panic. They can also vary in their length from a brief flash, to a constant ordeal. While anxiety, by its nature and definition, is an unpleasant sensation, it is not dangerous. This last point is the theme of this chapter. These pages describe the components (physical and mental) of anxiety in order that (1) you realize that many of the feelings you now experience are the result of anxiety and (2) you learn that these feelings are not harmful or dangerous.

Anxiety Defined

While a definition of anxiety that covers all aspects is very difficult to provide (indeed, whole books have been written on the subject), everyone knows the feeling that we call anxiety.

There is no one who has not experienced some degree of anxiety, whether—for example—it is the feeling upon entering a schoolroom just before an exam, or the feeling when one wakes in the middle of the night, certain of having heard a strange sound outside. What is less known, however, is that sensations such as extreme dizziness, spots and blurring of the eyes, numbness and tingling, stiff, almost paralyzed muscles, and feelings of breathlessness extending to choking or smothering can also be a part of anxiety. When these sensations occur and people do not understand why, then anxiety can increase to levels of panic, since people imagine that they must have some disease.

Fight/Flight Response

Anxiety is a response to danger or threat. Scientifically, immediate or short-term anxiety is termed the *fight/flight response*. It is so named because all of its effects are aimed toward either fighting or fleeing the danger. Thus, the number-one purpose for anxiety is to protect the organism. Back in the days when we were cave people, it was vital that when some danger faced us, an automatic response would take over, causing us to take immediate action (attack or run). Even in today's hectic world this response is necessary. Just imagine yourself crossing a street when suddenly a car speeds toward you blasting its horn. If you experienced absolutely no anxiety, you would be killed. Probably, however, your fight/flight response would take over and you would run out of the way to be safe. The moral of this story is simple: *the purpose of anxiety is to protect the organism, not to harm it.*

Systems of Anxiety

Anxiety manifests itself through three separate systems, any one of which can be primary in a particular person. The *mental system* includes the actual feelings of nervousness, anxiety, and panic and also thoughts such as "There is something wrong." The *physical system* includes all the physical symptoms such as dizziness, sweating, palpitations, chest pain, and breathlessness. The *behavioral system* includes the actual activities such as pacing, foot tapping, and avoidance. In panic attacks the physical system becomes the most important, since it is the physical symptoms that are most easily mistaken as indicating some serious disease.

The best way to think of all of the systems of the fight/flight response (anxiety) is to remember that they are all aimed at getting the organism prepared for immediate action and that their purpose is to protect the organism.

Physical System

Nervous and Chemical Effects

When some sort of danger is perceived or anticipated, the brain sends messages to a section of your nerves called the *autonomic nervous system*. The autonomic nervous system has two subsections or branches: the *sympathetic nervous system* and the *parasympathetic nervous system*. These two branches of the nervous system are directly involved in controlling the body's energy levels and preparation for action. Very simply put, the sympathetic nervous system is the fight/flight system that releases energy and gets the body "primed" for action, while the parasympathetic nervous system is the restoring system that returns the body to a normal state.

The sympathetic nervous system tends to be largely an all-or-none system. When it is activated, all of its parts respond. In other words, either all symptoms are experienced or no symptoms are experienced; it is rare for changes to occur in only one part of the body. This may explain why most panic attacks involve many symptoms and not just one or two.

A major effect of the sympathetic nervous system is that it releases two chemicals, adrenalin and noradrenalin, from the adrenal glands on the kidneys. These chemicals are used as messengers by the sympathetic nervous system to continue activity, so that once activity in the sympathetic nervous system begins, it often continues and increases for some time. This activity, however, is stopped in two ways. First, the chemical messengers adrenalin and noradrenalin are eventually destroyed by other chemicals in the body. Second, the parasympathetic nervous system (which generally has opposing effects to the sympathetic nervous system) becomes activated and restores a relaxed feeling.

It is very important to realize that eventually the body will "have enough" of the fight/flight response and will activate the parasympathetic nervous system to restore a relaxed feeling. In other words, anxiety cannot continue forever, nor spiral to ever increasing and possibly damaging levels. The parasympathetic nervous system is an inbuilt protector, which stops the sympathetic nervous system from getting carried away.

Another important point is that the chemical messengers, adrenalin and noradrenalin, take some time to be destroyed. Thus, even after the danger has passed and your sympathetic nervous system has stopped responding, you are likely to feel keyed up or apprehensive for some time, because the chemicals are still floating around in your system. You must remind yourself that this is perfectly natural and harmless. In fact this is an adaptive function. In the wilds, danger often has a habit of returning, and it is useful for the organism to be prepared to activate the fight/flight response.

Cardiovascular Effects

Activity in the sympathetic nervous system produces an increase in heart rate and the strength of the heartbeat. This is vital to preparation for activity, since it helps speed up the blood flow, thus improving delivery of oxygen to the tissues and removal of waste products from the tissues. There is also a change in the blood flow. Basically, blood is redirected away from places where it is not needed (by a tightening of the blood vessels) and toward places where it is needed more (by an expansion of the blood vessels). For example, blood is taken away from the skin, fingers, and toes. This is useful because if the organism is attacked and cut in some way, it is less likely to bleed to death. Hence, during anxiety the skin looks pale and feels cold, and fingers and toes become cold and sometimes experience numbness and tingling. In addition, the blood is moved to the large muscles, such as the thighs and biceps, which helps the body prepare for action.

Respiratory Effects

The fight/flight response is associated with an increase in the speed and depth of breathing. This has obvious importance for the defense of the organism, since the tissues need to get more oxygen in order to prepare for action. The feelings produced by this increase in breathing, however, can include breathlessness, a sense of choking or smothering, and even pains or tightness in the chest. Importantly, a side effect of increased breathing, especially if no actual activity occurs, is that blood supply to the head is actually decreased. While this reduction is small and is not at all dangerous, it produces a collection of unpleasant (but harmless) symptoms, including dizziness, blurred vision, confusion, a sense of unreality, and hot flushes.

Sweat-Gland Effects

Activation of the fight/flight response produces an increase in sweating. This has important adaptive functions, such as making the skin more slippery so that it is harder for a predator to grab, and cooling the body to stop it from overheating.

Other Physical Effects

A number of other effects are produced by activation of the sympathetic nervous system, none of which is in any way harmful. For example, the pupils widen to let in more light, which may result in blurred vision, spots in front of the eyes, etc. There is a decrease in salivation, resulting in a dry mouth. There is decreased activity in the digestive system, which often produces nausea, a heavy feeling in the stomach, and even constipation. Finally, many of the muscle groups tense up in preparation for fight or flight, and this results in subjective feelings of tension, sometimes extending to actual aches and pains as well as trembling and shaking.

Overall, the fight/flight response results in a general activation of the whole bodily metabolism. Thus, one often feels hot and flushed. Afterwards, because this process takes a lot of energy, the person generally feels tired, drained, and washed out.

Behavioral System

As mentioned before, the fight/flight response prepares the body for action—either to attack or to run. Thus, it is no surprise that the overwhelming urges associated with this response are those of aggression and a desire to escape from wherever you are. When this is not possible (owing to social constraints), the urges will often be shown through such behaviors as foot tapping, pacing, or snapping at people. Overall, the feelings produced are those of being trapped and needing to escape.

Mental System

The number-one effect of the fight/flight response is to alert the organism to the possible existence of danger. Thus, a major effect is an immediate and automatic shift in attention to search the surroundings for potential threat. In other words, it is very difficult to concentrate on daily tasks when one is anxious. Therefore, people who are anxious often complain that they are easily distracted from daily chores, that they cannot concentrate, and that they have trouble with their memory. This is a normal and important part of the fight/flight response, since its purpose is to stop you from attending to your ongoing chores and to permit you to scan your surroundings for possible danger. Sometimes an obvious threat cannot be found. Many humans, however, cannot accept having no explanation for something, and so they turn their search upon themselves. In other words, "If nothing out there is making me feel anxious, there must be something wrong with me." The brain now invents an explanation, such as, "I must be dying, losing control, or going crazy." As we have seen, nothing could be further from the truth, since the purpose of the fight/flight response is to protect the organism, not harm it. Nevertheless, these are understandable thoughts.

Panic Attacks

Up until now, we have looked at the features and components of general anxiety, or the fight/flight response. How does all this apply to panic attacks? After all, why should the fight/flight response be activated during panic attacks, since there is apparently nothing to be frightened of?

Following extensive research, it appears that what people with panic attacks are frightened of (i.e., what causes the panic) is the actual physical experience of the fight/flight response. Thus, panic attacks can be seen as a set of unexpected physical symptoms and *then* a response of panic or fear of the symptoms such as illustrated below:

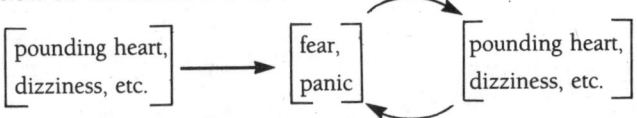

The second part of this model is easy to understand. As discussed earlier, the fight/flight response (of which the physical symptoms are a part) causes the brain to search for danger. When the brain cannot find any obvious danger, it turns its search inward and invents a danger, such as, "I am dying, losing control, and so on." This is illustrated below:

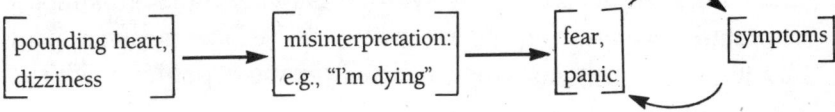

The first part of the model is harder to understand. Why do you experience the physical symptoms of the fight/flight response, if you are not frightened to begin with? There are many ways these symptoms can be produced, not just through fear. For example, perhaps you have become generally stressed for some reason in your life, and this stress results in an increase in production of adrenalin and other chemicals, which from time to time produce symptoms. This increased adrenalin might be maintained chemically in the body even after the stressor has long gone. Another possibility is that you tend to breathe a little too fast (subtle hyperventilation), owing to a learned habit, and this also can produce symptoms. Because the overbreathing is very slight, you easily become used to it and do not notice that you are hyperventilating. A third possibility is that you are experiencing normal changes in your body (which everyone experiences but most don't notice), and, because you are constantly monitoring and keeping a check on your body, you notice these sensations far more strongly than most people.

Even if we are not exactly certain why you experience the initial symptoms, we can assure you that they are a part of the fight/flight response and therefore are *harmless*.

Thus, our final model of panic attacks (simplified) looks like this:

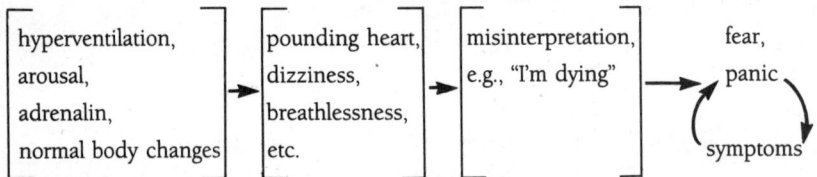

Obviously, then, once you truly believe (100%) that the physical sensations are not dangerous, then the fear and panic will no longer occur, and you will eventually no longer experience panic attacks. Of course, once you have had a number of panic attacks and have misinterpreted the symptoms many times, this misinterpretation becomes quite automatic, and it becomes very difficult to consciously convince yourself during a panic attack that the symptoms are harmless.

Anxiety Summarized

Anxiety is scientifically known as the fight/flight response, since its primary purpose is to activate the organism and protect it from harm. Associated with this response are a number of physical, behavioral, and mental changes. Importantly, once the danger has gone, many of these changes (especially the physical ones) can continue, almost with a mind of their own, owing to learning and other longer-term bodily changes. When the physical symptoms occur in the absence of an obvious explanation, people often misinterpret the normal fight/flight symptoms as indicating a serious physical or mental problem. In this case, the sensations themselves often can become threatening and can begin the whole fight/flight response over.

MYTHS AND MISINTERPRETATIONS

Going Crazy

Many people, when they experience the physical symptoms of the fight/flight response, believe they are "going crazy." They are most likely referring to a severe mental disorder known as schizophrenia. Let us look at schizophrenia to see how likely this is.

Schizophrenia is a major disorder characterized by such severe symptoms as disjointed thoughts and speech, sometimes extending to babbling, delusions, or strange beliefs (for example, that they are receiving messages from outer space), and hallucinations (for example, that there are voices in their head). Furthermore, schizophrenia appears to be largely a genetically based disorder, running strongly in families.

Schizophrenia generally begins very gradually and not suddenly (such as during a panic attack). Additionally, because it runs in families, only a certain proportion of people can become schizophrenic. In other people, no amount of stress will cause the disorder. A third important point is that people who become schizophrenic will usually show some mild symptoms for most of their lives (such as unusual thoughts, flowery speech, etc.). Thus, if this has not been noticed in you yet, then the chances are you will not become schizophrenic. This is especially true if you are over 25, since schizophrenia generally first appears in the late teens to early twenties. Finally, if you have been through interviews with a psychologist or psychiatrist, then you can be fairly certain that they would have known if you were likely to become schizophrenic.

Losing Control

Some people during a panic attack believe they are going to "lose control." Presumably, they mean that either they will become totally paralyzed and not be able to move, or they will not know what they are doing and will run around wildly, killing people or yelling out obscenities and embarrassing themselves. Alternatively, they may not know what to expect but may just experience an overwhelming feeling of "impending doom."

From our earlier discussion, we now know where this feeling comes from. During anxiety the entire body is prepared for action, and there is an overwhelming desire to escape. However, the fight/flight response is not aimed at hurting other people (who are not a threat) and it will not produce paralysis. Rather, the entire response is simply aimed at getting the organism away. In addition, there has never been a recorded case of someone "going wild" during a panic attack. Even though the fight/flight response makes you feel somewhat confused, unreal, and distracted, you are still able to think and function normally. Simply think of how seldom other people even notice that you are having a panic attack.

Nervous Collapse

Many people are frightened about what might happen to them as a result of their symptoms, perhaps because of some belief that their nerves may become exhausted and they may collapse. As discussed earlier, the fight/flight response is produced chiefly through activity in the sympathetic nervous system, which is counteracted by the parasympathetic nervous system. The parasympathetic nervous system is, in a sense, a safeguard to protect against the possibility that the sympathetic nervous system may become "worn out." Nerves are not like electrical wires, and anxiety cannot wear out, damage, or use up nerves. The absolute worst that could happen during a panic attack is that an individual could pass out, at which point the sympathetic nervous system would stop its activity and the person would regain consciousness within a few seconds. However, actually passing out as a result of the fight/flight response is extremely rare, and if it does occur, it is adaptive, since it is a way of stopping the sympathetic nervous system from going "out of control."

Heart Attacks

Many people misinterpret the symptoms of the fight/flight response and believe they must be dying of a heart attack. This is probably because many people do not have enough knowledge about heart attacks. Let us look at the facts and see how heart disease differs from panic attacks.

The major symptoms of heart disease are breathlessness and chest pain as well as occasional palpitations and fainting. These symptoms are generally directly related to effort. That is, the harder you exercise, the worse the symptoms, and the less you exercise, the better. The symptoms will usually go away fairly quickly with rest. The symptoms associated with panic attacks, on the other hand, often occur at rest and seem to have a mind of their own. Certainly, panic symptoms can occur during exercise or can be made worse during exercise, but they differ from the symptoms of a heart attack, since they can occur equally often at rest. Of most importance, heart disease will almost always produce major electrical changes in the heart, which are picked up very obviously by the EKG. In panic attacks the only change that shows up on the EKG is a slight increase in heart rate. Thus, if you have had an EKG and the doctor has given you the all-clear, you can safely assume you do not have heart disease. Also, if your symptoms occur in various situations and not only upon exertion, this is additional evidence against your having a heart attack.

11 In Vivo Desensitization: Contextual Analysis

Dr. Manuel Zane began one of the first phobia clinics in the United States at White Plains Hospital in 1972. He pioneered in the idea, now so widely accepted, that the anxiety is gradually diminished in the context of the phobic situation itself. His approach, for which he coined the term *contextual therapy*, is now more commonly called *in vivo desensitization*. He advocates using contextual therapy as a research tool to observe directly the rapid changes that take place in the phobic person while in the phobic situation.

This chapter presents the "Six Points of Contextual Analysis and Treatment" he developed with Doreen Powell. These six points incorporate the core ideas in desensitization, and they can serve either as a guideline for the therapist in the field or as a self-help reminder for the patient.

In Vivo Desensitization: Contextual Analysis

Manuel D. Zane

EXPECT AND ACCEPT YOUR PHOBIA

When you enter, or try to enter, the phobic situation, expect that you are going to become frightened and have physical reactions, whatever they may be in your case—rapid heartbeat, difficulty in breathing, butterflies in the stomach, weak legs, sweating hands, blurry eyes, dizziness, lightheadedness, and so on. It is your past phobic experiences that automatically trigger your physical feelings. It is your phobic thoughts about what you imagine is going to happen that make your physical and mental reactions get worse and accelerate. Try to recognize these negative, phobic thoughts when they start to come and then change them. Substitute more realistic thoughts for the negative ones. This is difficult to do and takes some working on, but with practice it can be done.

It is helpful if you can accept the fact that you have a phobia. Try not to get angry or upset at not being able to do what other people can do. Anger, envy, and embarrassment simply add other negative feelings to those with which you already must cope.

WHEN FEAR APPEARS, WAIT

This is very hard to do, but it can be accomplished with practice. When you find your fear level rising, stop, wait, and try not to run out or rush back to your place of comfort. Expose yourself to the fear little by little and stay with it. Remember that phobic people have a fear of the fear itself.

FOCUS ON THINGS IN THE PRESENT

Anticipatory thoughts of the phobic situation are usually negative and destructive. Try to stay with the present and not project ahead to what might be: generally, anticipatory thoughts are much worse than what actually occurs. Catch yourself running ahead when you start to say, "*What if* this should happen?"

LABEL YOUR FEAR LEVEL 1-10, AND WATCH IT GO UP AND DOWN

Number 10 is a fear level so bad that you almost cannot tolerate it; number 1 is the absence of fear. Many people, after being in a phobic situation, will tell you that they were up at a 10 the whole time. When you state your level of fear in the situation, you will find the level goes up and down and doesn't usually stay at a 10. When you are thinking about your level of fear, this is the first step in changing your thoughts. The reason is that, when you concentrate on what your fear level is, it is harder for the negative thoughts to get through. Thus you change your thinking.

DO THINGS THAT LOWER AND KEEP MANAGEABLE THE LEVEL OF FEAR

Each individual has to find his own ways to handle his fear in particular situations. Here are some examples of what some people have done to keep the fear level manageable. One person sings when he is driving his car. The sound of his voice is a comfort to him. Another person tells himself, "I will just let it be, I won't fight it. Let the feelings come, they are only feelings, I'm not going to faint. I haven't done so yet, and even if I do, so what." Another person keeps a picture of his family on the dashboard of his car. When he finds the feelings coming on, he quickly glances at the picture and asks himself, "What is so different between sitting here in my car and sitting at home in the living room?" He also touches the material of the seat of the car to bring his thoughts back to the present—to keep connected to the familiar environment. To touch familiar objects, to see and recognize familiar things, helps bring the fear level down.

TRY TO FUNCTION WITH FEAR

If you try to eliminate the fear altogether, you are fighting it and not letting it be. If you can accept it and let it be, it will decrease. Learning that you can do things to bring your fear level down is the first step to being able to cope in the phobic situation.

12 In Vivo Desensitization: Anxiety Coping Techniques

Jerilyn Ross has been active for many years in the field of phobia therapy. As a practicing psychotherapist, she draws upon her personal experience with overcoming a phobia to help others with the disorder. As an activist advocate for improved services to people suffering from phobias and related anxiety disorders, she has been particularly effective in conveying the phobic experience in the media and in public forums.

This chapter is taken from Jerilyn Ross's training manual for professionals and paraprofessionals who work with the phobic person in the field. The details of the in vivo approach given here are rarely available without hard-won first-hand experience. The author also addresses the pragmatic issues involved in structuring the therapeutic experience. Instructions are given for teaching the patient to use a daily log, motivating the patient to enter into and remain in phobic situations, creating positive attitude changes during the practice session, and offering a variety of anxiety-coping techniques.

In Vivo Desensitization: Anxiety Coping Techniques

Jerilyn Ross

When treating someone for a phobia, I believe a major part of the work must take place directly in the situation that is anxiety provoking. This is known as *in vivo* or *contextual* therapy. It involves gradually guiding the phobic person into the feared situation and teaching fear-reducing techniques while the phobic anxiety is being experienced. These techniques enable the person to deal with the symptoms, while developing confidence that the feared consequences of a panic attack will not occur. At the same time, the person learns how to change maladaptive thoughts and behavior patterns into adaptive ones. The patient is taught to define the thoughts and symptoms as they occur, to observe what is happening internally as these thoughts and symptoms appear and disappear, and to deal with anxious feelings in a positive way.

GOAL SETTING

A critical part of contextual therapy is helping the patient to set and work toward specific goals. Goals give the patient something concrete to strive for. They provide an opportunity to measure progress and to feel a sense of accomplishment, both of which are important for growth to take place.

While in treatment, the patient should be encouraged to set long-term (8- and 16-week) goals and short-term (weekly, daily, and sometimes even minute-by-minute) goals. The goals should always be specific: drive to Suzy's house, meet Tom for lunch at Restaurant X, go to a job interview. They should reflect what the patient really wants to do, since motivation is a key factor in accomplishing any goal. The goals serve as guidelines and milestones.

When setting the 8-week goal, ask the patient to consider: "If I were able to _____ , I would feel as if I were very much on the way to recovery." And in setting the 16-week goal, "If I were able to _____ , I would feel as if I were leading a normal life." The goals should focus on the *activity* rather than the *feeling*. Discourage the patient from saying, "After 16 weeks I would like to drive without anxiety." Explain that true growth comes when you are able to enter into and stay in the situation *in spite of* anxiety. I encourage patients to set long-term goals that may seem overly ambitious rather than ones that are very comfortable. I explain that they can always back off if they want to. One patient said to me at a final group session: "Sixteen weeks ago when I reluctantly set my 16-week goal as driving on the highway to my cousin's house, I thought I was crazy and so were you for encouraging me to set that as my goal. Now I do it without even thinking about it!"

Before choosing the long-term goal, I encourage the patient to think about it carefully. I suggest talking it over with a family member or friend. Most important, it must be a goal that the patient wants to accomplish. The goal should be formulated in a way that is specific and unambiguous, so that the patient knows very definitely when it has been achieved.

THE DAILY TASK SHEET

Overcoming a phobia is not always immediately rewarding. The opposite of feeling phobic is not necessarily feeling good. Also, phobias are often unpredictable, so that one can do something five times without feeling phobic and the sixth time have a panic attack. Because of these uncertainties, it is particularly important to attempt to make the process of overcoming a phobia as concrete as possible.

Often, progress not only seems slow but is unrecognized. One woman who had been in treatment for 16 weeks was upset during her last session because she was still unable to drive to her office alone. However, in looking back at a daily log, she was astonished to realize that 16 weeks earlier she had been not only unable to drive at all but barely able to leave her house, let alone hold down a full-time job. It was important for her to see this written in her own hand, since it was so difficult for her to acknowledge her own progress. Her experience reflected a common pattern of automatic "negative thinking," usually of a self-deprecating nature, that is common for phobic people and is a barrier to recovery.

The daily log or task sheet is designed to be used every day until the patient is no longer avoiding the phobic place, object, or situation. I constantly emphasize that patience and perseverance are essential for recovery.

To maximize the effectiveness of using a task sheet, I have the patient begin each week by setting a specific goal for that week and then breaking it down into daily tasks, noting the *day of the week* and the *specific task*. Specific tasks, for example, might be:

1. Drive to the grocery store alone.
2. Make a purchase in a specific department store.

3. Have lunch with a friend.
4. Get a haircut at the beauty parlor.
5. Ask one question at a business meeting.
6. Use an elevator to visit a friend on the fifteenth floor.
7. Attend a religious service.
8. Visit a museum.
9. Give a dinner party.
10. Use public transportation to visit a friend.

I then instruct the patient to make note of the following:

Who With

Will you do this task alone or with a support person? If the latter, who will that person be?

Highest Projected Level (HPL)

Think about and write down the anxiety level you "think" you will reach when you confront the phobic situation. Zero (0) level means "no phobic anxiety." Ten (10) is "absolute panic." The number given to the anxiety is a subjective rating.

Highest Actual Level (HAL)

After you have completed your task, write down the highest phobic level you actually reached. Note how it compares to your highest projected level. Usually the level that you actually reach is much lower than the one you thought you would reach. It is important to recognize this—for three reasons: (1) The next time you think about entering a phobic situation and you are afraid you will experience a high level of anxiety, you can recall that the last time was not as bad as you anticipated. (2) You can begin to develop trust that the anticipatory anxiety is almost always worse than the anxiety experienced while actually in the phobic situation. (3) Even if your level is high, you will notice how quickly it comes down.

How Long

What is the duration of time spent in the practice session? This does not mean how long you felt uncomfortable, but rather the length of the practice situation itself.

Physical Symptoms

Note, for example, rapid heartbeat, sweaty palms, feelings of disassociation, "noodle legs," difficulty breathing, etc. Notice how these vary from session to session.

Thoughts

Write down any thoughts—positive or negative—that either contributed to the phobic feelings or lessened them. Notice whether your thoughts involved magical or exaggerated thinking and, if so, what that did to your anxiety level.

What You Actually Did

The more specific you are, the better. For example: "Took the #2 bus to lunch with Sally at McDonald's."

Helpful Techniques

List anything that helped you stay in the phobic situation such as: counted backward from 100 by 3's, talked to the bus driver, counted the red cars on the highway.

Satisfaction Level (SL)

Although the temptation will be for you to rate yourself with a high grade only if you accomplish your task without feeling high levels of anxiety, it is important that you do just the opposite. That is: Consider the practice session a success if you accomplish your task *in spite of* the high levels of anxiety. Remember, the more you experience the high levels and are able to remain in the situation rather than fleeing from it, the more progress you will make in desensitizing yourself to the uncomfortable feelings.

During the time the patient is using the task sheets, it will be helpful to make a contract with a family member or other support person to review the task sheets at the end of each week. I instruct the patient to ask this person to be tough and insist the sheets be completed each week. I tell the patient, "This way, if you do slip up on your practice, knowing there is someone else who cares will make you think twice about skipping a practice session or not doing your homework. Make sure this person is aware of the courage it takes for you to complete your task, so you can feel free to share your excitement upon accomplishing a goal."

IN VIVO PRACTICE

Repetitive exposure to the phobic situation is a critical part of treatment. I present to the patient the necessity for contextual practice in the following manner:

> Phobic avoidance is a learned behavior. Of course, it was not learned or developed by choice. However, there was a starting point—your first panic attack—and you quickly learned that the way to avoid the terrible and frightening feelings associated with the phobic situation was to avoid it. So you naturally practiced avoiding the phobic situation. At first you made excuses to yourself: "I really don't have to drive on the highway to get to the store," or, "The train is more comfortable than the plane." You then began to learn how to change your life style so you could avoid dealing with the phobic situation altogether: taking a job where you could avoid public speaking, or shopping via mail-order catalogues. Each step, no matter how small, builds upon the previous steps. Without consciously trying you have mastered a new behavior—unfortunately, it is a negative behavior. You have taught yourself that by avoiding certain situations you will have fewer anxiety attacks. The result? A full-fledged phobia.

Now that you understand the technique that helped you learn to be phobic, you are ready to unlearn your phobia and replace the avoidant behavior with a positive behavior. The philosophy behind this is quite simple. You will start at whatever point you feel comfortable and begin by taking one step at a time, no matter how small, and building upon your accomplishments. As with an athlete in training, the frustrations, pains, and boredom will become secondary to the excitement of your progress. However, when you are first beginning your training, it is difficult to realize or trust this process of recovery. It can be as slow and subtle—but as profound—as the process of creating the phobia.

During your practice sessions you will be doing two things: (1) unlearning negative behavior and (2) learning to replace it with positive behavior. It is hard but rewarding work. Think about your favorite athlete. He or she did not become a winner by wishing away the pain and tediousness of developing strong muscles and stamina. However, when the athlete can foresee that the rewards will be greater than the pain, continued effort seems easier. You may have spent many hours, days, or even years wishing for the phobia to disappear. But as with the athlete, just wishing does not produce change. The hard work and commitment involved in learning to overcome a phobia are worthy of the respect given to an Olympic medal winner—and they should be treated as such. There is certainly nothing inherently pleasurable about exposing oneself to discomfort, either physiological or psychological. And it takes a tremendous amount of courage to do so. Therefore, in order to maintain the proper attitude for learning to overcome a phobia, it is crucial to keep the rewards in mind at all times, the most exciting being your new-found ability to lead a full and normal life without irrational limitations.

The necessity of practicing EVERY SINGLE DAY cannot be stressed enough. There is a direct correlation between the number of times a person practices going into the phobic situation and the amount of progress that is made. I sometimes see people who have had a phobia for only a short time, yet do not do as well as others who have been phobic for years. The differences in the clinical outcomes of people in treatment depend less on how long they had a phobia than on how much they practice in exposing themselves to the phobic situation.

Motivation in Practice: Practical Practice

It is important to structure the practice situation in a way that is both practical and motivational. The more the patient attempts practice situations with real rewards, the more successful he will be. Some examples of "practical" practice situations I have encouraged patients to set up are described below.

1. An elevator phobic accepted her boss's request that she move up to the ninth floor. Now she would have a real reason to use the elevator each day. This was a courageous step. Within a short period she was using the elevator regularly without experiencing panic attacks.
2. An agoraphobic woman who was afraid to drive alone accepted an interesting part-time job that was a reasonable distance from her home. Although driving was difficult at first, her motivation to get to the office overcame her fear of what could happen to her if she had a panic attack en route. Thus, she was forced to practice every day, and eventually she became comfortable with the trip.
3. A public-speaking phobic accepted the role of president of his synagogue and therefore had to confront the various committees and members on a regular basis. It was anxiety-provoking at first, but after a while his only complaint was that he had waited so long to accept the challenge.

These people did well not only because they entered the phobic situation over and over again, but also because (1) they were highly motivated, (2) they practiced on a continuous basis, and (3) they used the various techniques taught in the group and individual therapy sessions. As a result of their experiences in the phobic situation, they were able to see for themselves that their frightening feelings, however unpleasant, were not dangerous. This enabled them to stay in situations long enough to develop the trust that nothing would happen to them, no matter how close they felt they were to losing control.

They also realized that they did not have to remain a victim of phobic fear: there were things they could do to lower their anxiety levels.

Practicing versus Testing

In choosing a practice situation, it is important to make sure the person is really practicing and not just testing. In *practicing*, the person has chosen a specific goal and, by breaking down the steps and using the techniques to help stay in the situation, works toward achieving that goal. In *testing*, the person says, "I'll keep going until I have a panic attack and then I'll leave." I explain that testing is *not* helpful, because:

1. You are assuming a negative outcome before you begin.
2. You miss out on experiencing the sense of accomplishment that you feel when you reach a specific goal.
3. Your focus of attention is more likely to be on "future thinking" than on the present.
4. You are telling yourself that you can leave the phobic situation as soon as you feel your level rising, thus not allowing yourself to experience your level coming down without your having to leave.
5. You "reward" yourself by failing: you stop when you panic. This is an example of negative conditioning.

I then explain how practicing differs from testing:

1. Practicing is something you do voluntarily; testing is something that is done to you or that you "must" do.
2. Practicing is something that leads to a sense of mastery and pride. Testing leads, at best, to a sense of "having survived" and, at worst, to a sense of "having failed again."
3. Practicing is something you can control in terms of who, where, and what. It is desirable to practice setting goals that are a bit beyond where you feel comfortable—that way you continuously push back the restraining wall of the phobia. And once you set your sights on the farther peak, the nearer ones are suddenly more manageable.
4. Practicing leads to successes built on successes. Testing leaves you always passively back at square one.
5. Practicing is something you can share—with other phobic people, therapist, and family members. You can get encouragement and support. Testing is something that often must be endured alone.

Beginning the In Vivo Practice

The first step is difficult. Often the patient will procrastinate or manipulate the therapist and the situation to avoid getting started. I help the person get started by suggesting the following:

> Begin with something easy and manageable. As you progress to more difficult tasks, always remember: NO STEP IS TOO SMALL. Each step leads to the next, no matter how insignificant it may seem at the time.
>
> Begin each practice session with a definite goal in mind. The more specific the goal, the better. After you've established your goal, break down the steps you will need to take to reach it. If the first step is too difficult, cut it in half. Take a small step. And if that's too difficult, cut in in half again. Remember, no step is too small.
>
> If your goal is to go into the store and buy ten grocery items, begin by just walking into the store, picking up one item, and feeling good about it. If that is too difficult, just walk in and out of the store and feel good about that. If that is too difficult, just walk up to the door of the store and try to stand there for several minutes. If you feel you cannot do that, just get out of your car and walk within ten feet of the store. If that is too difficult, just drive into the parking lot near the store. Keep breaking down your steps until you find one that you can make. As you reach each step, wait a few seconds, take a deep breath, and take one more step. If necessary, take one step back, rest a few seconds, and then go forward again. If you feel foolish about only going as far as the entrance to the store, or only as far as the parking lot, think of the alternative: not to do anything at all. Take a deep breath and GO!

I tell the patient:

Keep in mind that the more uncomfortable you feel during the practice sessions, the more you are truly practicing and progressing. Think of it as taking the "bad medicine" to get better! As you continue breaking down the steps and moving forward, you want to always aim toward and remain in the "Discomfort Zone" (which will then become the "Progress Zone"). You are the only one who can determine where this line is for yourself; finding this "Discomfort Zone" and practicing in it is the most creative and the most important part of your practice. The longer and more often you can practice at this level, the more progress you will make. As Claire Weekes says, "Peace is on the other side of panic." Try imagining an inner voice advising you that every time you feel bad and continue to move forward instead of running away, you are getting stronger and healthier. Remember: NO PAIN, NO GAIN!

Coping with Situational Anxiety

I help the patient understand that the aim in contextual therapy is to stay in the phobic situation in spite of any bad feelings. I say:

> You want to set your goals, stay in the present, keep your primary thought focused on simple, manageable tasks, and stay connected to reality by carefully observing what is really happening at the moment. Once you have taken your first step, no matter how small it may seem, you have begun to make progress.

I emphasize in the following way the importance of staying in the phobic situation until the anxiety diminishes:

> In the past you have found that when you leave the phobic situation your anxiety level goes down. You are therefore tempted to leave as soon as you begin to feel uncomfortable, assuming that this is the only way to be relieved of your phobic feelings. If you *remain* in the phobic situation, you will find that your level will also go down, but you don't trust that yet. Each time you stay long enough to see your level come down without your having to leave, you reinforce the idea that nothing is going to happen to you. Intellectually you understand this, but the only way you will really believe and trust it is to experience it for yourself. This is difficult at first, but it gets progressively easier with constant practice.
>
> If you feel you absolutely *must* leave, try to "wait out" the panic and then leave. Let the feelings pass. The worst will only be a few seconds. Tell yourself that you will wait 20 seconds and then leave. If you are driving, you might say to yourself, "I'll pass one more sign or five more trees and then pull over." In the store you might say, "I'll look for one more item or ask someone one more question before leaving." In a high building you might touch three things or take two steps closer to the window before leaving. Then you may leave, rest awhile, and go back. It is very important for you to go back to a place where you felt uncomfortable as soon as you can. The longer you wait to return, the more difficult it becomes. Go back, step by step, any way you can—but GO BACK!

The more time you spend in the phobic situation, the easier it will become. Your body cannot physically maintain very high levels of anxiety for a long time. The panic attack itself rarely lasts longer than 15 to 25 seconds. No matter how anxious you feel, after a while your anxiety level will drop. It will go up and down, but the longer you stay, the more comfortable you will become. Therefore, you want to stay in the situation long enough so that you are reasonably comfortable before leaving.

Ideally, you should spend several hours at a time in the phobic situation. But, since this is not always practical, try to practice for at least one hour a day. You may have difficulty finding the time, but daily practice must be made a priority. You'll be pleasantly surprised at how much more time you have for everything, once you stop devoting so much time to worrying about your phobia.

Coping with Anticipatory Anxiety

For phobic patients the anticipatory anxiety can be a greater problem than the panic itself. To help them to cope with this, I distribute a list of "Helpful Hints":

1. When you find yourself thinking of what might happen ("future thinking") use the technique to STAY IN THE PRESENT. You are not in the phobic situation, so keep your thoughts focused on where you are at the moment, what is going on around you, who you are with, and so on.
2. When you begin to think of all the "what-if's," tell yourself, "So what!" Allow yourself to face the absolute worst. Say, "Okay, the worst that will happen to me is that I will go crazy, have a heart attack, crash my car, or make a fool of myself." Your phobia will not cause any of these things to happen to you, but by allowing yourself the thought of facing them, you are no longer trying to fight or control your feelings. The more you face and accept your fears, the less intense they will become.
3. Think about a time you thought you could not do something and were then surprised at being able to do it. Think back to how much more difficult it seemed before you actually did it, how it really wasn't that bad (you did survive), and how pleased you felt with yourself afterward.
4. Become aware of the discrepancy between your anticipated anxiety level and the level you actually reach while in the phobic situation. Each time you are about to enter a phobic situation, ask yourself, "What level do I think I will reach?" Then notice what really happens. After several experiences you will begin to see that the level of anxiety you actually reach is rarely as high as your projected level.

5. There is a tendency to "rehearse" the potential bad feelings over and over again, based on previous feelings or on "future thinking." It's as if you feel that the more conscious you are of these feelings, the better prepared you will be when the panic hits. Just the opposite is true. The less attention you give to your feelings and symptoms, the less vivid they become and, thus, the less frightening. When you find yourself "rehearsing," change that *primary thought*. STAY IN THE PRESENT. Remember, you want to let go of those phobic thoughts, so that they will eventually *die of neglect*!
6. To help disrupt the chain of anticipatory anxiety, you might try THOUGHT STOPPING. When you begin to anticipate a panic attack, give yourself the command, "STOP!" Say it to yourself or scream it out loud, but make sure you are firm about it. Say it *as soon as* and *every time* you have anxious thoughts about entering a phobic situation. Also, put a rubber band on your wrist and snap it every time your phobic thought recurs.

Hints to Stop Fears of Loss of Control

I help patients cope with frightening thoughts and impulses by presenting the following:

> Many people have experienced that sudden, overwhelmingly frightening, split-second feeling that they are going to lose control of themselves and do something that is harmful or humiliating to themselves or to someone else. One might suddenly feel a compulsion to jump while standing on a high balcony, a sudden urge to head into oncoming traffic while driving, an overwhelming urge to scream in a theater or at a business meeting, a fear of losing control and harming a child, and so on. This is a *common* experience.
>
> While these impulses seem very real and frightening when they occur, they are only "thoughts" and are in no way dangerous. You may not have control over which thoughts and feelings enter your mind, but you do have control over what you do with them. As overwhelming as these frightening thoughts and impulses may seem, remember that you do *not* really want to hurt yourself or someone else, or make a fool of yourself, and so you *won't*. These thoughts are similar to dreams—and we all know how creative and bizarre dreams can be. Remind yourself that you have never acted on these or similar thoughts. You never will! Phobic people have terrible *fears*. They do not do terrible *acts*.
>
> The more you *try* to lose your frightening thoughts and impulses, the more difficulty you will have in getting rid of them. The more willing you are to accept them as "frightening," but not dangerous, the more they will

begin to diminish. You can even learn to "enjoy" them just as you can learn to enjoy the creative process of your dreams—even your nightmares. Allow them to be there. Do not try to force forgetfulness. Tell yourself, "I've experienced this before and nothing happened. The scary thoughts have passed before and I know they will pass again." Allow yourself to face the "worst."

The "worst" will not happen; you know that intellectually. To really believe it you must allow yourself to experience it, no matter how scared you are. Try sitting in the middle of the theater when you are afraid of screaming and imagine yourself actually screaming. Stand on a balcony and imagine yourself jumping. Accept and even elaborate on the thoughts. Do you really want to? Of course not, and you won't. You won't drive into oncoming traffic, purposely drop a baby, hurt someone with a knife, or do anything that is out of control. The less you fight your thoughts, the less vivid they will become. Recall as often as necessary that thoughts are creative and often involuntary. We are not responsible for them any more than we are responsible for our dreams. Thoughts are *not* actions. You can control your actions. Once you truly accept these flashing thoughts and impulses, they will lose their nightmarish power, begin to become less important to you, and eventually disappear.

CONCLUSION

Treating a phobic patient with in vivo therapy can be as exciting and rewarding for the therapist as for the patient. Dramatic progress often occurs after just a few sessions. For best results it is most important that the therapist take the time to develop the patient's trust as well as demonstrate trust in the patient. Never try to trick or fool the patient. Allow for setbacks and display the same kind of understanding patience one would have while leading a child toward his first steps. To the patient, confronting a phobic situation is often that monumental!

13 In Vivo Desensitization: Action and Talking Therapy

Arthur Hardy developed the Terrap (Territorial Apprehension) program in the 1970s. It was a time-limited program of 16 weeks, each week covering a specific body of psychoeducational material as well as topics for group discussion and in vivo practice. Therapists learned the material of the Terrap program and started clinics around the country. These Terrap programs were often the only effective phobia treatment available outside the major urban centers. In this chapter Dr. Hardy discusses the development of the program and his observations on the most effective elements of the treatment.

The guiding concept, "Face the fear and the fear will disappear," neatly summarizes to the patient the need for in vivo desensitization. The chapter also emphasizes that "action therapy" is more effective than "talking therapy" for phobia disorders. This principle is reiterated in the literature on phobia therapy. Change takes place through actually approaching the phobic situation, armed with a new therapeutic orientation so that one can experience some measure of control of anxiety rather than feeling helplessly overwhelmed. Dr. Hardy emphasizes understanding and resolving feelings associated with the phobia, but as an adjunctive technique for more difficult cases, not as prerequisite for change.

In Vivo Desensitization: Action and Talking Therapy

Arthur Hardy

FEAR

In the treatment of anxiety, phobias, and the various panic disorders we work with the primary feeling of FEAR. Fear causes many strong physiological reactions. These are so strong they tend to override any other feelings, as well as inducing strange and often neurotic thinking and behavior. When the fear is left untreated, its intensity grows, interpersonal relationships suffer, marital problems develop, work problems arise, and usually a state of depression occurs. The person with these problems grows miserable to the point where life is, at best, difficult, and may not even seem worthwhile.

Fear itself is a normal, natural, useful emotion. It is essential to our survival. It is the body's warning signal that we are in danger of some kind, which our autonomic nervous system prepares our body to run away from in order to escape. This is an instinct we have inherited from our ancestors, whose daily survival was much more threatened than ours is today. If we are trapped, the reaction of flight-to-safety changes to fight-for-your-life.

Because fear is an instinctual reaction, it is not under our conscious control. To persons with phobias it seems that the reaction comes out of the blue, and they misattribute it to such things as going crazy, the early stages of a heart attack, or some other strange malady that has taken over their body and mind. Since they do not understand what is happening and do not know what to do, the reaction pervades and distresses many aspects of their lives. It often leads to adolescent suicides, alcoholism, depression, despondency, divorce, impoverishment, sexual problems, the breakdown of relationships, and the breakup of the family.

AVOIDANCE

The major thrust of the autonomic reaction is to direct the persons with phobias to AVOID the danger—to get to a safe place, a safe person, an area of security where they will feel safe and be able to recover from the shock of facing a danger signal. Thus, they establish what I call their *phobic nest*. The value of the phobic nest as a haven from anxiety is quickly learned, and the phobic becomes reluctant to leave its safety, fearing he may encounter a place, person, or situation that would trigger the dreaded danger signal and the attendant unwelcome physiological distress.

Avoidance increases the fear, which generalizes and spreads to anything in any way reminiscent of the original trigger stimulus. Avoidance also increases the sensitivity, which means that smaller and smaller stimuli are required to trigger the panic or anxiety reactions. With time, any stimulus even remotely connected with danger, no matter how small, can bring on a major reaction. Avoidance can then become a way of life, sometimes leading to the person's becoming housebound or parasitically attached to a "safe" person.

EARLY RESEARCH EXPERIENCE

Early in the 1960s I was working with Don Jackson, M.D., at the Mental Research Institute in Palo Alto, California. My training till then had all been psychoanalytically oriented. Using this approach with people who came to us for help with phobias, we found that many of them dropped out of treatment early, before they had made any progress dealing with their fears. We were interested, then, when a man came to MRI stating that he had cured himself of phobias and had helped a friend improve, and that perhaps he had discovered a method of helping many others with phobias.

This man's philosophy was that every person could do more with a safe person than alone, that people could always do a little more than they thought they could do, and that working with someone who had suffered from the problem and recovered would help more than working with someone who had never had the problem and therefore didn't understand the situation as well. His method was based on the approach *Face the fear and the fear will disappear* and was strictly behavioral.

I volunteered to observe this man's work with a phobic patient and then to report back to a committee formed to evaluate his methods. We worked together with an agoraphobic woman who we thought would be a very difficult patient. She had been housebound for seven years. Within an hour after we arrived at her home, we had her outside walking around the block. Her depression lifted, she now felt she had a chance to recover, her resistance to our suggestions disappeared, and she was anxious to have us come back the next day. We worked with this woman every day, nearly all day, for 8 days. By the end of this time she was able to leave her home on her own and to separate both from her husband and from us to accomplish assigned tasks. Her progress seemed a miracle.

During these eight days, the woman had relearned to drive and was driving by herself on the freeway to the Institute. She was going into stores, standing in lines, using escalators and elevators, and going over bridges. She also began talking more about things that had happened in her past that seemed to have a bearing on the problem. She seemed to have developed more insight into her difficulties than she had had when we first saw her.

The members of the committee could hardly believe my report, nor could they account for the rapid changes. Dr. Jackson thought it might be a transference cure due to my charisma. I reported this case to the Western Psychiatric Society and afterward I asked for comments on why this approach might work so well. All was silent until a psychiatrist in the front row said, "I don't know why it works, but if I ever get the problem, I'm coming to you."

TERRAP

Using what was learned from this agoraphobic woman and from similar cases, we began the Terrap program. Our motto became "Face the fear and the fear will disappear." We called this *exposure therapy*. It is now called *in vivo therapy*. We reasoned that, with our presence, patients had less tendency to avoid, and that facing the fears proved to the patients that things they feared were not as dangerous as they had thought. It seemed obvious that "doing" something was better than talking about it.

Example

At one point in our Terrap program we teach the participants that in some situations it is helpful to tell someone else about their problem with phobias. For example, it may be necessary to explain the phobia to a boss or a friend so that one's behavior can be understood. We give the participants a typed letter with a model explanation, and all the group members agree to talk to someone before the next meeting. However, it has been our experience that if we go no further than that, the group members somehow "forget" to talk to someone. On the other hand, when people practice in the group session by telling someone else in the group about the problem, the task suddenly becomes easier, and the members will manage to tell an outside person before the next session. Again, actually doing it is more effective than talking about doing it.

PSYCHOTHERAPY

With more experience in the treatment of phobias, we included other very effective approaches: education, relaxation training, assertiveness training, in vivo exposure, and cognitive therapy. However, these did not solve all the problems in mobilizing the phobic to try to face the fear. Often there were setbacks, unresolved issues from the past that needed to be faced, cases of self-defeating behavior that persisted even though the territorial difficulties had been overcome and the person could now move about more freely.

In the case of the first woman mentioned, her change was too fast. We paid no attention to the husband. The couple fought and then separated. Later we began to include spouses in the program, and our divorce rate greatly decreased. We realized that the spouses didn't understand the affliction; therefore, we added more education for the spouses, more discussion about feelings, more discussion about relationships, and communications training.

All this was helpful, but we still had problems. I decided to delve deeper. I put together a small group of people who had been through the basic Terrap program but who were still having difficulties. They set personal goals by developing a "want list." Then they started investigating their experiences of the past to discover any self-defeating thoughts or attitudes that prevented them from reaching their goals. In other words, we were hunting for insight into areas the patient was not fully aware of or did not realize existed.

Example

A patient was nearing the end of the program when I accompanied her to the market, a place in which she had previously experienced panic many times. She had improved, her self-confidence had increased, and she was relaxed in the store. As she stopped in front of a shelf of toys, she remarked that her sons loved "Star Trek," and she reached for a box of "Trekkie" paper dolls. Suddenly she became quite anxious, so we retreated from the dolls, she relaxed, and I encouraged her to talk about her experience. Spontaneously she recounted that she had bought her sons a toy oven the previous Christmas and had been severely criticized by her mother—the gift had been too feminine. She was fearful that her mother would criticize her again. We discussed this fear, and she decided she could deal with it.

A COMPLETE TREATMENT PROGRAM

As we gained more experience in treating phobias, I started to think about combining the separate treatment approaches into a sequenced program.

It did not seem advisable to use insight therapies early in the sequence. Insight therapies are "talking" therapies, not "action" therapies. They refer to the past, not to the present. The patient talks about his traumas from his past in order to gain insight into his difficulties in the present. Phobic patients, however, have become so sensitized to their own discomfort, both mental and physical, that they have learned to very skillfully avoid anything that might trigger this discomfort. Therefore, while talking in the therapist's office, they will avoid any subject that causes any anxiety or discomfort, thereby virtually assuring that the core of the problem is never reached. The therapy becomes frustrating for both the patient and the therapist.

The program appears to be most effective when it is begun with behavioral therapy in combination with cognitive restructuring. Education, relaxation training, in vivo exposure, assertiveness training, communication training, discussions about feelings and relationships, and a support group are all a part of this basic program. This basic program would develop quick changes that would give the patient mobility and hope of recovery. Appropriate medication could be used when and if necessary.

This basic program is enough for some patients. For others, who continue to experience major difficulties or frequent setbacks, involvement in insight-oriented psychotherapy appears necessary so that they can work through their self-defeating behaviors and attitudes. By the end of the basic program, patients have developed some trust in the therapist, and the fear of the reaction has become less intense. At this point, then, patients are less resistant to this therapeutic approach and more willing to become involved.

Given the patient's readiness to recover and willingness to work at it, this sequence effectively rehabilitates most of the patients who come for help with their fears and phobias.

14 Imaginal Desensitization

Reid Wilson came to the field of phobia therapy with an expertise in Ericksonian techniques of hypnotherapy and particularly in pain control. In this chapter he offers us a new look at visualization and hypnosis in imaginal desensitization. Today imaginal desensitization essentially has been replaced by a more effective and "high-powered" technique, in vivo desensitization—that is, exposure to the phobic situation in reality rather than in imagination. However, imaginal desensitization continues to have its place among the procedures of the phobia therapist. Often it is used in an office practice in which the therapist does not go out into the phobic situation with the patient, but rather discusses a set of exposure situations that will be approached by the patient between sessions (either alone or with a "phobic companion"). In this context it can be seen as a rehearsal to lessen anticipatory anxiety and to practice coping strategies before exposure to a phobic situation.

Hypnotherapy with phobias dates back to Freud's earliest work and is currently considered relatively ineffective. Yet it is clear from this chapter that the Ericksonian position provides some provocative and valuable new techniques. Dr. Wilson's perspective revitalizes both hypnotherapy and imaginal desensitization in providing some extremely sophisticated adaptations to our current understanding of effective treatment. This chapter also contributes a model for developing imagery in desensitization, and the relaxation exercise presented is a paradigm easily incorporated in nonhypnotic relaxation training.

Imaginal Desensitization

R. Reid Wilson

A guiding principle in psychotherapy is to identify and address the client's resistance to change before exploring the avenues of potential change. In individuals experiencing a panic or phobic disorder, such resistance can be readily identifiable.

For those whose problem developed from a spontaneous panic attack or a traumatic event, any consideration of facing the phobic situation can stimulate that dramatic memory. This recall reminds them of their perceived inability to cope with any such event in the future, since during their last attempts their loss of control (over their physiology or their circumstances) was of overwhelming proportions. They project this same failed strategy into their future, so that their view of coping with a similar situation tomorrow ends in failure as well.

Since these panic-prone individuals cannot perceive themselves successfully implementing coping strategies, when they do plan for challenging events, they mentally prepare for the worst possible scenarios. Since the mind responds to imagery in a way similar to reality, these imagined scenes stimulate increased anxiety. Thus phobic clients are in the proverbial "Catch-22": until they experience themselves successfully facing the panic-provoking situation, they remain fearfully immobile, yet they avoid facing the feared situation until they are certain they will succeed. They skirt confrontation until they can be guaranteed that they will experience "zero" anxiety. Thus avoidance becomes their primary pseudosolution.

This avoidance, however, is costly. When adopted as their response to anxiety, it leads to a more and more restricted lifestyle. And as these individuals limit their activities in response to irrational fear, this coping style reinforces low self-esteem, harsh self-criticism and depression.

As they enter treatment, these clients will often present rigid attitudes about their capabilities, their worth, their projected image in public, and their treatment options. Dogmatic themes reflecting the need for containment will surface: "I *must* hide my anxiety from others." "I *can't* let myself feel any anxiety." "If I don't control these feelings they will *run wild*." Underneath this position is often a loss of self-worth and a sense of hopelessness. Although not always stated openly in the treatment session, probing can reveal messages such as, "There is something inherently flawed about me," or "I don't have what it takes to cope with the world's pressures." Their hopelessness is reflected in their poor attitude toward the potential of treatment options and in their unwillingness to attempt new coping strategies: "I've had it too long." "I've tried everything; it's too ingrained." "This will never help; I can't improve."

Thus, the therapist seeking to treat clients with phobias, panic disorder, or agoraphobia must account for any powerful, traumatic memories of clients' past, the image and sensation of impending failure in the future, clients' psychic preparation for catastrophe, their strong investment in avoidance as the only safe and realistic option, and their restricted self-defeating attitude regarding their change potential. For clients who enter treatment with such a rigid frame of reference, cognitive-behavioral assignments alone can meet with resistance in the form of "forgetfulness," unwillingness to comply, brief or feeble attempts at the therapeutic strategies, canceled appointments, and treatment dropouts.

The use in treatment of imaginal exposure through brief hypnosis and visualizations offers many benefits in this difficult therapeutic relationship. The chief asset is the ability of these techniques to circumvent clients' resistance enough to allow them to entertain the possibility of change. This is accomplished through a special structuring of the therapist's language that encourages clients to become more receptive to presented ideas. Clients are gently guided through experiences that allow them to increase their control over physical and psychological responses before entering the actual fearful situation. This enables clients to build coping skills in less traumatic settings. If clients perceive that they can practice skills without suffering the "trauma" of anxiety, they become more willing to comply with the therapeutic request. Simultaneously, as they entertain the possibility of change through actively participating in a positive visualization, they begin the process of shaping: the gradual building up of a behavior by successive approximations toward the goal.

Consider the example of a client who wishes to overcome his fear of flying in an airplane. Perhaps he has flown successfully in the past but five years ago experienced a difficult flight and subsequently became frightened by the idea of flying again. A comprehensive initial assessment is important to identify the specific experiences, fears, and hesitations of each client, and a number of cognitive and behavioral interventions may be needed.

After an initial evaluation, suppose you assess that positive visualization would be a useful adjunctive tool. If imagery is to be beneficial within such a treatment, its function will be threefold: to develop clients' self-efficacy (their belief that they are capable of performing the task successfully) (Bandura 1977), to reduce clients' anticipatory anxiety, and to reinforce coping techniques that can be used during moments of anxiety.

The first therapeutic consideration should be how to reduce the chance that clients will resist your suggestions. Since pressure to perform will stimulate their fears, they are likely to respond to directives with resistance. For instance, a more traditional hypnotic approach to imagery for fearful flying might contain the following directives:

> Close your eyes now and begin to relax. Relax the muscles of your face, jaw, shoulders, and back. Just let go of tensions more and more. Now, I want you to see an image of yourself floating comfortably on a raft in a swimming pool. Just enjoy the warmth of the sun on your body. You're feeling so very comfortable now. Maintaining that sense of comfort, imagine yourself sitting on a plane, relaxed, enjoying a flight to your favorite vacation spot.

To receptive clients this approach is straightforward and supportive: you help clients access feelings of comfort and encourage clients to maintain those feelings as they place themselves into the fearful situation. However, if you ask a fearful flier to participate in this particular imagery, you will probably meet with resistance. Instead of comfort, the client will probably begin to experience anxiety, with images of himself feeling trapped as the plane door closes or feeling anxious as the plane passes into a stormy region.

PROBLEMS WITH TRADITIONAL IMAGERY

What is it about this approach that stimulates resistance? First is the theme of relaxation. For many panic-prone individuals simply the idea of relaxing is frightening, since one of their primary fears is of "losing control." "Control" means remaining consciously tense, braced, and vigilant. "Relaxing" means surrendering that conscious control over their body. This they will not purposely do until they experience an alternative method of maintaining control. In fact, as you suggest relaxation, they usually will respond to that "threat" with greater tension.

Second is the theme of being trapped. This traditional approach to imagery instructs clients in an authoritarian fashion to follow a specific path: close your eyes, relax your body, see an image, enjoy your flight. Such requests can stimulate a sense of being confined and restricted in thoughts, feelings, and actions. Once again, for some phobic clients the mere idea of having to perform in a specific manner will instantly stimulate anxiety and tension.

The third difficulty with this approach is the increased likelihood that you will lose rapport with clients. If you make a request that clients cannot perform, and if you continue to push for compliance, you will lose a basic therapeutic alliance. If you require that clients "relax" in order to proceed with the imagery, what happens if they don't feel relaxed at that moment? When you ask them to imagine themselves floating comfortably on a raft, what if they are afraid of water? If you state, "You are feeling so very comfortable now," when clients are actually tense and uncomfortable, what will happen to your rapport? While you are encouraging a pleasurable experience, these clients are probably experiencing failure and are subvocalizing this failure: "This isn't working; I can't do it; there is no way I can feel relaxed." In this paradigm, by the time you now tell clients to visualize themselves "sitting on a plane, relaxed, enjoying a flight to your favorite vacation spot," you have long lost therapeutic rapport.

These therapeutic mistakes are some of the primary reasons that clients will quickly abandon the use of visualization or will say, "I've tried hypnosis, but I'm not hypnotizable." However, if you define hypnosis to be a focusing of concentrated attention inward, all humans are capable of that skill. And, in fact, panic-prone individuals use a negative form of self-hypnosis to convince themselves that they will not change. They focus their concentrated attention inward to retrieve a memory image of failing at their task in the past. As the mind associates to an experience, it will respond physically, so clients now begin to notice sensations that they felt during that past event: their stomach gets tense and their heart begins to race. They next turn their concentrated inward attention to an imagined future time when they might attempt to face the same problem situation. Since they are now feeling tense and anxious and since they are calling up an image of an event in the future that is similar to the past traumatic event, they project their past behavior into this future situation, telling themselves, "I knew I couldn't do it."

IMAGERY THAT OFFERS CHOICE

A dilemma arises when attempting to balance clients' needs to remain consciously in control at all times, and the therapeutic need for clients to loosen conscious control in order to entertain novel solutions to old problems. Panic-prone individuals tend to create "rules" for interpreting and responding to anxiety-provoking situations: "Here is a restaurant. I have experienced panic in restaurants before; therefore, I might experience one today in this restaurant. I cannot cope with a panic attack; therefore, it is in my best interest not to enter this building." The deeper the clients' belief in this logic, the more difficulty therapists will encounter as they attempt to modify it. If clients remain controlled by this information-processing style, every event will be rigidly classified as either fearful or not fearful, and their response to "fearful" events will follow that same predictable pattern of anxiety and avoidance.

By building a new and different imaginal exposure paradigm that accounts for clients' needs to remain in control, to experience choices and options instead of feeling trapped, and to experience success and mastery instead of repeated failure, you can create brief hypnotic or imagery experiences that move clients closer to their therapeutic goals while simultaneously sidestepping resistance. This change in your therapeutic approach can assist clients in breaking through their rigid beliefs into creative problem-solving that allows them to freely and openly entertain novel ideas, in the same way that all scientists, mathematicians, musicians, and artists produce creative new themes to expand their technique. As these individuals suspend their need for linear logic, they gain access to their ability to notice resemblances and correspondences in seemingly unrelated objects or events. In this way they form a "gestalt" with new complex images to solve old problems.

One of the best methods for clients to accomplish this is to allow special kinds of *imagery*, not words, to do their creative thinking. These images can contain more information than cognitive statements (thus the expression, "a picture is worth a thousand words") and can hold more emotional impact, which makes concepts more concrete to the mind. Once a novel solution for an old problem is produced through imagery, *then* they can enlist the help of their cognitions to incorporate that change into their conscious daily living through specific rules or guidelines. In other words, this is a two-step process. In step one, complex imagery is used to generate options for change; in step two, clients choose among those options and select how to implement that solution.

PARADIGM FOR BRIEF HYPNOSIS

To move from theory to practice, here is one way we might use brief hypnosis and visualizations within a therapeutic session to assist clients in bypassing resistance and entertaining the possibility of change.

1. Select a therapeutic task that is the client's next appropriate step toward the treatment goal.
2. Identify the client's internal resources needed to accomplish this task.
3. Orient the client toward the task by indirectly discussing those needed resources.
4. Present one or more therapeutic images that are within the client's skill level, using option-oriented language. Suggest specific changes in the client's physiology, emotions, or images, while continuing to use option-oriented language.
5. Imply the client's ability to produce those changes in the future.

Returning to the example of the fearful flyer early in treatment, consider an initial therapeutic task (step 1) to be self-efficacy:

the sense that he can actually accomplish this goal through his own efforts. The image of success would certainly compete with his typical picture of considering taking a flight and becoming too upset or panicky to follow through. And it would be an invaluable resource, since one's ability to image positive change will have a direct impact on one's willingness to exert effort toward change.

The important internal resources (step 2) would be the client's willingness and ability to use imagery and to imagine a positive future. By discussing these resources in an indirect fashion and through asking rhetorical questions, you begin to stimulate the client's selective memories and images for these resources (step 3). This process plants the seeds for the next important step by enlisting the fundamental skills needed to produce a more complex therapeutic image.

SUCCESS IMAGERY

When selecting a therapeutic image for such clients (step 4), the therapist will need to design a task that stimulates the least resistance. If we ask the client to imagine "flying in comfort" before the client believes he can accomplish this feat, we will run into resistance. So, instead, ask the client first to see himself *already having succeeded at his goal of flying*, without yet considering *how* he will succeed. This circumvents the client's resistance ("I can't . . .") while setting the stage for more specific images supporting a self-efficacy belief ("What would it be like if I could . . .").

Let me illustrate the actual presentation of these steps to this hypothetical client. The illustration here begins with step 3: orient the client toward the task by indirectly discussing the needed internal resources. Keep in mind that the objective at this step is to begin to stimulate the client's ability to retrieve or develop complex imagery as it relates to the spoken phrases.

Therapist: As you have been talking, I've been developing a growing sense of just how much you would like to be rid of this whole problem, to not even think about how easy it is to get on a plane, and fly anywhere you want. . . . [*Pause*] Do you have any idea how you will feel when you have succeeded at this task?

Client: Well, I'd feel great . . . I'd feel a sense of freedom.

Therapist: You'll feel great, yes. And can you just sense how good you'll feel inside you as you step off a plane after a comfortable flight? . . . Because you have experienced that comfort before, haven't you? You used to fly with ease. Do you remember?

Client: Yes, I remember, but it seems so long ago.

Therapist: Yes, so long ago. And what I am really curious about is whether you can remember what it feels like to be comfortable, long before you ever had this hesitation? Looking back, what do you think it is like in your body when you are feeling comfortable, at ease?

Client: Well, I think my shoulders would be relaxed, I'd be breathing easily, my heart rate would be slow. And my mind wouldn't be racing.

Therapist: I can't tell whether you're feeling any of that right now. I wonder, is it possible for you to notice your shoulders relaxing? . . . And just let your breathing be nice and gentle as you listen to my words? [*Pause*] And it must be a good feeling to have your mind quiet down, since there's nothing you have to be working at right now. As though you're letting your body and mind have a break as I talk. [*Pause*] And wouldn't it be nice to be able to look ahead with these same feelings? . . . and having these feelings with you more often in the future? [*Pause*] Just imagine how things might seem different if you somehow could call up these feelings whenever you wanted to.

Here are my objectives for the client in the exchange above. Develop a feeling sense of what it would be like if this problem were behind you (first paragraph). See a glimpse of yourself getting off a plane with physical and emotional comfort by retrieving a memory of accomplishing that feat in the past (second and third paragraphs). Produce those sensations of comfort right now in this room, then imagine the results of having these feelings again in the future (fourth paragraph).

Even though I had concrete and specific goals, there was no pressure on the client to perform; it was as though we were simply having a casual conversation. Nonetheless, the content of my statements and questions makes certain presuppositions. For instance, the first question ("Do you have any idea how you will feel when you have succeeded at this task?") presupposes that the client *will* accomplish his stated goal. In order for the client to answer, he must conjure up an image of succeeding. At the same time, the indirectness of the question lowers the risk of conscious resistance, relative to a more direct request ("Imagine yourself now flying successfully"); therefore, the client more easily creates the picture in his mind. Next, I ask him to remember that this success is an experience he actually has in his repertoire of past successes. Rather than focusing on his comment that "it seems so long ago," I casually suggest he find out whether he can recall the memory of *physical* comfort, then experience that comfort now ("Is it possible for you to notice your shoulders relaxing?"). Finally, I present the rhetorical questions and comments regarding these comfortable feelings continuing into the future. In formal hypnosis, these comments would be called posthypnotic suggestions.

The client is now psychologically and physically ready to begin step 4, which will be the first direct request for imagery.

Therapist: While you're enjoying this physical comfort right now, I thought you might enjoy a brief little experience. As you continue to let those shoulders stay relaxed, and breathe easily, I wonder if you'd let your eyes close and try a little experiment? [*Client's eyes close.*]

Take a moment to pretend that you can drift through time into the future. And let yourself drift, as far into the future as you need to to imagine yourself in a time and place where you have long overcome this problem . . . where this difficulty is in the distant past . . . as many months or years or decades as you need to, and then just get to know what it is like to have succeeded. Here, now, in the future, you have the ability that you were seeking, the ability that you knew was inside you. All those problems between you and your goal have faded away because you have already reached your goal for some time. And you can now enjoy all the changes that come with attaining that goal. [*Pause*]

Let yourself fully experience how you feel now that you have made it. . . . And look around; how does your world appear to you now? . . . And who is around you: someone you know or someone new?

And what is the feeling of success like? . . . Does that feeling of confidence and pride influence the way you walk down a street? . . . Or hold your head on your shoulders? And if someone were looking at your face, would that person be able to see your sense of accomplishment? Would your smile, your eyes, reveal your good feelings?

So tell me, in a few words, while you continue feeling comfortable, what it's like to feel successful.

Client: Yes, I like it. I'm in Australia with my wife and, we're having fun on our own, without the kids!

If the client progresses as smoothly as this hypothetical one has, a second image can be suggested within step 4 that will take advantage of this current state of mind and move him one step closer to the current therapeutic goal of self-efficacy.

> Would it be acceptable with you if we tried another image? [*Client nods his head.*] Fine. Just let that image fade away as you focus on the comfort of your body here, and your nice easy breathing. . . . I would like you to see yourself having *just completed* your first flight, and the flights went *perfectly*, almost magically . . . beyond your dreams of success: no bumps, no difficulties, no tensions, just smooth as glass. And you are now stepping off that plane. [*Pause*] Let yourself begin to know what it feels like inside you to have accomplished this task. . . . As you are walking away from the plane, notice how this success is expressed in the movement of your feet. . . . And if some people are greeting you, I wonder if they will see the pride and relief and joy on your face. . . . And notice how *they* respond to your response. Really get to know how your body expresses your confidence, and absorb those feelings like a sponge.

This visualization capitalizes on the client's ability to experience success and moves that psychophysiological response closer in time to the feared task. However, three suggestions diminish resistance. First, the image is still of a time *after* the feared task, not during it. Second, the client is asked to imagine having completed a "magically perfect" flight. Third, the suggestions offered after the initial request for an image presuppose that the client is experiencing "success." In other words, in order for the client to comply to the indirect requests ("Really get to know how your body expresses your confidence . . ."), he must accept the premise that he has just succeeded in the flight. Instead of struggling to imagine flying comfortably, he must busy himself in the discovery of how his sense of success might influence how he walks or how other people might react when they see him smiling.

If, upon questioning, the client continues to express success in generating these images and physical responses, a third and final visualization can be presented.

> In a moment I would like you to imagine the entire process of taking a commercial plane flight, from calling the airlines for a reservation to

landing in some vacation location and enjoying your pleasures. I would like you to see yourself packing your clothes, driving to the airport, boarding the plane, taking the flight, and so forth. And I'd like you to experience that whole process—easily, comfortably, pleasantly—from start to finish, in 30 seconds. Go ahead and start now.

With about 10 seconds remaining in this imagery I would suggest to the client that he should soon see himself on the ground, enjoying his vacation. After the 30 seconds I would ask him to open his eyes and describe his experience.

This final visualization now takes the client through an imaginal experience of a successful flight sometime in the future. Two variables increase the likelihood that he will not have difficulty with this image. First, he has just had two visualizations giving him the feelings and the state of mind that support success: he has experienced himself long in the future with this success in his past, and he has seen himself take pride immediately after his first flight. Second, he is placed in a time bind: he has a great number of tasks to accomplish in his mind within 30 seconds of lapsed time. With all likelihood he will be so consumed by these elements that he won't have enough time or consciousness to become anxious. And he is reminded to end the imagery with the pleasant experience of his vacation.

Please note that the "30-second" guideline is not an absolute. A shorter exposure, such as the image of riding on an elevator or driving over a bridge, will require a visualization as brief as 10 seconds in order to maintain the therapeutic objectives.

This particular paradigm can be called "success imagery," since the emphasis is on the positive experience either during or after an accomplishment and not on confrontations or struggles within the task. Other variations of success imagery can be adapted for a variety of fears associated with panic or phobias, such as driving a car, grocery shopping, eating at a restaurant, riding an elevator or escalator, standing in line, or entering a crowd.

A few guidelines will assist you in their use. First, regardless of the task, the outcome picture should be something the client desires, for it will be this goal that motivates the client. When developing an outcome picture, help the client adjust the future images until they reflect a pleasing goal. Second, by using pauses of silence, give the client time after each suggestion to develop an internal response—physically, emotionally, and with imagery. The more you and the client take time to enhance each presented image—using colors, textures, sounds, physical sensations, and emotions—the stronger will be the influence of the image. And, third, embellish your suggestions using option-oriented language to reduce resistance.

These visualizations given below are presented as though they were verbatim instructions to the client, but they are only illustrating the general flow of the imagery. In the next section you will learn how to enrich these directions in ways that enhance client responsiveness.

Illustrative Imagery—Option One

Imagine yourself in some comfortable, safe place. Let yourself remain there for a few minutes, enjoying the pleasant experience. Continue in that scene until you can feel your body reflecting your comfort and sense of safety. Take a mental scan through your body; notice how that comfort feels.

Now, while you maintain that feeling, call up the image of your task. This transaction is an important one. Only see the *picture* of the task in your mind; turn off the sound and turn off the feelings associated with the picture. You should take on the role of a detached observer of the scene, as though you are the director reviewing the film clip. Keep your sense of bodily comfort from the previous scene.

While you are feeling physically relaxed, watch yourself, on that screen, simply float through the task. Don't bother making your actions realistic. Literally see yourself gliding through the entire experience, as if you are comfortably floating on a pocket of air. Do it with ease. Face no threatening moment. Have no difficulties. End your scene by reaching your goal and *enjoying it* when you get there. Spend as much of your imagery time enjoying your goal as you took to reach your goal.

As you complete that task in your mind, return to your first scene of that comfortable, safe place. Spend a few minutes experiencing that comfort in your body and mind again.

Option Two

Follow the same process as in Option One, and add these instructions.

> If, at any time, while you are viewing your task, you feel sensations of discomfort, take a mental eraser and wipe away that scene completely. Return your comfortable, safe scene to the screen. Stay in that scene as long as you need to in order to regain your sense of ease. Then, maintaining those comfortable feelings, return to floating through your task from the beginning.
>
> You can stop that task image as many times as you like, taking as long as you need to regain your sense of comfort. You don't even need to get through the task in your mind the first few times that you try it here. Consider that you are "playing" with these ideas and images. It doesn't really matter how far you get in any particular session.
>
> It is important, however, that you take time to end each imagery session feeling at ease. When you are ready to stop, return to imagining your comfortable, safe scene until you feel that comfort reflected in your body.

Option Three

Feel free to reduce the number of steps or change any particular step to create a process specifically designed for the client's task. It is unnecessary to go through all steps every time.

This session will require that clients first write down their answers to the questions below. Have them keep the sheet of paper in their lap.

1. What is my task?
2. When will I do this?
3. How long will I take?
4. What worried thoughts do I have about this task?
5. What self-critical thoughts do I have about accomplishing this task?
6. What hopeless thoughts do I have about this task?
7. What can I say (in place of those negative thoughts) to support myself during this task?

8. How can I increase my sense of safety while working on this task?

   A. Call up your success image. Give yourself a clear, positive goal. Take a nice calm breath as your body responds to that image.
   B. Now, let that image fade away as you visualize yourself briefly somewhere in the middle of your task. See yourself totally in control of the situation, smoothly handling the scene even if you can hold onto that sense for only a few moments. Take another nice calm breath as you let that image fade away.
   C. Glance down at your answers to question 4, "What worried thoughts do I have about this task?" Take your answers one at a time. Look at your first answer, then close your eyes and repeat that one statement or question in your mind. If you can, visualize a few of the key words of that worried thought at the same time. Now, take a calming breath as you let that thought, and those words, fade from your mind. Don't bother responding to the thought, or replacing it with a positive thought. Simply let it fade out, and let any of your associated tensions fade away. Return to that sense of calmness to your body. Completely dissolve that negative thought without responding to it.
   Once you have returned to that state of calmness and ease, glance down at your next answer.

Proceed in the same fashion as above. After completing this process for each of the client's answers to question 4, use this same method with each answer to questions 5 and 6.

   D. Spend as much time as you need to again develop your quiet mind and body. Consider this a "rest period": no work, no effort, just drifting comfortably, letting your body soothe itself.
   E. Now turn your attention to question 7, "What can I say to support myself during this task?" Reflect on your statements one at a time. Close your eyes and recite the first one to yourself. Think only about the statement, not about your task. Let the statement sink in. Let your body respond as though you believed the statement. Get to know how your body feels as it is supported. After you are satisfied with your response to that first statement, recite that second statement, let it sink in, and notice your body's response as you let yourself believe the statement to be true, if only for a few moments. Continue using this process with each of your supportive statements.

You may find that as you reflect on these statements a new and different supportive stance rises up in your mind. Reflect on that sentence and learn from it. If you like how your body feels as you attend to it, jot down the new sentence for a later use.

F. Begin to mentally rehearse your task, Start with any active preparatory steps you might want to take to increase your sense of safety. Then, see yourself moving through each stage of the task in the way that you have planned. Envision yourself at the beginning of the task, in the middle, and as you are finishing it. Finally, see yourself enjoying the completion of that task, smiling to yourself at the accomplishment.

G. Take a few minutes to become quiet and calm, without having to work on any task. Use this time to focus on a pleasant image, to experience comfortable body sensations, or to meditate on a calming word.

Suggest to the client that "you can continue to practice your success imagery a little bit each day, as many times as you need to, in order to have confidence in your ability to begin practicing the task itself."

OPTION-ORIENTED LANGUAGE

One of the therapist's most important goals in treating panic and phobic disorders is to assist clients in breaking through rigid, avoidance-oriented patterns of problem-solving in order to experience conscious competence in responding to stressful events. Imagery, especially success imagery, provides a safe therapeutic step toward producing new, competing, internal responses to the old fear-producing cues.

To maintain rapport with an individual who fears becoming trapped or losing control, the therapist must word these visualizations in such a way as to support the client's freedom and choice. (Fortunately, such option-oriented language structure also promotes the creative problem-solving style that I spoke of earlier.) In the general field of clinical hypnosis, technique has been slowly shifting away from a direct, dominant style of suggestion to an indirect permissive style (Erickson and Rossi 1980).

Based on this shift, five simple linguistic changes can significantly diminish the likelihood of client resistance to brief hypnosis and visualizations.

Questions and Rhetorical Questions

The simplest way to avoid resistance is to avoid requesting change. Good hypnotic technique involves suggesting change without requiring it. Questions and rhetorical questions serve this function of directly stimulating clients' curiosity while indirectly orienting them toward the possibility of changing. In order to respond to most questions, the mind must first consider the question. It is in the *consideration* that you gain the therapeutic advantage. For example, the direct request, "Relax your body now," might become:

> Do you think that there are times when your body is less tense than others? And during those times when *your body becomes less tense*, might you notice it? Have you ever just flopped down in a chair, *letting your body feel like a rag doll*? Do you think, during those times, that your *shoulders loosen and drop* a little? Is it like telling your legs they're on a break, that they can *go ahead and become loose and relaxed*, while you *focus on something pleasant*, like how nice it is just to *sit and unwind*?
>
> And, I wonder, what would it be like right now if 100% of your attention was on *letting yourself be physically comfortable*? Would you shift your body at all? Would your *breathing become nice and easy*?

Whether the client responds orally to each question or simply contemplates it, the therapist must pause long enough after each in order to allow a mental response. In this way, a direct or rhetorical question turns into an indirect suggestion. Notice how in the first paragraph of the example the client is asked about past experiences with relaxation. As he associates to the questions in a positive manner, he is more likely to begin ideomotor responses: physical responses to the ideas suggested within the questions. By the second paragraph the client is oriented toward the suggestions and becomes more susceptible to a mention of current relaxation.

Review now the phrases in italics in those two paragraphs.

Here, embedded within the questions, are the direct suggestions to produce physical and mental relaxation. While the conscious mind is somewhat distracted by the questions, these suggestions influence with less resistance. To increase the impact of these phrases, they can be spoken a little more slowly and quietly than the rest.

Qualifiers

Any time we give an explicit instruction or direction to a client, we invite resistance as well as compliance. *Qualifiers* are words or phrases that limit or modify the meaning of another word or phrase. In this context we want to modify the message, "Do/think/feel this." Any direct suggestion can become an indirect suggestion by adding qualifiers such as: *might, maybe, may, can, a little, somewhat, probably, can wonder,* or *don't know if.* Introductory phrases will offer the same benefit: *I wonder if. . . ? Do you suppose. . . ? Is it possible. . . ?You might be surprised if. . . ? I'm curious what it would be like if. . . ? I don't know if. . . .*

Here is an example of qualifiers with a client who is fearful of entering stores and restaurants. The embedded suggestions (indicated by italics) are designed for the client to feel physically relaxed while imaging a scene of sitting in a car outside a restaurant.

> I wonder if you can *imagine* what it might be like if you were able to *sit outside that restaurant in your car.* I don't know if you could *reassure yourself that you are safe.* Do you suppose, if you only had to sit there and not even get out, that you could *feel physically comfortable?* Maybe, if you *feel safe,* you could see yourself *breathing easily, gently.* Perhaps *your hands are relaxed in your lap.* If you want to right now, you can *let your shoulders relax,* too. And the *muscles of your forehead may loosen* a bit.

Negative Adjectives or Adverbs

Adding a negative to a statement can increase an internal search through the cortex for information by adding some brief confusion. It also can overtly support a resistance to change while covertly encouraging a mental association to the idea. In some cases it even challenges clients to produce the suggested change by suggesting that they are not yet ready or able to change. Negatives would be any words with the prefix of *un-*, *a-*, *im-*, *miss-* or *ex-* and adverbs such as *not*, *won't*, *never*, *can't*, or *couldn't*. Examples are:

> It's unnecessary to be *totally relaxed*.
>
> You don't have to *picture yourself having accomplished it perfectly, feeling as in control* as you would like to.
>
> It might be impossible for you to *imagine your hands loosening their grip on the steering wheel*, yet. You can't quite say what the *control* will feel like.
>
> I'm not sure whether or not you can remember *experiencing that success in a completely satisfying way* before.

All Possible Alternatives

With these suggestions the therapist gives the client a variety of options within a narrow field of endeavor, whether it is regarding images, emotions, physical sensations, or behavior. While the client experiences a sense of choice, almost all the choices are of a therapeutic nature. For instance, if we want the client to access a memory or a feeling of power in order to maintain that subjective state as he enters a fearful scene, we might say:

> Everyone has his own sense of *what personal strength feels like*. You may remember a time when you were *feeling powerful*. It could have been a few days ago in some conversation, or a few months ago as you experienced some change in your life. Or perhaps it was years ago, when you were a teenager, or a child, *feeling that energy of accomplishment or pride*.
>   I don't know *what it feels like inside of you when you are strong*. Does it feel as though it comes from one physical place, like your heart or your chest? Or perhaps you feel it throughout your body, *like a warmth or an energy field*. Or you may only *notice* the results of *your power*, by the way you hold your head, or stand, or your facial expressions, your tone of voice. You might not even *know what your strength is like as you feel a sense of power*.

Implications

Implications encourage clients to consider the possibility of change without challenging their rigid conscious beliefs. They do this by including phrases that presuppose change. For instance, the question, "As you begin to improve, I wonder how many new behaviors you will become comfortable with?" presupposes, first, the the client *will* improve and, second, that he will learn new behaviors as he improves.

One structure for implications stems from "if . . . then" thinking, such as

> Now, if you *create a voice inside you that supports your efforts*, then you will *notice* just *how good you can feel*,

or

> If your *breathing becomes slow and gentle* here, then your *thoughts* might *quiet*, too.

Neither statement directs the client to respond, but both will stir the client's associations and mental process regarding the suggested behaviors. To create such statements, choose two behaviors, one that the client is already experiencing or could easily experience, and another, more relevant therapeutic goal. Use an introductory phrase such as, "Before . . . ," "As soon as . . . ," "While . . . ," or "After . . . ." Use a phrase to link the two behaviors, such as ". . . then you can . . . ," " . . . it will remind you of . . . ," " . . . you might experience/notice . . . ," " . . . the problem will . . . ," or " . . . your feelings will. . . ." ("As soon as you begin to get comfortable in your seat, then you can think about what you would like to have when you leave this session today.")

A second method of generating implications is to speak in more abstract terms regarding change. Instead of directly addressing how the client should modify his own behavior, speak of other people:

> One thing many clients have found useful is to *remember back to experiences years ago, before the problem ever existed* . . . to *remember breezing through a grocery store without a moment's hesitation,*

or

>Each person can *overcome obstacles* at his own, safe pace.

Questions can also be posed that imply resources or behavioral options available for the client. For instance,

>As you *image yourself approaching the restaurant door*, which of your many skills might you use to *respond to your tension*?

or

>As you *see yourself walking up to that restaurant*, will you *take a nice, slow, calming breath*, or will you *tell yourself that you can manage this task and feel the relief* that comes with that knowledge, or will you just *forget all about your worries* and *enjoy your friends*? Maybe you will do something entirely different that will help you feel *safe and confident*.

VISUAL REHEARSAL WITH OPTION-ORIENTED LANGUAGE

Consider another example of the five-step design, described previously, for incorporating a brief hypnotic or visualization experience into a treatment session. Suppose the therapeutic task (step 1) is for the client to begin using a special breathing technique to assist him in remaining calm as he enters an anxiety-provoking situation, such as a restaurant. The internal resources he will need (step 2) are: to sit comfortably and visualize a scene, to perform that breathing process, and to respond physically to that process.

Assume that we have indirectly discussed these internal resources with the client (step 3). Here is a hypothetical transcript of steps 4 and 5 of such a brief visualization, using all the styles of option-oriented language: questions and rhetorical questions, qualifiers, negative adverbs and adjectives, all possible alternatives, and implications. It will begin by assisting the client in becoming physically comfortable and oriented toward the hypnotic experience. The client will then associate a special breathing pattern with a sense of emotional and physical comfort. Finally, the client will visually rehearse successfully using that breathing technique in two different scenes. Again, italics will indicate the embedded suggestions.

> We have talked quite a bit about your desire to *remain calm* in a variety of situations. Truly, all of us deserve to *feel a sense of being settled,* to be able to call "time out" and just *rest.* I guess resting could mean different things to different people. It could mean *not having to think very much,* simply *letting your mind be quiet.* No work. No effort. Or it might be *letting your legs get heavy and relaxed,* as they do after a good workout. Perhaps resting means to *rest your eyelids, your jaw, your shoulders, your chest.* Take a moment here to see what parts of *you can begin to rest.*
>
> And as you continue to notice what it is that changes in your body while you *let go of muscle tensions,* you may be able to discover that your *breathing has slowed* to a *gentle rate.* And do you ever wonder just how *your breathing helps relax you?*
>
> If you want to feel a few more of *those muscles loosen,* you can try something. In a moment I am going to ask you to take a nice long gentle inhale and then let it out ever so slowly through pursed lips. So slowly you could count from one to eight as you exhale. And as you let the air flow out easily, perhaps you will notice *your body becoming heavier and heavier, more and more relaxed.* And after you finish exhaling, just let yourself breathe gently, easily, from your abdomen.
>
> Now on your next inhalation, take that long deep breath, filling your lower lungs, then your upper lungs. Fine. Now ever so slowly begin that gentle, long exhale. And you don't even need to notice how *your body begins to melt, to loosen, to feel so much at ease* as you *let go more and more.*
>
> You'll probably find that you don't even need to pay attention to your breath now. Your body is totally capable of performing that simple task, just as it does for you every night as you sleep quietly. But you might notice with each *gentle exhalation* now you're *feeling more and more comfortable, more and more safe.* And physically you might notice a number of things: how *relaxed your stomach can feel,* a sense of *heaviness in your arms and legs,* or perhaps a *pleasant kind of tingling* somewhere in your body. I don't really know.
>
> And after your next exhalation, take another one of those nice long deep breaths . . . then very slowly exhale. And as you are exhaling, you can find out if your body wants to *feel* any *more comfortable* or whether it

feels just fine with this degree of *comfort*. When you are ready, tell me in a few words what you are aware of now. [*If client responds positively, then continue.*]

Fine, and let's refer to that breathing pattern as a Calming Breath. As you continue, do you suppose you could think of any times in your day when this kind of feeling of *comfort and safety* would come in handy? And if you do think of a *nice time* to *retrieve this feeling*, just nod your head gently. . . . Fine. Go ahead and see yourself during that time . . . and when you are ready, let yourself have that nice Calming Breath . . . and notice what happens.

If you *feel physically at ease*, find out just how things look to you. And any time you notice even a twinge of tension [*as client is exhaling*], let yourself have another *nice deep inhale* . . . and a *gentle, slow exhale*, as your body responds naturally to your desire for *physical comfort and ease*. Find out whether you notice [*use client's description of physiological changes after Calming Breath from above*].

It might even seem as though the scene stops and waits for you to *feel comfortable* again before it proceeds. Otherwise, continue to move in that scene, noticing whatever or whoever interests you, while you explore whether or not you *enjoy feeling safe, trusting your body*. And tell me in a few words what you are noticing right now. [*Listen and respond to client's experience.*]

Fine. Now, if you are interested, you might want to consider one other image here. Would you like to? [*Wait for client agreement.*] Pretend for a minute that this simple breathing can bring you a sense of *physical ease and comfort*, just as you describe. I'd like you to pretend that as you take that deep inhalation, and let it out slowly, you will remember just how you feel today. Would that be all right with you?

In a moment, I'm going to ask you to see yourself entering a restaurant that would have, in the past, felt uncomfortable. But this time, consider allowing your body to take charge of itself. Simply see yourself in a moment, walking into that restaurant and taking that nice long inhale and that easy, gentle, slow exhale that is a Calming Breath to your body. And then find out how you like it when your body responds to that Calming Breath by [*again use client's description of physiological changes after Calming Breath*].

So go ahead and begin to unfold that scene now.[*As you see client take that deep inhalation, continue.*] And just allow your body to respond, without work, without effort, and maybe even to your surprise. As you continue to *feel safe*, continue to drift through that scene with a knowledge that that Calming Breath is there when you need it. Otherwise, just *enjoy your comfort*, and the taste of that food, or the good company around you. And any twinge of anxiety can be a cue for you to let your body take care of itself with that Calming Breath.

Take all the time you want to *enjoy* your meal, then pay your bill and walk comfortably out to the parking lot. And give me a nod when you are there.

[*After head nod*] Speaking of enjoyable experiences, wouldn't it be nice if sometime soon you discovered that without even thinking about it you found yourself taking a Calming Breath, or noticing those *comfortable feelings in your body*, or, without even thinking, doing something that you once were avoiding? All because, in some way, a person can *begin to trust the body*. And the more you *trust the body*, the more you will be surprised at your *comfort* and your *control* in the coming weeks.

Now I doubt that you'll come in next week and say that you have been *having no symptoms* all week. That would even surprise me! But I wouldn't be surprised if you tell me next week about one time or another that you suddenly notice *how comfortable you can feel*.

But for now you can just notice what it's like to let a little light in your eyes as you begin to adjust to this room again.

CONCLUSION

The advantages of this special form of imaginal exposure have been outlined throughout the chapter. The common denominator of most of these benefits is that such visualizations enable clients to be more receptive to presented ideas. The therapeutic relationship can then be used to explore with greater frequency experiences that are outside of clients' usual frame of reference. In turn, as clients become capable of envisioning positive change in their lives, this encourages them to take responsibility for their own actions in the future.

In addition, at certain moments during imagery sessions there can be blending of conscious understandings and expectations with unconscious participation. New unconscious insights and learnings can be immediately gratifying to clients' conscious needs. As described in Bandura's self-efficacy theory, the client can acquire a sense of confidence that he or she will have adequate resources to cope with the phobic situation. Even this benefit alone makes imaginal exposure a significant technique in the treatment of anticipatory anxiety and phobic avoidance.

REFERENCES

Bandura, A. (1977). Self-efficacy: Toward a unifying theory of behavior change. *Psychological Review* 84:191-215.

Erickson, M. and Rossi, E. (1980). The indirect forms of suggestion. In *The Collected Papers of Milton H. Erickson*, vol. 1, ed. E. Rossi, pp. 452-477. New York: Irvington.

SUGGESTED READINGS

Erickson, M. (1954). Pseudo-orientation in time as a hypnotherapeutic procedure. *Journal of Clinical and Experimental Hypnosis* 2:261-283.

—— (1964). An hypnotic technique for resistant patients: The patient, the technique and its rationale and field experiments. *American Journal of Clinical Hypnosis* 7:8-32.

Erickson, M., and Rossi, E. (1976). Two-level communication and the microdynamics of trance and suggestion. *American Journal of Clinical Hypnosis* 18:153-171.

Mott, T. (1982). The role of hypnosis in psychotherapy. *American Journal of Hypnosis* 24:241-248.

Wilson, R. (1985). Interspersal of hypnotic phenomena within ongoing treatment. In *Ericksonian Psychotherapy*, vol. 2, *Clinical Applications*, ed. J. Zieg, pp. 179-184. New York: Brunner/Mazel.

—— (1987). *Don't Panic: Taking Control of Anxiety Attacks*. New York: Harper and Row/Perennial Library.

—— (1987). *Breaking the Panic Cycle: Self-Help for People with Phobias*. Rockville, MD: Phobia Society of America.

15 Breathing Control

Attention to hyperventilation and breathing control are not part of most programs, but these techniques are fast becoming an integral component of the treatment package. The rapid results achievable using only very simple interventions can be astonishing. There is increasing evidence that overbreathing and disruption of breathing may be major contributors to anxiety in many patients. Several workers, such as Dr. Lum in England and Dr. Fensterheim in New York, have been calling attention to the importance of this element in the anxiety disorders for the past 10 or 15 years, but it is only in the past 3 or 4 years that the effectiveness of breath control has been accorded research attention by such groups as that of Dr. Barlow in Albany and Drs. Salkovskis and Clark in England.

Breathing Control

Jonathan H. Weiss

INTRODUCTION

The diagnosis and treatment of hyperventilation can be crucial to the control of many symptoms, psychological and physical, that will otherwise resist the therapist's best efforts. There are no accurate estimates at this time of the prevalence of hyperventilation. However, it is believed to be so widespread among children and adults that almost every therapist is likely, knowingly and unknowingly, to have encountered patients in whom this problem was significant.

Hyperventilation and certain of its symptoms were described in the literature of antiquity. In medieval times one could read of "melancholik folke, lovers and all those which are busily occupied in some deep contemplation; silly fooles likewise, which fall into wonder at the sight of any beautiful and goodly picture (and) are constrained to give a great sigh." In the early part of the twentieth century Hofbauer (1921) coined the term *hysterical tachypnea*, a label that carried a theoretical bias and grouped overbreathing with the "conversion" or (a much-misused term [Weiss 1974]) "psychosomatic" symptoms. Kerr and colleagues (1937) then introduced the descriptive, theoretically neutral term we use today and paved the way for further observation and theoretical formulation.

Since then we have learned much that is important about hyperventilation. We have found, for example, that it is not always an expression of anxiety or heightened arousal but can be a faulty breathing habit developed under conditions having nothing to do with heightened emotion. We have learned that hyperventilation can be a cause as well as a consequence of anxiety. We have learned that hyperventilation can trigger or exacerbate both functional and organic physical syndromes of which it was thought to be a symptom or in which it was not noticed to have played a role at all. Most important, we have learned more about how to probe for its presence in emotional and physical symptoms and how to control it so that those symptoms can be effectively treated.

In this chapter I will define hyperventilation, discuss the physical and psychological symptoms associated with it, suggest techniques that can be used to make the diagnosis, and then describe how hyperventilation is treated. My purpose is to provide the working clinician with useful, "how-to" information rather than to discuss the science of hyperventilation research. Readers who are interested in the latter are urged to read Lum (1981, 1985, 1987) and the recent monograph by Fried (1987).

DEFINITION OF HYPERVENTILATION

Hyperventilation is an increase in ventilation in excess of the body's metabolic needs. Quick, deep breathing during exertion is normal and adaptive, but such breathing at rest causes too much carbon dioxide to be exhaled and lost from the blood. Lum (1981) suggests that, in predisposed people, the change in level of carbon dioxide, rather than the absolute level it reaches during hyperventilation, is the operative variable. He calls the condition *fluctuating hypocarbia* (1987).

Hyperventilation occurs in a variety of forms. Most familiar is the acute pattern of rapid, deep breaths with gasping inhalation and noisy exhalations seen, for example, in people during attacks of panic. The person in acute hyperventilation seems to be suffering from air hunger and may report, in fact, that he cannot get enough air. Shoulders and chest heave exaggeratedly, and breathing appears almost convulsive. This form of hyperventilation is dramatic in appearance and is probably what most people imagine when they think of hyperventilation.

Overbreathing, however, also occurs in a much more subtle form that involves less dramatic changes in rate or depth of breathing. It is based instead on an incorrect balance between the use of the muscles of the chest and of the abdomen for breathing. If the reader will place one hand on his belly and the other on his chest and breathe normally, he will notice (unless he has been practicing abdominal breathing) that both the belly and chest expand and contract during each breath. The movement of the belly reflects the working of the diaphragm, and the movement of the chest results essentially from the use of the muscles that raise and lower the rib cage. In normal breathing under relaxed conditions, the ideal ratio of abdominal to chest movement is about four or five to one, and breathing rate is about twelve to fourteen breaths per minute. (To see relaxed breathing that is primarily abdominal, the reader needs simply to watch a person asleep.) If there is more thoracic movement than the 10% to 15% suggested by the ideal ratio, or if the rate exceeds fifteen breaths per minute, assuming the person is not exerting himself, overbreathing is probably taking place, and more carbon dioxide is being lost than is optimal for normal physiological functioning.

The subtle form of hyperventilation is by far the more common. Many people have learned to breathe with the muscles of the thorax excessively. To look at them one would suspect nothing, since there is no labored, frantic heaving as there is in the acute form. Nor do these people feel that their breathing is abnormal or uncomfortable. They appear to have adapted to a chronically lowered level of carbon dioxide in the blood, and for the most part they have few or no problems. However, these people are at risk for symptoms triggered by relatively small additional changes in their breathing. A cough, a sigh, a sneeze, laughter, reading aloud, or even a deep breath taken in surprise or in response to going out on a hot or cold day can put the chronic low-level hyperventilator over the threshold for symptoms.

Chronic hyperventilation can be a habit acquired in the course of a lifetime for a variety of reasons not connected to heightened emotions. Some people, for example, are taught that it is desirable to stand straight with their bellies tucked in and their chests puffed out. Although this may look good, it forces a tightening of the abdominal muscles and an excessive reliance on the thoracic apparatus for breathing. Other people wear tight clothing that forces them to constrict their abdomens and to breathe with their chest muscles. (During the later nineteenth century fashionable women were corseted to the point of nearly total immobilization of their abdomens. Fainting was not uncommon.) Still others work at jobs that require them to bend over a desk or workbench, thereby constricting their abdominal muscles and interfering with their normal use for breathing. And people with respiratory allergies or asthma may learn to overuse their chest muscles for comfortable breathing.

Between the extremes of acute hyperventilation and chronic low-level hyperventilation are intermittent episodes of overbreathing that may occur during emotional excitement or during emotionally innocuous events such as speaking aloud, bouts of respiratory allergy or infection, spells of very hot or very cold weather, exposure to smoke or strong smells, wearing tight clothing, or working in cramped conditions. Intermittent hyperventilation can also occur in people who start to breathe more deeply and rapidly in response to exertion and then, for some reason, continue to do so after their metabolic needs for it are over. Stimulant drugs may also trigger hyperventilation as part of sympathetic arousal.

PHYSICAL SYMPTOMS OF HYPERVENTILATION

Hyperventilation can affect any of the body's physiological systems. This is probably a simple reflection of the fundamental role adequate air exchange plays in the regulation of blood chemistry, which, in turn, affects all of the body's functions. The presence of physical symptoms in the clinical picture presented by a patient, whether or not the patient relates them to the problem for which he is seeking help, should alert the clinician to the possibility of hyperventilation. This possibility is too often vastly underappreciated, even by physicians. Huey and Sechrest (1981) report that in 150 patients who were ultimately determined to be hyperventilators, the original (incorrect) diagnoses included:

Cardiovascular:	coronary heart disease
	rheumatic heart disease
	congenital heart disease
	acute rheumatic fever
	cor pulmonale
	paroxysmal auricular tachycardia
Respiratory:	asthma
	emphysema
	"respiratory tract infection"
G-I:	cardiospasm
	peptic ulcer
	cholecystitis
	cholelithiasis
Neurological:	epilepsy
	brain tumor
	poliomyelitis
	CVA
Musculoskeletal:	fibrosis
	myositis
	arthritis

Endocrine: islet-cell tumor of the pancreas
pheochromocytoma
hyperthyroidism
hypothyroidism
insulin reaction
"glands"
Psychological: "nerves"
"functional _____"
Other: allergies

Lum (1985) suggests that somewhere between 10% and about 30% of all visits to doctors are for symptoms due to hyperventilation. Lum has also noted that when physicians are trained to look for hyperventilation in their patients, the frequency of the diagnosis and of referrals for breathing retraining increases sharply.

The following list (Lewis 1959) shows the symptoms that have been reported to be triggered by hyperventilation:

Cardiovascular: palpitations
tachycardia
precordial pain
Reynaud's syndrome
Respiratory: bronchospasm
breathlessness
"air hunger"
chest pain
G-I: dysphagia
dyspepsia
epigastric pain
"spastic colon"
diarrhea
globus
esophageal reflux
burping
heartburn

Neurological:	paresthesia
	dizziness
	disturbance of vision
	disturbance of hearing
	blackouts
Musculoskeletal:	muscle pains
	tremors
	cramps
	tetany
General:	exhaustion
	lethargy
	weakness
	sleep disturbance
	headache
	anxiety
	panic attacks
	phobic states
	excessive sweating

To this list could be added: nausea, vomiting, dry mouth, tinnitus, and hallucination.

Pitts and McClure (1967) suggest that a number of diagnoses—neurocirculatory asthenia, vasoregulatory asthenia, nervous tachycardia, effort syndrome, neurasthenia, Da Costa's syndrome, vasomotor neurosis, nervous exhaustion, and irritable heart syndrome—are all the same phenomenon differently named. The phenomenon, they suggest, is related to hyperventilation.

It is crucial to remember that the symptoms brought on by hyperventilation are *real*, even though they may not be due to an organic pathology. Patients who hyperventilate are not malingerers, nor are their symptoms conversion phenomena. The absence of an organic pathology does not mean that there is no physiological basis for the symptoms. Conversely, hyperventilation can occur in people who do have an organic disease. In those instances, the symptoms due to hyperventilation can either be independent of the illness or be the symptoms of that illness triggered or aggravated by the hyperventilation. For example, in a patient with asthma, hyperventilation can precipitate or aggravate an attack of symptoms. It can also bring on secondary symptoms such as anxiety, headache, and so on.

In patients with a physical illness, such as asthma, controlling the hyperventilation may help reduce the frequency or severity of the illness symptoms, such as asthma attacks. It should also help control the secondary symptoms. However, since most illnesses can also be affected by other factors, treatment for those factors will continue to be necessary.

Hyperventilation can relate to physical symptoms in three ways that can be schematically represented as follows:

1. There is no organic pathology and the reported symptoms can be traced to episodes of hyperventilation.

   hyperventilation ⟶ physical symptoms

2. There is an ongoing physical illness whose symptoms are being triggered or aggravated by hyperventilation; secondary symptoms may also be precipitated.

   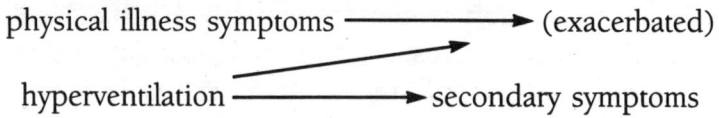

3. The symptoms of the physical illness trigger episodes of hyperventilation, which then affect the symptoms in a positive feedback loop. Secondary symptoms can also occur in this pattern.

   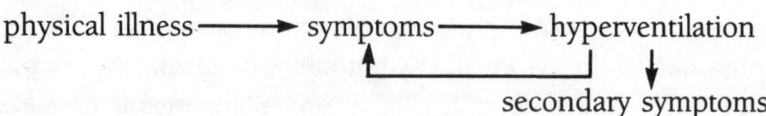

PSYCHOLOGICAL AND BEHAVIORAL SYMPTOMS OF HYPERVENTILATION

Just as one sees patients with physical symptoms that are due to hyperventilation, one also sees people with emotional or behavioral problems that have their roots directly or secondarily in faulty breathing habits. The direct effects of hyperventilation have been reported to include tension, free-floating anxiety, panic, depersonalization, derealization, depression, impulsive behavior, distractibility, nightmares, obsessions, and hallucinations. The secondary effects of hyperventilation include anxiety, depression, fear of dying, and dependency.

A case that illustrates the direct effects of hyperventilation is that of a young woman whom I had treated successfully for agoraphobia and who returned some years later seeking help for marital problems. These problems, it appeared, were exacerbated by the patient's barely controlled rages in response to even minor provocations. After each episode of rage the patient found herself unable to understand why she had reacted so strongly. She would resolve to control herself better in the future but was unable to do so. I decided to check the possibility that hyperventilation had something to do with the rages. I instructed the patient to overbreathe voluntarily and, within moments, she detected the onset of anger. Attention to abdominal breathing, especially during arguments, helped her to control her outbursts, and treatment then turned to other sources of the marital difficulties.

An example of the secondary effects of hyperventilation is a patient who was obsessed with the thought that he was going crazy. This thought both frightened and depressed him. Other than this obsession about insanity the patient showed no signs or history of psychological disturbance. He worked at a job he enjoyed, had a girlfriend with whom he was happy, and had realistic plans for the near-term future. As it turned out, the patient was a hyperventilator of long standing who had experienced rapid heartbeat, dizziness, and various muscle tensions for many years but had always ignored them. Shortly before his obsession started, however, one of his sisters died, an apparent suicide. After her death the patient learned that she had been diagnosed schizophrenic some time before. Now the hyperventilation-induced symptoms began to take on ominous meanings. The patient feared that he was showing the signs of impending schizophrenia and was doomed to follow in his sister's footsteps. The more he worried, the more frequent and intense the bouts of symptoms seemed to become. He reached the point where he was seeing an internist on an "emergency" basis almost once a week. Tranquilizers were tried but with little effect, and this frightened the patient even more.

I explained to the patient my hypothesis about hyperventilation and told him that in all likelihood he was misinterpreting the symptoms of overbreathing as symptoms of mental illness. This alone, as he later told me, proved to be enormously reassuring. I then proceeded to teach him how to relax and how to breathe abdominally. As the patient found that he could control his symptoms, his obsession about going crazy subsided. A call to his doctor confirmed the patient's report that he was no longer seeking emergency medical care as he had previously. In about three months, during which time the patient worked at his exercises extremely diligently, the problem was essentially cured and treatment was terminated.

In some patients, the secondary symptoms can become functionally autonomous, and treating the hyperventilation will not be enough.

For example, a patient of mine was terrified that he was growing a brain tumor because he experienced numbness, pain, and tingling on one side of his face and head. Extensive medical workups, including a CT scan, were negative but failed to reassure him. We demonstrated to him that we could affect the symptoms in the office by systematically changing how he breathed, and then we had him observe in real life how his symptoms were affected by tension and ensuing changes in his breathing. This demonstration began to persuade him that the problem was not what he feared. However, he had been worried for so long that, even after breathing retraining had significantly relieved the physical symptoms, it was necessary to work with a flooding approach in order to desensitize him to the obsessive thoughts.

Another patient whose major hyperventilation symptoms were nausea and dizziness was controlled by breathing retraining. However, he had become phobic to those sensations, so that when they were brought on, for example, by standing up too quickly or gagging on a piece of food, he became anxious. A course of desensitization was needed.

Patients with a history of panic can misinterpret the effects of hyperventilation as prodromal symptoms of panic and respond to them with a full-blown attack of panic that is, in essence, a self-fulfilling prophecy.

A young man I treated had his first panics after using illicit drugs. He subsequently became intolerant of even innocuous changes in bodily sensations, such as a stuffy nose when he had a cold. He was a chronic hyperventilator. Whenever he crossed the threshold and developed lightheadedness or dizziness he "knew" that a panic was on its way and, within a few minutes, would work himself up into a full-blown attack.

The effects of hyperventilation appear to be nonspecific—that is, they vary from person to person and maybe even within one person across time. Nevertheless, certain fears appear with some regularity in hyperventilators. They are variations on the theme of dying: a feeling of doom and an accompanying anticipation of dying; a fear of a fatal illness such as cancer or heart disease; and a fear of the death of somebody close to the patient. Fensterheim (1983) suggests that the first fear is a direct consequence of the physiology of hyperventilation. That is, sympathetic dominance is manifested by such sensations as muscle tension, sweating, and cold extremities, which lead to, or are experienced as, anxiety, fear, panic, or feelings of doom and depression. The second fear may be based upon the patient's misinterpretation of bodily cues, as in the cases I described above, or a reaction to repeated medical examinations that have failed to yield a satisfactory explanation or treatment—that is, no news is bad news. The third fear may be based upon a pattern of dependency that develops as a secondary consequence of the patient's symptoms. This is similar to what happens in phobic patients who acquire a "partner" without whom they cannot function and who they are, therefore, afraid of losing.

DIAGNOSING HYPERVENTILATION

As I have pointed out, there is a large discrepancy between the incidence of hyperventilation and the frequency with which it is diagnosed. Compernolle and colleagues (1978) have suggested five reasons for this discrepancy.

First, clinicians expect to see tetany as the primary symptom of hyperventilation, when, in fact, it is relatively rare. In its absence, the diagnosis frequently is not made.

Second, patients are usually seen between episodes of hyperventilation rather than during them. They tend to remember and describe the symptoms that most frightened them, such as chest pains, and fail to mention such symptoms as dizziness, paresthesia, numbness, air hunger, and so on that might be suggestive of hyperventilation. Unless the clinician specifically inquires about those symptoms, the diagnosis may be missed.

Third, the patient's avoidance of those situations in which he has learned that hyperventilation can occur may become the focus of his concerns. A diagnosis of phobia may therefore be made unless a careful assessment is carried out of the antecedents of the avoidance.

Fourth, because the symptoms of hyperventilation include impulsive acting out, exaggerated reactions that can appear to be bizarre, and hallucinations, a diagnosis of a major emotional or thought disorder may be made.

Fifth, hyperventilation has been given different names, such as *effort syndrome* and *neurocirculatory asthenia*, that suggest different etiologies. The name the clinician chooses, then, may orient him to a different body system than another name he might have chosen.

Finally, hyperventilation can be, as noted, subtle. Unless one is aware of the different forms hyperventilation takes, the diagnosis can be missed.

Besides the diagnostic problems described by Compernolle and co-authors, two others should be borne in mind. First, because hyperventilation can be triggered by a variety of antecedents, its symptoms are not infrequently attributed to the situations in which they occur rather than to the overbreathing itself. For example, if hyperventilation occurs during an argument, its symptoms may be taken as evidence of a fear of loss of control, as anxiety in the absence of appropriate assertiveness, and so on. If the overbreathing is noticed at all, it may be taken as further evidence of "underlying" anxiety.

Second, because hyperventilation can be subtle and have more than one antecedent, patients may not have noticed any pattern to the onset of their symptoms and may describe them as coming "out of the blue" (Fensterheim 1983). This leads to frequent misdiagnosis of the condition as hysteria.

I will illustrate some of these problems with two brief case descriptions:

Case History 1

> A young man in his mid-twenties had been referred to an anxiety disorders clinic by the most recent in a series of doctors whom he had consulted for treatment of "food allergies." The patient had suffered for years from chronic physical symptoms, including headache, running nose, stiffness in his back and joints, stomach cramps, indigestion, and rapid pulse. The symptoms were attributed by several doctors, traditional and nontraditional, to an exquisite sensitivity to almost every food other than the vegetables

and chicken that he largely subsisted on. His treatments had ranged from desensitization shots to exclusionary diets to, most recently, flower extracts. Each treatment appeared to offer some temporary relief. None achieved a cure. The doctor who made the referral, however, could find no evidence for allergies that would explain the clinical picture. He decided that he was dealing with an anxiety or psychosomatic disorder.

When I interviewed the patient he expressed skepticism about the usefulness of seeing a psychologist. He recited the findings of his numerous workups in a manner that suggested he was daring me to challenge the physical basis of his symptoms. He denied any emotional or behavioral triggers or aggravants of his symptoms and denied that he was particularly tense. The patient spoke in a breathy, nasal voice that he attributed to his latest bout of "allergies." He was very tall and thin and sat hunched over, partly because of a pronounced scoliosis, for which he had had surgery. His breathing was irregular, punctuated by sighs, and was clearly thoracic. I called this to his attention. To my surprise, he immediately acknowledged that he was a hyperventilator. I asked how he knew this, and he replied that several of his doctors had commented on his breathing and had called it hyperventilation. What advice had he been given regarding his breathing? "Calm down." I suggested that this might have been an oversight and explained a little about the effects of hyperventilation. The patient reacted with scorn. How, after all, could breathing cause food allergies? I replied that he was probably correct and that it would be extremely difficult to demonstrate any effect of his breathing on his symptoms. Would he, nevertheless, be willing to try some deliberate overbreathing? (I will describe this procedure in detail below.) The patient smiled as if he would be glad to show just how far off the mark I was and said he would try anything I suggested. I showed him how I wanted him to breathe and asked him to report any symptoms he might experience. He started to breathe as I had indicated, and within a minute he reported that he was starting to feel achy, congested, and dizzy. He also reported that his heart was racing.

Treatment was by means of breathing retraining, and the patient reported after a while, and with obvious reluctance, that he was able to tolerate more foods and that some of the stiffness in his back had eased. However, since he had started his flower extract treatment at about the same time, he insisted that it was, at best, a combination of those extracts and the breathing that was doing the trick.

Case History 2

A woman in her early forties consulted me at her husband's insistence, after more than two years of psychotherapy had failed to alleviate her symptoms. She told me she had been diagnosed as "borderline" and had been on major tranquilizers. Her complaint was of a pronounced sensation of heaviness in her head and a concomitant fear that she would not be able to hold her head up. She had seen a neurologist, an orthopedist, and a radiologist in addition to her psychiatrist, and no evidence of an organic disorder had been found.

As we talked, I observed that the patient sighed frequently and that her breathing was shallow and primarily thoracic. Checking by means of the technique I will describe below, I found that my impression was correct. Since nothing else seemed to account for her symptoms, I discussed with her the possibility that hyperventilation might be involved. Like the young man described above, this patient responded with skepticism. The problem, she said, could not be that simple. In her other therapy she had been exploring the meanings of her symptoms, and that made sense to her even if it did nothing to alleviate them. She agreed only reluctantly to have me demonstrate abdominal breathing and to try it during the next week.

When she returned for her second appointment, the patient said she had been practicing the abdominal breathing and a relaxation exercise that I had shown her and that, for the first few days, her symptoms did seem to improve. Now, however, they were back in full force and she was feeling discouraged. I reasoned to myself that she could not have mastered abdominal breathing in one week and I assumed that she had slackened off, despite the noticeable improvement. I told her, therefore, that learning was never a smooth process and that ups and downs were par for the course. I hoped that she would continue to practice for the next three weeks while I was on vacation, and I told her I would call her when I returned.

Three weeks later I called the patient. She told me with no little amazement and gratification that her symptoms were clearly getting better and that she was practicing diligently. My contacts with her thereafter were mainly by phone, and she continued to do well.

These examples hint at the various guises under which hyperventilation makes its appearance. In neither instance did the patient come in asking for help with his or her breathing, even though one patient had been made aware of his hyperventilation. In neither case was the hyperventilation dramatic and acute but rather chronic or intermittent low-level. In each case there would have been sufficient reason to pursue a different behavioral formulation and treatment plan. In all likelihood, however, the plan would have failed. At the very least, it would have been less efficient than the breathing management appeared to be.

To make the diagnosis in an office interview one can begin by simply asking, "Do you hyperventilate?" With surprising frequency the patient will answer, "Yes, I do," or "My doctor has told me that I do." In most instances, however, it will be necessary to elicit information about the effects of breathing changes by a detailed inquiry into the events that precede the onset of the patient's symptoms. One should be sure to ask specifically about the effects of such "respiratory behaviors" as laughing, coughing, sneezing, crying, shouting, reading aloud, sighing, and so on. One can also request that the patient keep a symptom log in which the events that precede and accompany the onset of symptoms are recorded.

One should ask what the patient has noticed about how episodes of symptoms end and what has brought relief. One looks for things that might restore normal breathing, such as lying down or taking a nap. One looks also for evidence that exercise has been associated with either relief from an episode of symptoms or a decrease in the frequency of episodes. This is because increased activity brings the metabolic needs of the body in line with the hyperventilatory breathing and thereby restores equilibrium.

The patient's medical history can also be a source of clues to the presence of hyperventilation. Physical symptoms that have resisted treatment or for which no clear physical basis has been established, and "doctor shopping" in a futile search for relief, should be regarded as such clues. If the patient is in treatment for physical complaints, a call to the doctor may elicit other clues. It may also help to alert the physician to the possibility of hyperventilation in his other patients.

During the interview the clinician will want to look for signs of hyperventilation by noticing the rate, depth, and regularity of the patient's breathing as well as the patient's tendency to breathe thoracically rather than abdominally. Should anything that the patient says, or the way he breathes, suggest hyperventilation, then more systematic observations of his breathing should be undertaken. Devices are available for making precise measurements of various breathing parameters. For most clinical purposes, however, they are largely unnecessary. Watching the patient carefully is enough, once one knows what to look for.

The patient should be seated comfortably, slouched with his chin resting on his chest. One of the patient's hands should be placed on his abdomen with his pinky just above the navel. His other hand should be resting across his chest just below the collarbone. Belts or clothing that constrict the abdomen should be loosened.

The patient is told to close his eyes and to breathe comfortably for a few minutes. I have noticed that many people find it hard to do that without becoming self-conscious and altering their breathing in the attempt to breathe "naturally." I have found it useful, therefore, to distract the patient by having him count backward in his head from 100 by threes. In less than a minute the patient usually settles down and observations can be made. What one wants to observe are the ratio of abdominal to thoracic breathing, rate and depth of breathing, and breathing irregularities.

The relative movements of the abdomen and chest are easy to see by watching the rise and fall of the patient's hands. In normal breathing the ideal ratio of abdomen to chest movement is about four to one. As far as rate is concerned, somewhere between twelve and fourteen breaths per minute is desirable. Anything over twenty breaths per minute is likely to be shallow and primarily thoracic. (During acute hyperventilation, the rate can exceed thirty breaths per minute.) Finally, as regards regularity of breathing, the clinician will want to note sighs, gasps, coughs, throat clearings, forced audible exhalations, breath holding, and abrupt changes in rate or depth of breathing.

If the patient's breathing is normal during the period of observation, an additional check should be carried out. The patient is asked to imagine something stressful or to remember his last episode of symptoms. Patients who breathe normally under the distraction instruction may begin to hyperventilate when they think of something stressful. If that happens, the patient is instructed to switch to a pleasant scene, and the time it takes for his breathing to return to normal is noted. Yet another check can be carried out by having the patient read or recite aloud.

When irregular or primarily thoracic breathing has been observed I have found it very useful to describe this to the patient and then to demonstrate it for him by reproducing his pattern myself. I then show him what relaxed abdominal breathing looks like. In order for the clinician to do this, of course, he must master abdominal breathing himself.

It will do little harm, in ambiguous cases, to lean toward a diagnosis of hyperventilation as part of the overall formulation. Teaching patients who are not in fact hyperventilators to be aware of abdominal breathing will have no negative effects. Underdiagnosing the condition, however, will perpetuate the problem for which the patient is seeking help.

The clinician can choose to have the patient hyperventilate voluntarily in the office as an acid test of whether such breathing affects the patient's symptoms. Symptoms triggered or exacerbated in this way can then be controlled by one of several techniques that will be described below. The demonstration can be quite dramatic. Compernolle and co-authors (1978), in fact, see this procedure as extremely reassuring to the patient and believe that it makes the patient highly receptive to the clinician's further interventions. Fried (1987), however, cautions against voluntary hyperventilation on grounds that it carries risk for patients, such as those with a history of coronary disease or seizure disorders. I have concluded that the risks involved in voluntary hyperventilation are not worth taking. As I suggested above, if hyperventilation is suspected, breathing retraining can do no harm. Furthermore, if there are beneficial effects, then, retrospectively, this will suggest the correctness of the diagnosis.

If the clinician opts for having the patient hyperventilate in the office, the procedure is as follows. The patient is told that an attack of hyperventilation will be deliberately induced. Compernolle and co-authors (1978) suggest that the exact procedure for doing so not be described in advance, so that the patient's anxious anticipation can aid in the production of a full-blown attack. The patient is then told to inhale deeply and rapidly and then to exhale forcefully, and to repeat this at least twenty times a minute. The patient can be standing or, if there is a history of fainting, lying down. Rate and depth are monitored by the clinician, and feedback is given until the desired rate and depth are achieved. The patient is then told to report the moment he begins to feel any of the symptoms for which he is seeking help.

According to Lum (1987), some symptoms will take longer to appear than others. However, when symptoms happen, it is usually within a minute or two. They can happen almost immediately. In any event, the provocation should not be continued for more than 4 minutes. If symptoms are reported, the provocation is stopped, and the patient is instructed to breathe abdominally or to breathe into a small paper or plastic bag kept on hand for that purpose until the symptoms subside. For most people this will be in about 3 minutes. For some, however, a longer recovery period is required and should be allowed for. People who during provocation do not develop the symptoms for which they are seeking help will probably report dizziness and lightheadedness anyway. This is perfectly normal and will pass rather quickly, once hyperventilation has stopped.

In summary, interview, observation, and provocation are used to investigate the possibility that hyperventilation is involved in the problem the patient brings in. Where these produce ambiguous findings, it is suggested that the clinician be rather over- than underinclusive in his diagnosis of hyperventilation. There are no ill effects related to breathing retraining, so a definitive diagnosis is not, strictly speaking, a necessity.

TREATING HYPERVENTILATION

There are three techniques that patients can learn to control hyperventilation-induced symptoms. Two are ameliorative and are used to control acute episodes of hyperventilation. The third corrects the patient's faulty breathing habits so that it prevents hyperventilation and its effects.

Ameliorative Techniques

Rebreathing

Hyperventilation is believed to cause symptoms because of an excessive loss of carbon dioxide from the blood relative to the patient's metabolic needs. The goal of rebreathing, therefore, is to arrest the loss of carbon dioxide during episodes when the patient's rate, depth, or pattern of breathing are off. To do this, the patient simply breathes into a small paper or plastic bag held in place over his mouth and nose. The patient does this for several minutes, removing and "shaking out" the bag every twelve breaths or so in order to prevent the depletion of oxygen from the air he is breathing. Patients can carry a bag with them in order to be prepared in the event of an episode of symptoms. The rebreathing technique is effective but purely ameliorative. It will do nothing to prevent the onset of symptom episodes.

Voluntary Exertion

Since hyperventilation is a matter of an excessive loss of carbon dioxide relative to the patient's needs, rapid, deep breathing during exertion will not have the same effect as it will when the person is at rest. Voluntary exertion, therefore, attempts to bring the patient's needs into line with the way he is already breathing, hoping thereby to restore equilibrium and alleviate symptoms.

The patient is instructed to engage in some form of moderately strenuous exercise when he feels the onset of his symptoms. Jogging in place, climbing stairs, or an isometric exercise are examples. The patient does this for about 3 minutes, by which time a noticeable improvement should have occurred. The technique should work especially well for patients who report that exercise has been associated with a reduction in their symptoms in the past. Like rebreathing, it is a purely ameliorative technique and will do nothing to correct the patient's faulty breathing habits or prevent the onset of symptoms.

Rebreathing and voluntary exertion should be taught early on, so that the patient will be able to cope with episodes of symptoms while he is learning to prevent them.

Breathing Retraining

Breathing retraining involves four steps: (1) making the patient aware of how he breathes and how his chest and abdomen feel when he is breathing thoracically and diaphragmatically, (2) teaching the patient to breathe primarily with his diaphragm, (3) teaching the patient to breathe rhythmically, at a normal and comfortable rate, while he is at rest, and (4) teaching the patient to breathe diaphragmatically while active or under stress.

There is no strict timetable to follow in accomplishing these steps. Some patients catch on quickly and progress smoothly in a matter of weeks. Others will take a year or more of supervised practice to reach the point where abdominal breathing is a habit. Few patients fail to learn to breathe diaphragmatically at all. Similarly few fail to report at least some relaxing effect of the retraining early on and some relief of their symptoms soon thereafter.

Building Awareness

The first step toward this goal is taken when the patient's breathing is observed and the results of the observation are fed back to him. The patient's attention is directed toward the relative movements of his two hands and toward irregularities that occur spontaneously or when stressful images are brought to mind. The therapist then demonstrates what, by contrast, diaphragmatic breathing looks like. The patient is urged at that point to try to copy the therapist's breathing. If he is successful, it will be very encouraging to him. If he fails to breathe abdominally, on the other hand, it will underline for him how deeply he has come to rely on thoracic breathing.

Some patients can be taught to breathe abdominally while they are sitting up. Many, however, find it easier to get abdominal movement while they are lying supine or in a fetal position. Whatever the patient's position, he is instructed to place one hand on his abdomen and the other across his chest, as described above. The therapist can place his own hand on the patient's hand and put pressure on the patient's abdomen while he is trying to breathe abdominally. Or, if the patient is supine, a heavy book can be put on his abdomen so that it provides a resistance against which the patient tries to breathe. The purpose is twofold. First, the pressure provides feedback to the patient as he moves his abdomen against the resistance. Second, the abdominal muscles may be strengthened by the requirement to work against that resistance.

If the patient has difficulty getting abdominal movement at the start of retraining, there are several ways in which he can be helped. First, while standing or sitting, he is instructed to put his hands on his hips with his thumbs almost touching behind him. He can also try to get his elbows as close together as he can behind him. If the reader will try this, he will find that the muscles of his chest are essentially locked and that the only way to breathe is abdominally. The patient is instructed to breathe this way for a few minutes and to study how the abdominal muscles feel.

A second way to facilitate abdominal movement is to have the patient get down on all fours. In this position, the abdomen is free to move, the chest is somewhat restricted, and abdominal breathing almost always happens as if by itself.

Throughout these maneuvers the patient can be encouraged to imagine that the air he inhales is going directly from his nose to his belly. He might visualize a balloon filling and emptying as he inhales and exhales.

When patients are getting started in breathing retraining, it is not unusual for them to report some discomfort. There are several reasons for this. First, they may be trying too hard to expand the entire abdomen, and they need to be told to concentrate on the upper part of the abdomen, between the navel and the rib cage. Second, simply focusing on breathing, which is normally done without conscious control, feels awkward and unnatural. It typically leads to some disruption in breathing. This is only temporary, however, and patients should be encouraged simply to bear with it until it passes. Third, it may take a while for the patient to settle into a comfortable rhythm and rate. In the meantime he may experience some air hunger. This is to be expected, and the patient can be forewarned and supported through it. Finally, the patient is using abdominal muscles that may have been underutilized, and this is likely to produce some temporary strain. The patient should be encouraged not to work those muscles too hard at the beginning, and he can be assured that the muscles will grow stronger with practice.

On rare occasions, patients will be encountered who simply cannot gain control of their abdominal muscles. For them the rebreathing or exertion techniques may have to serve the purpose of controlling symptoms when they occur. Or biofeedback, using end tidal carbon dioxide as the dependent variable, can be tried in hopes that the patient will discover some means of his own to achieve a proper balance.

Although it may seem unlikely, it is true that some patients have trouble telling their inhalations and exhalations apart. They become confused about when they should be expanding the abdomen and when they should feel it contracting. These patients can be helped by having them fill their lungs with air and holding their breath for about 10 seconds. When they let the air out all at once, they are instructed to focus on how the chest and belly feel as they "collapse."

Teaching Abdominal Breathing

Assuming that the patient can distinguish between inhalation and exhalation and can get abdominal movement reliably, the next step is to shape a thoracic/abdominal ratio of about four to one. For this the patient can be seated comfortably or lying in the supine or fetal position. He is reminded to breathe through the nose and to visualize his breath going directly into his abdomen. Care should always be taken to see that the patient's shoulders and arms are fully relaxed. Often, even if the patient appears relaxed, reminding him to let go of his shoulders and arms is followed by noticeably more loosening up. The patient is then asked to try to let his chest remain as motionless as possible and to breathe only with the muscles of the abdomen. The therapist's job is to observe, give feedback, and reinforce progress.

Achieving a Relaxed Rhythm and Rate

When the patient can breathe primarily with his abdomen, the focus shifts to achieving a rhythmic pattern of about twelve to fourteen breaths per minute. The patient should be told that it is possible to hyperventilate even abdominally if the rhythm, rate, or depth are pushed.

To begin establishing a relaxed rate, the patient is instructed to breathe along with the count given by the therapist: "Breathe in-two-three-four; out-two-three-four; pause and relax—in-two-three-four; out-two-three-four; pause and relax"—and so on.

The therapist should start his count somewhere close to the patient's rate and gradually shape it to the desired twelve to fourteen breaths per minute, giving support and reinforcement along the way.

After I have counted about ten to fifteen breaths, I usually suggest to the patient that he count in his head along with me. After another ten breaths or so, I tell the patient that I am going to leave out parts of the count and he is to fill in the gaps silently. In that way I gradually fade myself out and shift the timing to the patient, while I check on rate, depth, rhythm, and so on. If the patient changes the rate or starts to breathe irregularly, I will pick up the count until regularity has been restored and then let the patient try on his own again. It is useful to put the counting on tape so that the patient can practice on his own at home. I usually tape about 3 minutes of my counting aloud and another 3 minutes of the fading-out procedure.

Abdominal Breathing during Activity and Stress

The goal of breathing retraining is to re-establish abdominal breathing as the norm rather than as a technique to be used at certain times only. The typical sequence to follow in pursuit of this goal is as follows: abdominal breathing while lying down; sitting up; standing; walking slowly; walking at the patient's normal gait; walking more rapidly or climbing steps slowly. At each point in the sequence the patient is monitored, and feedback and reinforcement are given by the therapist. The patient can, to some extent, self-monitor by practicing whenever possible in front of a full-length mirror.

With regard to abdominal breathing under stress, the therapist and patient can construct a hierarchy of stressful scenes and then have the patient practice abdominal breathing as he progresses through the hierarchy, much as happens in systematic desensitization. The patient can then be instructed to attend to his breathing during in vivo stressful experiences and to try to breathe abdominally during mild stresses at first and then progressively more intense ones. With patients who have never been trained to relax systematically, I have found a modified Jacobson technique, or some form of imagery technique, to be a useful supplement to breathing retraining. Scripts for various relaxation techniques are readily available for the therapist to use.

Whatever has been accomplished during a training session can be given as a practice homework assignment. I usually ask for two 15-minute practice sessions a day. I find, however, that few patients are willing to put that much time into practicing. I suggest, therefore, that if they do not practice in 15-minute blocks, they try to practice four or five abdominal breaths each time they do some particular activity that is recurrent during the day. For example, the patient can tie practicing to phone calls, opening a book, going to the refrigerator, and the like.

EFFECTIVENESS OF TREATMENT

The success of breathing retraining is largely a function of the patient's motivation to master it. Given that motivation, together with adequate practice, the large majority of patients can be expected to benefit. Lum (1981) has reported that 70% of patients treated in his clinic over the years were completely symptom free after retraining, 25% had minor residual symptoms, and only 5% failed to benefit at all. Those figures, of course, were based upon observations of people who had no organic illness. In patients with physical illness the number of people who will be symptom free as opposed to less symptomatic will be smaller.

For example, I have seen people with chronic physical illness for whom breathing retraining provided a means of coping with their illness, even though no cure could be expected. The same will be true to some extent for patients who have significant emotional problems. Treating the hyperventilation will be one component of a more comprehensive treatment plan.

Treating hyperventilation is a satisfying experience for the therapist. Not only do the majority of patients show benefits as regards their symptoms, but they give the therapist an opportunity to see frustration and pessimism turn to confidence and optimism. This is an experience that every therapist will value.

REFERENCES

Compernolle, T., Hoodguin, K., and Joele, L. (1978). Diagnosis and treatment of the hyperventilation syndrome. *Psychosomatics* 19:612–625.

Fensterheim, H. (1983). *Hyperventilation: Magnifier and maintainer of phobias.* Paper presented at the Fourth Annual Conference of The Phobia Society of America, White Plains, NY.

Fried, R. (1987). *The Hyperventilation Syndrome.* Baltimore: Johns Hopkins Press.

Hofbauer, L. (1921). *Atmungs—Pathologie and Therapie.* Berlin: Julius Springer.

Huey, S. R., and Sechrest, L. (1981). Hyperventilation syndrome and psychopathology. Center for Research on the Utilization of Scientific Knowledge, Institute for Social Research, University of Michigan, manuscript.

Kerr, W. J., Dalton, J. W., and Gliebe, P. A. (1937). Some physical phenomena associated with anxiety states and their relationship to hyperventilation. *Annals of Internal Medicine* 11:961–992.

Lewis, B. I. (1959).Hyperventilation syndrome: A clinical and physiological evluation. *California Medicine* 91:121.

Lum, C. (1981). Hyperventilation and anxiety state. *Journal of the Royal Society of Medicine* 74:1–4.

——— (1985). Hyperventilation and pseudo-allergic reactions. In *PAR, Pseudo-allergic Reactions: Involvement of Drugs and Chemicals*, vol. 4, pp. 106–119. Basel: Karger.

——— (1987). Hyperventilation syndromes in medicine and psychiatry: a review. *Journal of the Royal Society of Medicine* 20:229–231.

Pitts, F. N., and McClure, J. N. (1967). Lactate metabolism in anxiety neurosis. *New England Journal of Medicine* 277:1329–1336.

Weiss, J. H. (1974). The current status of the concept of a psychosomatic disorder. *International Journal of Psychiatry in Medicine* 5:473–482.

16 Bibliotherapy

Dr. Weekes, an Australian psychiatrist, was the first to write self-help books on phobias. Despite her geographical and historical isolation, her books, with quaint titles such as *Peace from Nervous Suffering* and *Hope and Help for Your Nerves* are widely read and are regarded as among the most comforting, supportive, and useful of self-help books. It is not uncommon to find a copy of one of Claire Weekes's books in the handbag of an agoraphobic, to be read at difficult moments, or merely carried as a talisman against overwhelming panic.

This chapter gives a sense of the tone Dr. Weekes strikes that achieves such wide patient acceptance. Her key concepts are "first and second fear" and "floating through." She advocates facing the anxiety, experiencing it, and accepting it. Only by this means, without distractions, does the patient learn the dimensions of the panic and become able to tolerate it without fears of disintegration.

Bibliotherapy

Claire Weekes

Agoraphobia—the condition in which a patient suffers incapacitating anxiety in public places or anywhere outside his own home—is a common syndrome affecting thousands of people in Britain. Optimism in treating it is contrary to much current opinion. However, after many years of practice with a special interest in the anxiety state of which agoraphobia has often been a major symptom, and especially after the results of my last 10 years' experience concerned almost exclusively with treating agoraphobic people, an optimistic approach is in my opinion justified.

A brief outline is offered here of my method of treating agoraphobia. The special difficulty of treating the disorder is that inability to travel to the doctor's office is often so much part of the agoraphobic's illness that he may rarely, perhaps never, succeed in making the journey. In these circumstances, offering a satisfactory program of treatment and in addition giving the frequent encouragement and reassurance the agoraphobic patient needs present special difficulties; while to treat a patient adequately at home is surely asking too much from a busy practitioner.

The treatment described here overcomes these difficulties. It does not require the personal presence of the doctor. It is available when needed (which may be many times during one day) either at home, or away from home when the patient's agoraphobic fears are at their worst. In addition, the cost is negligible.

Treatment is in the form of two books (Weekes 1962, 1972), two long-playing records (Weekes 1967), quarterly magazines sent to 1,800 agoraphobic men and women in Great Britain and Ireland during the four years 1969–1972, and a cassette (Weekes, n.d.) for a small portable tape player. This remote "control" (perhaps "direction" would be a more accurate word) has made it possible to treat people living in distant parts of many countries.

The books are available in most libraries, the recordings and cassette are available from Charlotte Radeau, Living Growth Foundation, P.O. Box 48751, St. Petersburg, FL 33743, and the quarterly magazines (1969–1972) have been published in book form (Weekes 1972). In psychiatric clinics in Great Britain where the recordings are used, patients are encouraged to bring their tape recorders and make copies, and no objections are raised. The condition is explained to the patients in the following way.

EXPLANATION TO PATIENTS

Understanding by the patient of the cause of agoraphobia is essential for successful treatment, and the key lies in understanding the state in which the nervous reaction to stress is unusually intense and swift. This I term *sensitization*, and I explain that when mildly sensitized, nerves feel on edge and little things upset too much, too easily. Severe sensitization can be more disturbing, even alarming. An ordinary spasm of fear may be felt as an "electrifying" flash of panic, which may come in response to no more than the shock of a slamming door, or, more bewildering still, for no apparent reason other than thinking of it. A slightly quickly beating heart may feel like an acute attack of palpitations, irregular beats like a sudden descent in an elevator, a mild attack of faintness like impending death, and so on. Such intense responses so impress the sufferer he thinks they must be unique to him. He rarely recognizes them as part of the usual pattern of stress exaggerated.

Sudden severe sensitization can follow the shock of physical stress, such as a severe hemorrhage, a difficult confinement, or a surgical operation. Gradual sensitization may accompany continuous domestic stress or debilitating illness—anything that puts a patient under stress for a long time.

I also explain to patients that where a special problem has started the illness and helps to keep a person sensitized, understanding sensitization and knowing how to cope with it are themselves steps toward recovery, because the sufferer may become as much concerned with the state he is in as with the original problem. Sensitization resolves naturally if not kept alive by bewilderment and fear. Bewilderment acts by placing a sensitized person constantly under the strain of asking himself why he is like this, why he cannot be his old self, and what could happen next. The more he struggles to be the person he was, the more exasperation and tension he adds and so the more stress. While in his bewilderment he feels he cannot adequately direct his thoughts and feelings, he stands vulnerable to fear, which seems to overwhelm him before he has time to reason with it.

Sensitization, bewilderment, and fear are three reactions leading to an anxiety state of which agoraphobia, when present, is the most crippling symptom. Often the first attack of the disorder in a man or woman takes the form of panic or palpitations or severe dizziness or a feeling of weakness or collapse while out of doors. Such an attack probably follows any of a variety of stresses. If a woman (almost 90% of agoraphobic patients are women) has had a frightening attack of palpitations or a weak "turn" or panic while away from home and yet one day manages, in spite of this, to walk as far as the supermarket, how natural when immobilized in a long line at the checkout to be suddenly smitten with the fear of having one of her spells. The panic and mounting tension that follow may so stiffen her muscles that she may feel unable to move and may cling desperately to the nearest support.

After a few such attacks, she either avoids supermarkets—or any place where she feels restricted by a crowd—tries to take someone to shop with her, or becomes finally housebound when she discovers that "paralysis" may strike anywhere away from the house. When patients understand severe sensitization, what may have seemed incredible behavior becomes a more understandable human reaction.

PRACTICAL APPROACH

Some therapists search for a deep-seated cause for agoraphobia, believing that unless this is found and treated, the illness cannot be cured. In my experience, while finding an original cause for sensitization has been intellectually interesting, it has rarely been essential for cure. Agoraphobia persists because the habit of fear—and, because of this, sensitization—remain. This must be cured. The sensitized person has become afraid of so much. He sits near the door in a restaurant, at the back of the hall at a meeting, always leaving a way open for quick escape should, as he thinks may occur, his fear grow beyond him.

After relieving a patient's bewilderment by adequate explanation of his illness, I follow with a program of treatment based on the four principles of facing, accepting, "floating," and letting time pass. Many people sink deeper into their illness by doing the opposite. The nervously ill person notices each symptom with alarm and withdraws from it, afraid to examine it too closely for fear of making it worse. He may agitatedly seek occupation to try to force forgetfulness. This is running away, not facing. He may try to cope by tensing himself against unwelcome sensations, trying to "get the better of them." This is fighting, not accepting. "Floating" implies going along with the feelings without resistance, as if floating on the sea, submitting to the undulation of the waves. The thought of floating lessens tension that may inhibit action. Letting time pass is an important concept, since so many patients worry because much time has passed and they are still ill. They are impatient with time, and this impatience increases tension and anxiety.

COPING WITH PANIC

To help the patient cope with panic I explain that when he panics he feels not one fear, as he supposes, but two separate fears—a first and second fear. First-fear comes to any of us in response to danger. It is normal in intensity and passes with the danger. However, the "electric" flash of first-fear the sensitized person feels is so out of proportion to the danger causing it, he recoils and as he does so he adds a second flash—fear of the first fear. He may be more concerned with the feeling of panic than with the original danger. And because sensitization prolongs the first flash, the second flash may join in and the two fears seem as one. Though he may have no control over the first fear, and this is often true, with practice he can learn how to control the second fear—and it is the second fear that is helping to keep the first fear alive and keeping him sensitized and ill.

The agoraphobic person hemmed in at the school meeting has only to feel trapped to experience first-fear and then to immediately follow with second-fear and an urge to escape from the building. As the panic grows, he feels his mind go numb and is sure "something terrible" will happen. He does not understand that it is the second-fear he adds himself that may finally drive him to seek refuge outside.

To cope while inside the hall he should practice seeing panic through with as much acceptance as he can muster (usually aided by sedation in the early stages of treatment). It is important for him to appreciate that his body has a limited capacity to produce panic, so that panic always comes in a wave, which will pass if he waits. If he remains seated and tries to relax to the best of his ability, even lets his body slump in the seat and is prepared to let panic do its very worst, it will not mount. His sensitized body may continue to have flashes of panic from time to time, but these will be bearable and he will be able to see the function through. The realization that they have been bluffed by physical feeling has been enough to cure some people.

The patient should be taught the difference between true acceptance and just "putting up with." "Putting up with" means bearing panic with clenched teeth, hoping that it will "get it over quickly" and not come again. True acceptance means recognizing second-fear (which can be prefixed by "Oh, my goodness" and "What if?"), and adding as little as possible. It also means learning to regard panicking as yet another opportunity to practice coping with it until it no longer matters. This can be done. I have watched many agoraphobics come through panics to lasting cure in this way, even those who thought courage was not their strong point.

However, before a patient should be expected to face and accept his nervous symptoms (not only panic), they should be fully explained to him. While I hesitate to make the following elementary suggestions, I am reminded of the many anxious patients who have complained that they had never previously been given such explanations, and who began to recover afterward.

SPECIFIC SYMPTOMS

For example, I keep crackers in my surgery for the nervous person with difficulty in swallowing solid foods and hence with a habit of avoiding eating in public places. At the sight of a dry cracker he usually recoils. I then suggest that he chew, not swallow. As soon as the softened, moistened cracker reaches the back of his tongue, his swallowing reflexes take over and some of the cracker is automatically on its way down. When the patient understands that he needs only to chew and that swallowing will look after itself, some of the fear and tension go and swallowing becomes easier.

Again I hesitate to discuss such a common symptom as hyperventilation. However, I am reminded of a young girl sent to me by her general practitioner because she had been breathing shallowly almost constantly for a year. She entered my office in distress. I explained the respiratory center's automatic control of breathing, how it worked during sleep and unconsciousness. To illustrate its action I asked her to hold her breath as long as she could. When she found that she was soon forced to take a deep breath almost against her will, she appreciated the control beyond her control and saw the folly of her struggle. Some months later her doctor reported that she was cured. He had thought of every treatment except simple explanation. Every nervous symptom has explanation. It is not enough to say it is "only nerves."

RESPONSE TO TREATMENT

In my opinion dependence on constant medication to tranquilize nervous symptoms or on learning how to avoid having them—for example, avoiding waiting in a line—carries the danger of leaving the patient vulnerable to the return of symptoms at any time, in any place. Dr. Isaac Marks has stressed the disadvantages of the unexpected return of panic after weeks of present-day treatment of agoraphobia by medical desensitization (Marks 1969). A patient must be taught to cope with his symptoms. If a technique needs a name, perhaps mine could be called *coping through understanding*.

There are many ways to help understanding beside those already mentioned—for example, stressing the difference between testing and practicing. The thought of testing brings tension, whereas the thought of practicing holds no urgent demand. Also, testing followed by failure brings an acute sense of defeat, whereas failure while practicing means merely the necessity to practice again.

Again, it helps the sufferer to understand that the symptoms of stress are part of life and that the illness is their exaggeration in his sensitized body, not simply their occurrence; that therefore cure lies not in their complete elimination, as he probably believes and hopes, but in their reduction to normal intensity.

RELAPSE

Even months after a patient is desensitized and thinks he is cured, the sudden return of his symptoms in an exaggerated way in response to stress can so shock the sufferer he may think he has "slipped right back." He should be taught to understand the traps memory can set and try to accept the setbacks it may bring, until he knows the way out of setbacks so well that he no longer fears the way in. Indeed the definition of recovery should include having setbacks and knowing how to cope with them, so that neither doctor nor patient becomes too discouraged by them.

In this short chapter I have not mentioned the complications sometimes associated with agoraphobia: indecision, suggestibility, loss of confidence, feeling of unreality, feeling of disintegration, obsession, and depression. These too may develop following a set, logical pattern, and this pattern, with treatment, is discussed in my books and recordings.

Finally, I stress that repetition of advice is the crux of treatment of the agoraphobic. He finds achievement difficult because he remembers past failures and how he felt then, so that when he thinks of facing similar experiences, his reactions are automatically those of withdrawal, fear, and despair. With enough repetition of the right advice new association paths are established, which ultimately replace the old automatic flashback reactions of panic and withdrawal when the patient is stressed. I call this *right reaction-readiness* and know of no better way of establishing it than by using records and cassette tapes, which can not only be played immediately before the patient sets out to practice but also while he is out.

RESULTS

In 1970-1971, questionnaires were filled in by 528 agoraphobic people in Great Britain and Ireland whom I had treated for periods varying from a few months to 6 years using the method outlined above, without any personal contact. Of these, 60% had been agoraphobic for 10 years or more and 27% for 20 years or more, so that most could be classed as chronic agoraphobics. For their present illness 65% had had treatment from one or more psychiatrists and 30% from their general practitioner alone. Previous treatment had included almost every known orthodox method. This group offered a challenge to treatment without the personal supervision of a doctor.

Of the patients aged 14-29, the results were satisfactory or good in 73%; of those aged 30-39 similar good results were found in 67%, and in those aged 40-49 in 55%. Of the older and therefore more difficult group aged 50-74, good progress was made by 49%. As so many of these people were chronically ill (only 27 had been ill for less than 3 years), the chances of spontaneous recovery irrespective of treatment were negligible.

REFERENCES

Marks, I. M. (1969). *Fears and Phobias*. London: Heinemann.
Weekes, C. (1967). *Hope and Help for Your Nerves* (record album). Charlotte Rudeau, Living Growth Foundation, P.O. Box 48751, St. Petersburg, FL 33743.
—— (nd). *Moving towards Freedom and Going on Holiday* (cassette). Charlotte Rudeau, Living Growth Foundation, P.O. Box 48751, St. Petersburg, FL 33743.
—— (1972). *Peace from Nervous Suffering*. London: Angus and Robertson.
—— (1962). *Self Help for Your Nerves*. London: Angus and Robertson.

17 Marital Therapy

There is a considerable literature on the role of the family in agoraphobia and in other phobias. The psychodynamic literature notes that the agoraphobic expresses both sides of her conflict in the symptom. For example, a wife who limits her husband's freedom excessively by her fears of uncontrollable panic if not with him, might express both sides of the separation issue—both her intense dependency and her rage. The concept of secondary gain brought by the symptoms is also frequently noted in the psychodynamic literature, as in the case of the unassertive agoraphobic wife exerting control over her husband through her symptoms. Though this concept is rarely found in today's literature on phobias, the tangle of interdependencies in agoraphobic relationships has led many therapists to work directly on the marriage as a means of ameliorating the phobic symptoms.

This chapter explores the diverse facets of treatment of the family. Dr. Friedman promotes marital therapy as an adjunct to in vivo desensitization. The marital or other crucial dyadic relationship is seen as providing a primary source of resistance to therapeutic change and is addressed specifically to revise that limitation. This has the added benefit of lowering the dropout rate; it addresses the needs of the patient and at the same time does not make the spouse feel at fault. The chapter provides an excellent format for sensitivity to the plight of the phobic partners.

Marital Therapy

Steven Friedman

MARITAL THERAPY AS AN ADJUNCT TO BEHAVIORAL TREATMENT OF AGORAPHOBIA

In vivo desensitization treatment for agoraphobia, based on a social learning model, has met with remarkable success (Emmelkamp and Kupiers 1979, Mathews et al. 1981). The treatment, often implemented in a group setting, involves educating the patient to the nature of anxiety, fear, and the "fear of fear" cycle, teaching the patient various coping skills, and gradually exposing patients to different anxiety-producing situations, while they learn how to cope with the resulting anxiety (Chambless and Goldstein 1980).

While behavioral treatment of phobic states is generally found to be effective for 75% of the patients, this rate is for patients who agree to and complete the treatment. When initial dropouts and early terminators are considered, the overall effectiveness may be lowered to 51% (Barlow and Wolfe 1981). While additional success in the behavioral treatment of agoraphobia may be achieved by further study of in vivo techniques, the integration of systems theory with a behavioral model provides for a more comprehensive treatment. Such an integrated approach helps decrease dropouts by engaging the family in a supportive role during the early part of the treatment process and potentially allows for more intensive treatment when clinically indicated.

The role of the patient's family in this syndrome continues to be a source of controversy in the behavioral literature (Barlow et al. 1984, Cobb et al. 1980, Goldstein 1970, Hand and Lamontague 1976). A range of clinical reports suggests that agoraphobia is typically triggered by marital distress (Milton and Hafner 1979). It is argued that the symptom formation resolves or at least contains an emerging marital conflict in a highly enmeshed family by binding the spouses in a "compulsory marriage" (Fry 1962). Also widely noted is the impression that the inadequacies and covert symptomatology of spouses is obscured by the identified patient's phobia. In such a view any effective treatment for the phobia poses a threat to the equilibrium that the symptom has purchased. The evidence for this view is inconclusive and often contradictory (Agulnik 1970, Barlow et al. 1981, Cerny et al. 1987, Hafner 1977, 1982, Mathews et al. 1981).

To decrease the dropout rate and improve the overall efficacy of in vivo exposure I have found it useful to apply a family systems approach to complement the behavioral model. This perspective has helped clarify the ways in which phobics tend to embroil others, especially their spouses and their therapists (Friedman 1985, 1987), in transactions that reinforce their phobias.

Whatever the cause of disharmony in phobic families, it is clear that once established, this disharmony can function as a significant reinforcer for the agoraphobic syndrome. It can be hypothesized that much of what has been observed in phobic marriages can be understood as a consequence of the phobia. Agoraphobics tend to "draw out" particular responses from others. The resulting transaction does indeed "cause" the phobia, in that it functions as a persistent reinforcer. This pattern will have a profound effect on any therapeutic intervention.

I will outline a treatment approach that is adjunctive to the usual in vivo exposure for the individual patient (Emmelkamp 1982). This approach may help resolve the contradictory advice given in the behavior literature, which suggests including the family as agents of change (Mathews et al. 1981), or excluding them because family therapy will make things worse (Emmelkamp and Van Der Hout 1983). Indeed the treatment I will describe might well be termed *psychoeducational marital therapy for agoraphobia* (e.g., Anderson 1983).

Such an approach steers a middle ground between viewing phobic symptoms solely within an individual or family context. To take a completely individual approach in the treatment of agoraphobia would be to ignore family system issues that are present in many cases. At the same time to view phobic symptoms primarily from a systems point of view can lead one to look for family dynamics that may not be present in every case. In addition, it is quite clear that at present a broad-based behavioral treatment is the psychotherapeutic treatment of choice for working with agoraphobics, and a systems perspective may enhance but should not replace this approach.

THE INTERPERSONAL MANEUVERS OF THE AGORAPHOBIC

Chambless and Goldstein (1980) hypothesized that frank agoraphobia in adulthood emerges when a person with the agoraphobic predisposition experiences a traumatic life event. Any life event that makes the outer world more dangerous, or the home less safe, can trigger the illness. Thus familial events, such as marital conflict, are only one of a series of phenomena that can result in agoraphobia. Other such crises may include the birth of a child, graduation, promotions, deaths, and so on.

Regardless of what event triggers the acute onset of panic and avoidance, once a person has become agoraphobic there is a tendency to regard significant others as either safety-producing companions or as cruelly indifferent, even punitive individuals. The marital partner may then be "pulled" into shadowing the patient and thereby alleviating the patient's anxiety but reinforcing the phobic behavior. Conversely, the partner may become punitive and reject accompanying the patient, which would increase anxiety and similarly reinforce the phobic avoidance. Commonly these patterns of response alternate, leaving both the phobic patient and partner embroiled in a circular transaction associated with declining marital satisfaction, mutual resentment, and entrenched symptomatology.

As noted, in response to such urgent polarized requests from the agoraphobe, significant others tend to respond in a parallel polarized manner. It is important to underscore the point that requests for help from the agoraphobe are often polarized between these two extremes of either "care for me" or "cure" me. These requests, polarized as they are between complete "dependence" or "independence" (Guidano and Liotti 1983), result in family members' responding in an equally polarized manner. The spouse may act in an either a totally nurturing manner, thereby encouraging a dependent role, or a cold, pushy, rejecting manner, thereby encouraging an unrealistic independent role. When family members enact either of these two polarized roles, the phobia becomes further entrenched. To be a safety-producing companion is to reinforce or reward the phobic behavior and erode the patient's capacity to master separation anxiety. On the other hand, to become a spokesman for a traumatic degree of separation also fosters the need to cling to companions and safe places. Despite the pathogenic impact of either response, the urgency of the phobic's requests makes an alternate or neutral response quite problematic. Thus a response of silence, or an attempt to "leave the field" as the phobic expresses anxiety will be experienced as abandonment. An expression of understanding, on the other hand, can be received as a sanction for avoidant behavior.

Observations of the marital relationship have invariably shown an alternation between these patterns of responses. Followed over time, however, there is a marked tendency for the relationship between phobic and spouse to become increasingly unhappy and hostile. The phobic behavior is then met by the companion with the very withdrawal and consequent threats of separation that heighten the phobic anxiety (Bowlby 1973). This cycle may become structured and can act as a powerful resistance to treatment. The resistance to change in agoraphobics and the complications of their interpersonal relationship has been alluded to in the literature (i.e., Hand and Lamontague 1976).

The readiness with which the companion will respond in these polarizing maneuvers is certainly dependent upon the companion's own personality and situation. For example, a covertly phobic spouse, with no extrafamilial involvements, is more likely to embrace the role of nurturing companion and to discourage the patient's efforts to venture out alone. Similarly a spouse without strong dependency needs of his or her own and a favorable job situation is more likely to "push" counterphobic behavior and to be unsympathetic to the patient's pleas. Only with strong support can the "normal" spouse resist these pulls. The treatment strategy that will be outlined is aimed at providing the spouse with the necessary support to resist the phobic's "pull," countering it instead with alternative behavioral responses that can lead to a gradual diminishing of the phobia. The method described here is aimed at developing a collaborative set in couples before and during the behavioral treatment of the agoraphobic patient.

TREATMENT APPROACH

Since it is assumed that the phobia has reshaped and rigidified marital interaction, the initial family intervention focuses on clarifying the phobia's impact on the family and offering the treatment as a way out of the phobic "double bind." This interview is meant to help develop the collaborative set with the agoraphobic couple.

Stage One: Initial Family Contact

Goal: Joining with the Spouse by Keeping the Focus on the Patient

Since most agoraphobes are unable to travel alone, almost all arrive with their spouses. We introduce ourselves to both members of the couple, but we initially exclude the spouse and take a detailed individual history from the patient. We purposely exclude the partner for the major part of this initial session to highlight our focus on the phobia and the in vivo exposure treatment. The central focus of this initial evaluative session is on the phobic and not on the partner. Any role the spouse may have in either the etiology or maintenance of the symptoms is explored in a later session.

In this initial evaluation we do a general behavioral assessment, which focuses on the detailed aspects of the symptomatology, the onset of the illness, its course, and so on. However, at the end of this evaluation we invite the partner in for a few minutes. At this point we discuss with the two of them the nature of the patient's disorder and briefly attempt to get "information the partner has to offer about the phobia." It has routinely been our experience that at this point the spouse is usually eager to either give information about the patient or blame the patient for the illness. Invariably spouses feel constrained by the time limitation, and we set up a "special appointment so that you can fill us in on your observations of the phobia." We make it explicit that they will be "part of the treatment team" and that "history giving" is their first contribution. This session focuses on information gathering and not on "blaming" anyone for the development of the symptoms.

We have found that spouses have long histories of negative contacts with mental-health professionals. They have either been ignored and left to fend for themselves in an intolerable situation or treated in a covertly as well as overtly hostile fashion. Including the spouse in the treatment team is an alternative to either excluding them entirely or labeling them as part of the problem. In this way a therapeutic alliance is facilitated and resistance to marital treatment, if later indicated, will be minimized. Traditional family systems interventions that frame the symptom as metaphor and solution for dysfunctional family structure are contraindicated in this model (Stedman and Murphy 1984).

Case Example

Mrs. A., a 32-year-old Italian-American housewife, presented to the clinic with an 8-year history of agoraphobia. Her symptoms had worsened over the past 8 months, and she could not leave the house except in the company of her husband. Mr. A. entered the first session obviously ill at ease. He began by saying that he had already had "marriage therapy" and "didn't want any more." We informed him that this was not "marriage therapy," but that as the closest observer of his wife he might be able to provide further information. We told him that our success rate was higher when the spouse was part of the treatment team. We also told him that we would be glad to offer specific suggestions about how to "help his wife get better." Nonetheless, we stressed that the main treatment would be the in vivo exercises and that we would be glad to tell him all he wished to know about this treatment. At this point Mr. A. appeared to relax. Answering a question that hadn't been asked, he said, "I don't see how they could have blamed me for her phobia. She had it before I met her. All the other therapists did was add insult to injury."

As this case example illustrates, the crux of our approach is to enlist and encourage the cooperation of the spouse in our treatment. We have found that this is possible only when we take the onus of the agoraphobic's problem, and "cure," off his or her shoulders. We let the spouse know, in no uncertain terms, that they are not the patient, that they (the spouse) will not be "blamed" or "belittled," and that we respect their knowledge about the agoraphobic and their problems. We let the spouse know that we will look to them for their help in providing comprehensive treatment.

Stage Two: The Structured Family Interview

Goal: Reframing the Dysfunctional Transaction

The second session is a semistructured interview (see Table 17-1), that includes both partners. In this session we review the spouse's understanding of the cause and meaning of the phobia and the impact of the phobia on the marriage. While many

---

TABLE 17-1 The Semistructured Family Interview

1. Introduction
   Explain that the purpose of the family interview is to:
   a) Secure information about the phobia to help the treatment.
   b) Learn how the phobia is affecting each family member.
   c) Answer questions about the phobia and its treatment.
2. The symptoms
   a) Ask the patient to describe the symptoms, their time course, and what makes them better or worse.
   b) Ask each family member individually their observations of the symptoms, their time course, and what makes them better or worse.
   c) Ask the patient and each family member what they think causes the phobia.
   d) Ask the patient and each family member what solutions they have tried.
   e) Ask about a family history of phobias and other emotional problems.
3. The Impact on the family
   a) Ask each family member (including patient) what behavioral and emotional changes have resulted from the phobia.
4. The impact of change
   a) Ask each family member (including patient) what positive results would occur for the family if the patient's symptoms got better.
   b) Would there be any negative effects of improvement?
5. Recent stresses
   Especially at time of symptom occurrence.
6. Explain treatment
   In vivo work and any family involvement.
7. Answer questions
   About the phobia, the treatment, and family involvement.

spouses are quick to deny a loss of love for the spouse, we emphasize the negative effect the agoraphobic syndrome has on the marriage and other family members. The stated therapeutic goal of the session is to "help the family with the phobia." An attempt is made to understand the onset of the phobia, as well as the subsequent unfolding within the marriage.

Our focus during this evaluation helps the family develop cognitive clarity about the phobic process by delineating, first, the onset of the phobia and, second, the impact of the evolving phobia on the relationship. This division is rarely made by marital partners themselves. That is, they tend to confuse the onset of the phobia, which may occur from extrafamilial sources as well as intrafamilial forces, with the subsequent unfolding of the phobia within the marriage.

The goal of the evaluation is to determine the degree to which the spouse is responsive to the phobic symptoms. Some spouses can remain relatively calm and supportive through the most dramatic displays of panic and avoidance. Others will send for an ambulance at the first sign of a palpitation. Still others will become enraged at any indication that the spouse is experiencing anxiety. A partner will often discover that the question of who is imprisoned by the symptoms becomes increasingly moot as the entire family becomes concerned and preoccupied with the patient's fears. Often partners who are hostile to the patient can easily become solicitous when they sense the genuineness of the patient's symptoms and the degree to which the symptoms are out of the patient's conscious control.

The greater the phobic companion's responsivity to the symptoms—positive or negative—the more intensive is the marital treatment that we will prescribe. However, in this interview the aim is to reframe the spouse's response in a positive manner.

Spouses who clearly covertly encourage avoidant behavior are labeled "sensitive," "caring," and "soft-hearted." Spouses who more or less belligerently espouse facing the phobic situation immediately are termed "action oriented," "very strong-minded people," or "very anxious to help the patient get over this quickly." Clearly relabeling a spouse's approach in this manner is experienced by the spouse as supportive and ego syntonic and will often result in a very positive therapeutic alliance. In addition, the agoraphobe is encouraged to view their spouse's approach to their problem in a more positive manner. At the same time we are laying the groundwork for the agoraphobic to work on their symptoms in our in vivo group, with their partner's support and encouragement but to be realistic and not to rely on their partner to "cure" or always care for them.

However, we point out to the family that neither response, the overly "soft" or "hard" approach, has been helpful and, in fact, both invariably reinforce the syndrome. It is then suggested that much of their recent marital distress can be traced to these "well-meaning efforts" of the spouse to help. Ultimately we suggest and discuss ways in which the spouse and patient can experiment with alternative interactions.

Case Example 1

A year before presenting at the clinic, Mr. B. lost his job, shortly after his employer died. Mr. B. had become increasingly distraught as he failed to find alternative employment. His symptoms began apparently in response to his job loss and the death of a boss whom he "loved." His wife became frustrated and resentful at having to carry the financial burden of the family. She tended to ignore Mr. B. at home as she became "fed up" with telling him to "just forget about your fears and go out." In the initial evaluation Mr. B. claimed that his symptoms and agoraphobia were caused by his wife's "coldness," even though the marital distress had begun after the onset of Mr. B's increasing phobic avoidance.

During the interview the sequence of events was clarified, and it was suggested that "Mrs. B. was trying to help in the best way she could think of." Mrs. B. piped in, explaining her approach. She had "gotten off" alcohol after 10 years by going "cold turkey," and she wished Mr. B. could do the same with his phobia. We suggested that since her efforts had not worked and since she had accumulated a great deal of experience trying to help Mr. B., we would appreciate her "joining the treatment team." We suggested that we would meet biweekly to review our "respective strategies."

Case Example 2

Mr. C. was a computer programmer who, after receiving a promotion, began having panic attacks and subsequent difficulty traveling to work. His wife, who had no friends of her own and was "stuck home" alone with their 2-year-old infant, was very "understanding." In fact, Mr. C. claimed his wife "wants me to stay home. If I feel a slight twinge of panic she will say, 'You have all that sick leave built up. Why don't you use it?'"

Mrs. C. vehemently disagreed with this formulation and pointed out that "just last week I screamed at you for an hour to go to work and even poured ice water on you to get out of bed."

Again, we clarified the sequence of events and pointed out that Mrs. C. was generally a "very caring and soft-hearted person who tries to help by not pressuring you in any way. However, she is only human, and when she suddenly realizes you can lose your job, she panics. She then will do anything to get you going."

Clarifying the sequence of events in the development and maintenance of the agoraphobic symptoms, as in these two cases, is helpful in defusing a great part of the marital tension that exists in these families. We have found that the atmosphere in the family can often change quite dramatically from a hostile punitive one with much mutual resentment to an atmosphere of collaboration between the partners. There is the implicit message in our approach that the agoraphobic's problem resides, for the most part, in the agoraphobe but that the symptoms touch everyone in the family. The family can become hostile or overly solicitous, but it is "normal" for patients and their spouses to fall into these extremes.

A purely individual perspective, either psychoanalytic or radically behavioral, that focuses solely on the patient and ignores the spouse, often leaves the spouse with the feeling that he/she is being left behind. Spouses can often feel slighted, and consequently in very subtle ways they undo any treatment success. At the same time a pure systems approach can implicitly, or explicitly, blame and disparage the spouse. Clearly these extreme approaches, which in our experience most mental-health professionals adopt either overtly or covertly, damage the relationship between the spouses and enhance the collaborative working alliance among patient, spouse, and treatment team. After this initial session both patient and partner often feel that their own viewpoints have been acknowledged and understood by the therapist. This alliance paves the way for any further interventions.

Stage Three: Education

Goal: Cementing the Alliance

We then offer the couple in this session a "private tutorial" on agoraphobia and its treatment. Our goal is to decrease marital conflict and encourage the feeling that they are indeed part of the treatment team. We review the symptoms of a panic attack (the heart palpitations, dizziness, weakness in the legs, rapid breathing and pulse, and so on) and their relative invisibility to the outside observer. We outline "normal responses" to the panic attack, such as returning to a safe place or person that guarantees immediate relief. We explain the "fear of fear" cycle, in which the anticipated anxiety leads to progressive avoidance and ultimately to a spiral of increasing anticipatory anxiety and panic attacks.

We address a great deal of our education toward the spouse. In our experience, the patients are quite aware at this point in their illness of the role of the panic, their avoidance, and the "fear of fear" cycle. Though they might not have labeled it quite this way, they can readily understand it with reference to their own experience. It is the spouses who are mystified by apparent sudden changes in their partner's behavior.

We then describe as part of the syndrome the characteristic responses of others. Just as the agoraphobe has symptoms, so does the companion. For example, companions themselves can become anxious and hostile when the panic attack begins or when it is anticipated. We term these "sympathetic responses" that express their identification with the patient and are designed to help the patient overcome the phobia.

We make the spouse's response a part of the patient's illness. That is, we say that it is "part of agoraphobia for the spouses to react in either an overly 'infantilizing' way or to respond with an 'indifference and hostility.'" At this point, we ask the spouses what responses they have noticed in themselves when the patient was anxious. Our attitude to the spouse's production is one of understanding. We are constantly reframing these responses as an inevitable part of the agoraphobic syndrome—inevitable, because the spouse both desires to help the patient and yet feels helpless to respond in any way other than the overly infantilizing or the overly angry ways. At this point we suggest to the spouse that our treatment will help him/her learn alternate ways to respond to the patient's anxiety.

For example, with Mr. and Mrs. B. we found it helpful to point out that while "being strong-minded was necessary to overcome alcoholism, in dealing with panic attacks and agoraphobia a strong mind is not sufficient." We explained to Mrs. B. that in "overcoming agoraphobia you need to learn many things. You need to learn ways to use various coping mechanisms, such as slow breathing, relaxation exercises, and different cognitive strategies, and then to very gradually learn to use these techniques in overcoming the phobia. We will teach you (Mrs. B.) how to be helpful in this difficult, almost impossible situation."

I believe that this approach, while similar to the one described by Mathews and colleagues (1981), goes beyond just using the spouse as a "therapist's aide." These authors, in fact, through the use of written manuals, attempt to minimize therapist time and involvement. While this approach will work with some couples, it has been our experience that simple instructions for self-exposure may not be enough. We have found in our work with patients, particularly those who have been symptomatic for over a year, that the marital system has developed a homeostatic balance, and any attempt to change the status quo evokes the usual homeostatic response of families to restore a threatened equilibrium. In our approach the therapist enters the system and attempts to change the equilibrium between the two partners. He does so by the nature of his interventions. These interventions are framed in a psychoeducational manner. This framework serves to minimize the resistance that may be expected in more direct attempts to change the marital system.

The evaluation of the relative's hyperresponsiveness to the patient's symptoms is often ongoing, but in situations where the spouse does not appear to have become intensely involved in the patient's phobia, no further interventions are necessary with the family. Instead, the spouse is told that the patient will be given exercises in in vivo exposure groups, which will require his/her cooperation, and we assume he/she will be involved in a positive manner.

During the in vivo group experience the therapist and group will generate homework assignments that can be done alone or with the aid of the spouse. We encourage spouses to follow the lead of their phobic partner. For example, if at all possible, we encourage them to respond with assistance if directly asked. If they observe the patient not practicing assignments, their task is to only *once* gently remind the patient of the necessity for continuous exposure and practice. The attitude that we encourage the spouse to adopt is very much our own—one of understanding toward the symptoms and phobic avoidance coupled with gentle encouragement to change. Ultimately only the patient has the responsibility and ability to change. As behavior therapists we often help structure for our patients gradual separations, rather than encouraging avoidance or pushing counterphobic behavior. We encourage spouses to adopt this attitude and approach with their phobic partner.

In our experience couples have universally responded with relief and gratitude to this routine initial evaluation. Both patient and partner feel understood and leave the sessions with a sense of unity as well as an understanding of their possible roles in the treatment. In our in vivo exposure group, as noted above, we continue to encourage the patients to involve their spouse as "a more cooperative and teaching partner."

In this initial evaluation we also attempt to elicit the couple's prediction about the effects of successful treatment on their relationship. Uniformly we have found couples can only think of "good effects." Commonly described is the sense of having more freedom, the ability to do things together more frequently, and the strength, if need be, to attempt to do things on their own. However, we do not accept blind cheery optimism. We at times playfully suggest that there may be some "very bad things happening temporarily to your relationship."

We describe this "potential crisis" to the couple as a normal phenomenon experienced by all our couples. We explain that ultimately all of our couples successfully negotiate this crisis point. We point out to the family that by the nature of their characteristic polarized responses they have been discouraged from finding a "more middle-ground position." We suggest to them that during the course of the treatment their relationship may need to be altered, because they have been caught in these responses for a number of years. In addition, we believe such statements tend to co-opt possible sabotage. However, in cases where clinically indicated, the couple is immediately invited to weekly or biweekly "couple meetings to identify the patient's problematic areas at home and devise tasks to overcome them." We should emphasize that this way of joining with spouses has led to almost universal spouse acceptance of subsequent participation in our more intensive marital treatment.

Case Example

Mr. and Mrs. A., when asked the question described above, insisted that "it would be wonderful to feel a sense of freedom and relief." Mr. A. felt that he would be quite happy becoming assertive and phobia free, while the patient felt that "our relationship can only get better." However, Mrs. A. was extremely attractive and an openly seductive woman. She dressed in a style that was much younger than her stated age. She also exhibited flirtatious behavior with both the therapist and members of our staff. The therapist playfully suggested that "if your wife really got better and you went to work, you wouldn't always be sure that she was home. She is a lively and intelligent woman and if she didn't have this fear, who knows what fun she could have." Mr. A. carefully and somberly considered this statement, though he didn't openly comment upon it. Mrs. A. on the other hand was quite visibly pleased and laughed seductively at this comment.

Stage Four: In Vivo Exposure Group

Goal: Changing the Relationship by Keeping the Focus on the Patient

For the majority of our patients the primary and often only treatment will be our in vivo exposure group. During these group sessions patients are taught a variety of coping skills and are accompanied while they face their fears. Since the nature of in vivo exposure suggests slow, gradual adaptation to previously feared situations, the patients are encouraged to enlist the support of their spouse, extended family, and friends in practicing skills and tasks learned in the group treatment as well as in trying out new, novel stimuli.

Through the course of treatment part of the group discussion will often focus on members' reports on the reactions of significant others to their new behavior. It has been our experience that by and large most spouses may initially have trouble adjusting to a more independent and assertive spouse, but they will ultimately reward and appreciate a less phobic partner.

Stage Five: The Couple Tasks (When Indicated)

Goal: Changing the Relationship through Graded Separations

For those families who upon initial evaluation seem hyperresponsive to the patient's symptoms and seem to require more than our psychoeducational approach, as well as families for whom severe marital conflicts are uncovered by our in vivo exposure, the family is instructed in this segment of the treatment to discuss areas of difficulty that they encounter at home. These meetings are often assigned biweekly. For example, a spouse may complain that the patient refuses to accompany him to an important business gathering, or a patient may complain that the spouse "bullies me" or "just walked out on me." These issues then become the topic of the session. On the other hand, the family may want to talk about other, more overtly conflictive matters. Mr. and Mrs. C., for example, wished to focus on the fact that Mr. C. seemed to prefer his mother over his wife. The therapists deemed it "not immediately relevant though undoubtedly very important." The focus of the session returned to the question of how Mrs. C. could help Mr. C., the phobic, return to work. In other words, the focus remains on specific behavioral operations rather than on substantive but often illusory family dysfunctions. It has been our experience that focusing on "meaty" family issues is often nonproductive. At times the patient will want to discuss these red herrings in order to avoid the difficult in vivo exposure work. At other times spouses can attempt to utilize these very same issues to keep the patient from making further progress, which he may find threatening. Ultimately we find the approach outlined here more productive in making behavioral progress as well as in helping the couple, in the long run, to very gradually realign their relationship. Often in this segment of the treatment we teach communication training and problem-solving skills (Arnow et al. 1985). However, these interventions are always focused upon the implementation of the in vivo exposure.

These couple sessions are assigned in addition to our in vivo exposure group. The purpose of the communication and problem-solving training is to enhance the couple's ability to negotiate tasks. During the session the therapist uses his or her knowledge both of behavioral principles (such as the use of a graded hierarchy in systematic desensitization) and of the particular family dynamics to suggest a number of couple tasks. The couple is then encouraged to negotiate over these tasks. Each session ends with an explicit family task. The task is designed to steer a midground between discouraging and overencouraging efforts at separation. We tend to err on the side of excessively slow change.

The therapist will also encourage the spouse to support the increasingly independent behavior demonstrated by the identified patient. Throughout the course of treatment we routinely urge the couple to "predict possible sabotages in the treatment," and in this way we limit these crises. We also support and empathize with the role of the partner who now has to deal with an increasingly assertive and at times aggressive spouse.

We encounter two manifestations of resistance to our tasks. Either the couple does not comply with the task, or they overcomply. In either case we make explicit their difficulty with the task. In the first case we suggest that we have been too ambitious and work out the next task with that in mind, reaching for even less separation. In the latter case we make vigorous efforts to slow them down and suggest that they may be moving toward the overambitious "pushing" side that landed them in the difficulty to start with.

In certain of the most difficult cases we have found it helpful to use traditional paradoxical methods of prescribing the pathogenic transaction (Selvini-Palazzoli et al. 1978).

Case Example

Joan and Barbara were two sisters who had lived together for 7 years. Joan's severe agoraphobia elicited extremely angry responses from Barbara, who saw it as a manipulative attempt to "ruin my life." During treatment, Barbara responded to the assigned tasks by often saying, "I'm too sick to help her, I have my own problems." Nonetheless, Barbara religiously came to the sessions and proceeded to sabotage the most careful of plans. Her anger subsided and she became more cooperative after it was suggested that three times a week for 15 minutes she "yell at your sister to tell her how she is ruining your life." We offered this as a way in which she could "get it off her chest" and resume her basically helpful ways. The next week Barbara reported that she couldn't comply with the task, since Joan had improved.

Where the relationship between spouses is particularly aggressive or where the fact that the patient is attending a phobia clinic is perceived as a threat to the marital relationship, we found that co-therapy offers several advantages. In co-therapy one therapist can specifically side with the spouse and give voice to his/her anger at the phobic behavior and his/her distress at being left out of the group in vivo experience. When the spouses cannot agree on appropriate homework assignments and remain polarized between an overly fast or an overly slow approach, one co-therapist can be labeled the "slowpoke" and the other co-therapist the "mover." The therapists may then adopt the posture of fighting between themselves and model a final graded transition.

CHANGES IN THE MARITAL RELATIONSHIP AS A RESULT OF TREATMENT

We have found that "successful" treatment of the presenting agoraphobic nearly always has a profound effect on the family system. This should not be surprising, since the nature of phobic symptoms must at the very least effect family members' ability to travel, socialize, or otherwise engage in activities outside the home (Friedman 1988).

As others have noted (i.e., Cerny et al. 1987), in most cases we have found that the marital system eagerly accepts these changes. Couples will often report major improvements in their relationship. However, we have found it almost impossible to predict, before actual treatment, which marriages will hold up well and which may begin to crumble.

We, like others (Hafner 1977, 1982, Hand and Lamontague 1976), have seen a number of dramatic cases where successful treatment of the agoraphobia, usually a female agoraphobic, has led to the development of severe emotional turmoil and/or phobic symptoms in the initially nonsymptomatic spouse. In all of these cases in our initial evaluation we had been able to trace the onset of the phobic symptoms to a conflict or stress within the family. However, I must stress that we have also seen a large number of cases where, while the onset of phobia symptoms seemed to be traceable to such family conflicts, behavioral treatment of the phobic symptoms, with minimal family interventions, has led to an alleviation of both the phobic symptoms and the family conflict.

Another scenario we have seen is that after our treatment, perhaps months later, couples will recontact us and request traditional marital therapy. Again, it is very difficult to successfully predict which couples as a result of behavioral treatment will worsen or later need more intensive family treatment. In our clinical practice utilizing the approach we have described we are able to develop an alliance with the couple that allows for clinical flexibility. It seems to us that this clinical flexibility is important in maximizing our ability to successfully treat agoraphobia.

Our phobia clinic has been in operation for 5 years. During this time we have evaluated well over 200 clients. Of the cases we have seen in treatment only about 25% have become involved in the more intensive family treatment we have described in this chapter. The vast majority of our cases have required just our initial family intake interview and psychoeducational approach with occasional family sessions. This approach has helped cut our dropout rate from 25% to below 5%. We have had only five cases where families have refused to become even minimally involved, and four of these patients, while showing some initial improvement in the in vivo exposure group, dropped out during the course of treatment.

CONCLUSION

The initial psychoeducational sessions help to develop a collaborative alliance with the couple in dealing with the agoraphobic symptomatology. These sessions also help minimize the resistance for marital treatment when indicated during the course of the behavioral treatment. In addition, where the intake interviews suggest that behavioral treatment will lead to dramatic and stressful changes in the family or where the treatment will encounter severe resistance, we routinely recommend family treatment of the type and manner described in this paper.

REFERENCES

Agulnik, P. (1970). The spouse of the phobic patient. *British Journal of Psychiatry* 117:59-67.

Anderson, C. M. (1983). A psychoeducational program for families of patients with schizophrenia. In *Family Therapy in Schizophrenia*, ed. W. R. McFarlane. New York: Guilford Press.

Arnow, B. A., Taylor, C. B., Agras, W. S., and Telch, M. J. (1985). Enhancing agoraphobia treatment outcome by changing couple communication patterns. *Behavior Therapy* 5:452-467.

Barlow, D. H., Mavissakalian, M., and Hay, L. R. (1981). Couples treatment of agoraphobia: Changes in marital satisfaction. *Behaviour Research and Therapy* 19:245-255.

Barlow, D. H., O'Brien, G. T., and Last, C. G. (1984). Couples treatment of agoraphobia. *Behavior Therapy* 15:41-58.

Barlow, D. H., and Wolfe, B. E. (1981). Behavioral approaches to anxiety disorders: A report on the NIMH-SUNY, Albany research conference. *Journal of Consulting and Clinical Psychology* 49:448-454.

Bowlby, J. (1973). *Separation: Anxiety and Anger*. New York: Basic Books.

Cerny, J. A., Barlow, D. H., Craske, M. G., and Himadi, W. G. (1987). Couples treatment of agoraphobia: A two-year followup. *Behavior Therapy* 18:401-415.

Chambless, D. L., and Goldstein, A. (1980). The treatment of agoraphobia. In *The Handbook of Behavioral Interventions: A Clinical Guide*, ed. A. Goldstein and E. Foa. New York: Wiley.

Cobb, J. P., McDonald, R., Marks, I. M., and Stern, R. (1980). Marital versus exposure therapy: Psychological treatment of co-existing marital and phobic-obsessive problems. *European Journal of Behavioural Analysis and Modification* 4:3-17.

Emmelkamp, P. M. G. (1982). In-vivo treatment of agoraphobia. In *Agoraphobia: Multiple Perspectives on Theory and Treatment*, ed. D. L. Chambless and A. J. Goldstein. New York: Wiley.

Emmelkamp, P. M. G., and Kupiers, A. C. M. (1979). Agoraphobia: A followup study four years after treatment. *British Journal of Psychiatry* 134:352-355.

Emmelkamp, P. M. G., and Van Der Hout, A. (1983). Failure in treating agoraphobia. In *Failures in Behavior Therapy*, ed. E. B. Foa and P. M. G. Emmelkamp. New York: Wiley.

Friedman, S. (1985). Implications of object-relations theory for the behavioral treatment of agoraphobia. *American Journal of Psychotherapy* 39:525-540.

——— (1987). Technical considerations in the behavioral-marital treatment of agoraphobia. *The American Journal of Family Therapy* 15:111-122.

——— (1988). The family environment of agoraphobics: Assessment and change in treatment. Unpublished manuscript.

Fry, W. (1962). The marital context of the anxiety syndrome. *Family Process* 1:242-252.

Goldstein, A. J. (1970). Case conference: Some aspects of agoraphobia. *Journal of Behavior Therapy and Experimental Psychiatry* 1:305-313.

Guidano, V. F., and Liotti, G. (1983). *Cognitive Processes and Emotional Disorders*. New York: Guilford Press.

Hafner, R. J. (1977). The husbands of agoraphobic women: Assortative mating or pathogenic interaction? *British Journal of Psychiatry* 130:233-239.

────── (1982). The marital context of the agoraphobic syndrome. In *Agoraphobia: Multiple Perspectives on Theory and Treatment*, ed. D. L. Chambless and A. Goldstein. New York: Wiley.

Hand, I., and Lamontague, Y. (1976). The exacerbation of interpersonal problems after rapid phobia-removal. *Psychotherapy: Theory, Research, and Practice* 13:405-411.

Mathews, A. M., Gelder, M. G., and Johnston, D. W. (1981). *Agoraphobia: Nature and Treatment*. New York: Guilford Press.

Milton, F., and Hafner, J. (1979). The outcome of behavior therapy for agoraphobia in relation to marital adjustment. *Archives of General Psychiatry* 36:807-811.

Selvini-Palazzoli, M., Boscolo, L. Cecchin, G., and Prata, G. (1978). *Paradox and Counterparadox: A New Model in the Therapy of the Family in Schizophrenic Transaction*. New York: Jason Aronson.

Stedman, J. M., and Murphy, J. (1984). Dealing with specific child phobias during the course of family therapy: An alternative to systematic desensitization. *Family Therapy* 11:55-60.

18 Systems Therapy

Dr. Platt describes in this chapter a program that uses principles of systems theory to improve the outcome in phobia therapy. The marital relationship itself is the primary therapeutic tool. The leading idea is that a small change in a frozen system can release the process of change, which is then supported and promoted by the therapist.

As Dr. Platt notes, research does not provide unequivocal support for marital therapy. Yet, perhaps because of the obvious discord often seen in couples, one partner of whom is phobic, those interested in systems theory and marital therapy have found fertile ground in which to make a contribution. In the general eclecticism of treatments of the anxiety disorders, an understanding of the system in which the symptoms are being expressed is a valuable perspective. Needless to say, the focus of systems theory is on the interpersonal, rather than the intrapsychic or strictly behavioral, context. In this case Dr. Platt reminds us that the phobia might serve a dynamic purpose for the spouse as well as for the patient, and further, that regardless of the dynamic origin, the interaction becomes self-perpetuating.

Systems Therapy

Richard Platt

In 1981, Barlow and Mavissakalian projected that future directions in the treatment of phobias would incorporate a focus on the interpersonal context. This projection was based on a growing appreciation of the influence of interpersonal relationships on the development and maintenance of phobic disorders. In a report on the treatment of agoraphobia, for example, Emmelkamp (1974) noted that the agoraphobia appeared to play an important part in the marital relationship. Other reports (Hand and Lamontague 1976, Milton and Hafner 1979, and Barlow et al. 1984) examine the role of the patient's family in this disorder in efforts to elucidate the system's dynamics. Researchers (Mathews et al. 1981, Emmelkamp and Van Der Hout 1983) reached often contradictory conclusions about what to do with this systems information. Mathews suggests including the family as agents of change, while Emmelkamp and Van Der Hout suggest excluding them. This latter report cites evidence that improvement in the phobia leads to a deterioration of family relationships, noting that the phobia serves a function for the spouse.

While a clear direction for incorporating family dynamics in phobia treatment has not been established, efforts continue.

Barlow and colleagues (1984), using a couples group in the treatment of agoraphobia, found success rates in the range of 75%—similar to those reported by Matthews and co-authors in 1977, with one crucial difference. In the couples treatment, dropout was as low as 5%, compared with dropout rates of 25% to 50% found in noncouples treatment (Chambless and Goldstein 1982).

Relevant to incorporating systems dynamics in the treatment of childhood phobia, reports (e.g., Stedman and Murphy 1984) describe modified in vivo and imaginal desensitization procedures where both the therapist and one or both parents are in the role of encouraging a relaxation response in the face of increasingly anxious situations. This report notes that the parent in this therapeutic role is discouraging prior dependency interactions and is thus increasing a healthy differentiation between child and parent.

Perhaps the area of greatest research on childhood phobias relates to school phobia—the fear of attending school. In this area, there is almost universal involvement of the parents in the treatment process. Similar to the way adults are taught a supportive role with their phobic spouse or friend, parents are taught how to coach their child to attend school (Du Pont 1983, Marks 1978, Ross 1982).

The most recently reported study of a treatment effort including interpersonal relationships is the work of Friedman (1987). Friedman outlines a five-stage psychoeducational–marital approach, of which the first stage is designed to create a collaborative relationship between the therapist and the spouse of the phobic person. Subsequent stages of treatment teach the couple about the mechanisms of phobias and about the graded-exposure approach to desensitization. Friedman, like Barlow, found that including the partner helped to nearly eliminate dropouts. In addition, Friedman concluded that spouse support in exposure practices helped to minimize the avoidance to exposure. One final point, with reference to the Friedman report: a small percentage of spouses refused to become even minimally involved in the treatment. Addressing this particular situation from a systems perspective is an area for future research and is further discussed later in this chapter.

In short, while researchers continue to ask and answer questions about the role of the family in phobia treatment, reports suggest improved treatment results with the family involved in the therapy. Generally, systems approaches solicit the support and assistance of significant family members so that relationship issues will be made part of the phobia treatment and in vivo exposure practices will be more difficult to avoid.

The remainder of this chapter presents a systems approach to the treatment of phobias that is a modification of the interactional model of the Mental Research Institute in Palo Alto (Watzlawich et al. 1974, Weakland et al. 1974). We clarify the MRI approach in specific application to treating phobias and incorporate understanding of family dynamics with families that are either willing or unwilling to participate in the treatment.

This specialized application of the interactional model was developed over the past 10 years at Focus: A Private Mental Health Center in Albany, New York. The use of the interactional model has led to an appreciation that phobic family systems can be distinguished along several distinct categories of interaction. In addition, specific treatment strategies are required in each category. The work presented delineates these categories of phobic interaction, their respective treatment strategies, and the use of the interactional model as the framework.

The fundamental premise of the interactional model is that regardless of origin, problems, such as symptoms (panic attacks) or behavioral patterns (avoidance), persist only if they are maintained by current and ongoing interactions between the symptom bearer and others. For example, panic attacks in an agoraphobic woman may, in part, be maintained by her husband's hostile attitude about the nature of her panics. His view that she is weak and ineffectual can undermine her confidence to confront phobic situations, thus contributing to her highly anxious state. A corresponding premise suggests that if this problem-maintaining behavior is changed or eliminated, the problem will be resolved, regardless of its nature, origin, or duration (Weakland et al. 1974). If the husband's attitude could be shifted to one of understanding the difficulty, his agoraphobic wife would feel less self-critical and more inclined to attempt anxious situations. The specific procedures of assessment, case planning, and treatment follow from these two key concepts.

Within the context of this model, problems are best understood as difficulties between people. For example, while many people have anxiety attacks, only some individuals develop a phobic pattern to handle them. Phobic individuals almost universally try to avoid situations that they think will create more anxiety or panic attacks, or they spend a great deal of time and energy preparing themselves for the uncomfortable situation. In some situations, spouses, parents, and friends offer reassurance that is designed to prevent the discomfort but may unwittingly support it. In other situations, they act in a demanding way attempting to get the phobic person to take action, adding additional anxiety. The difficulties between the significant other and the phobic person become the treatment problem: the task of therapy is to change the interaction between the spouse or parent and the phobic person. The therapist takes deliberate action to alter the interaction as effectively and efficiently as he can.

We have found that the work proceeds most efficiently when it remains simple in its scope and is directed toward achieving a concrete and minimal goal. Minor changes in overt behavior or in how the patient thinks of his behavior are often sufficient to initiate progressive changes—a principle called the *ripple effect*. In addition to its goal orientation and problem focus, therapy is limited in its duration, usually to fifteen sessions. In summary, this therapy approach:

- Remains focused on a solution
- Establishes a minimal goal for treatment
- Occurs within a limited number of sessions

PRINCIPLES OF ASSESSMENT AND TREATMENT

In order to devise effective interventions, the therapist needs a clear understanding of the behavior that is maintaining the problem. The assessment procedures obtain information on *what* the significant others do about the problem as well as on their beliefs about the efficacy of their actions. The therapeutic strategy is most effective when it is presented in a manner consistent with the client's own assumptions, beliefs, values, and unique motivation. For example, a husband who accompanies his wife into a phobic situation may do this based on the belief that some harm will come to her if she panics and is alone. He will be more amenable to changing his behavior with her if the nature of the changes suggested take into account this motivation to have no harm come to her.

The individual who is most bothered by the problem is identified as the "complainant." This is not always the identified phobic patient. The intervention is directed toward the complainant, who, as the person most upset about the situation, is the person most ready for change (for example, the mother of a phobic child).

The family are also assessed as to their tendency to comply with or to oppose instructions. These "compliant" or "oppositional" postures determine the strategy of how the interventions are designed (Rohrbaugh et al. 1981).

Behavior may be altered on occasion by telling the parties directly to do, or to not do, something specific. Such occasions are rare in therapy, however, since common-sense solutions are often the very behaviors perpetuating the problem. Paradoxical interventions are frequently used to circumvent the seeming logic of the family system. For example, a phobic symptom may be encouraged in order to lessen it or to bring it under control.

Another related treatment approach is called *the dangers of improvement*. This method challenges an "oppositional system" to change by presenting the rationale for the inadvisability of such change. Similarly, the therapist might restrain change in order to help people change.

ASSESSMENT PROCEDURES

The treatment facility must be sensitive to discovering persons in the system who are involved in interactions that have an impact on the phobia. The family or other significant members of the phobic person's life are invited to the initial assessment appointment. If resistance occurs, the assessment is arranged with whoever will attend the appointment. It is made clear that this initial meeting is solely for evaluation and not for immediate solutions to the problem.

The question "What is the problem?" is posed to those people present. As the participants tell their story, the interviewer determines who is the complainant. This may often be assessed from the initial telephone contact—for example, "I'm calling for an appointment for my wife. She has been suffering from this phobia for years and the situation is beginning to drive me crazy."

Information is elicited about how the phobia interferes with daily life, the nature of the phobic symptoms, past treatment efforts, and what changes might constitute improvement in the problem. At the end of the assessment session the interviewer maintains a neutral role with regard to the information and avoids creating early expectations for change.

The strategy for treatment is determined by several specific factors, summarized below into four interactional categories.

INTERACTIONAL CATEGORIES

Category 1: "Other" not significantly involved in problem maintenance

In this category of interaction, the significant other is not doing anything identifiable to maintain the phobia. This person will often take a positive role in the treatment and makes a good candidate for a "phobia coach" or "therapy aide" in the desensitization process.

Category 2: "Other" enables phobic behavior

In this category of interaction, the significant other facilitates the phobic in avoiding phobic situations. For example, a husband is "overprotecting" when he accedes to his phobic wife's wishes not to attend social gatherings. This enabling behavior might be based on a belief that he is protecting her from anxiety or embarrassment, or that he is avoiding marital conflict by not insisting.

Category 3: The phobia enables the "other" to be "stronger"

In this category, the significant other benefits from being in a superior position to the phobic. This benefit may take the form of feeling healthier, more capable, more competent, or more valuable by virtue of being needed. The nonphobic partner might give advice or reassurance to the phobic with the covert implication "I know better" or "This is how strong people handle a situation." For example, a husband whose wife will not leave home without him may feel threatened if she does not need him in this role, or may feel jealous if she is out of the home alone.

Category 4: Mutually enabling behaviors (mutual protection)

In this category of interaction typically both individuals have significant psychological distress. The equilibrium in the system is such that the phobias prevent problems in the nonphobic partner, and the nonphobic partner's problems help prevent further stress for the phobic. The nonphobic most frequently exhibits an anxiety disorder, depression, psychosomatic illness, sexual dysfunction, or chemical dependence. An example of this category, cited here, will be expanded upon later in the chapter. An agoraphobic woman married to an alcoholic man was unable to be home alone or drive alone. He drank only at home. In taking care of her, his drinking was by necessity structured and limited; at the same time, his alcoholism allowed her to feel helpful to him.

In summary, the assessment phase of treatment in the interactional model is used to determine not only the nature of the phobia itself but also the behaviors of significant others as these behaviors relate to the phobia. In addition, the assessor attempts to determine the underpinnings of people's behaviors—that is, to understand their beliefs about the phobia, the phobic person, and the phobic person's needs. The complainant is also determined. Finally, an initial statement of what would indicate improvement—a goal—is solicited. Based on this information, the category of interaction is determined, and treatment planning commences. The four categories and their respective treatment approaches are presented in Table 18-1.

TREATMENT OF THE INTERACTION

Category 1: "Other" not significantly involved in problem maintenance

Treatment in this category involves helping the significant other(s) to assume a positive role as a therapeutic adjunct or coach. The individuals in this category usually comply with direct instruction to achieve the desired goal. Once this shift into the "coach" role is achieved, the treatment proceeds with educational material concerning the "fear of fear" cycle of thinking and the teaching of coping skills. A goal is established with the phobic and family, which the therapist should insure is concrete, observable, and within the reach of the patient. This first-step goal should also be one that is an important step to the patient. Treatment may then progress in a step-by-step behavioral program of in vivo desensitization with the spouse as "therapy aide," moving toward the agreed-upon goal.

TABLE 18-1 Interactional Categories of Phobic Problems

Category 1	Category 2	Category 3	Category 4
"Other" not significantly involved in problem maintenance	"Other" enables phobic behavior	Phobia enables "other" to be "stronger"	Mutually enabling behaviors; mutual protection
Treatment plan: Teach "other" to be "coach"; in vivo exposure for phobic	Treatment plan: Directly reverse enabling behaviors; instruct supportive exposure	Treatment plan: State dangers of improvement and restrain from change	Treatment plan: Start with dangers of improvement, move to "no change"

Concrete aids such as maps, journals, and cards printed with helpful techniques are useful in organizing the work. Usually, treatment sessions are arranged weekly for the first 6 to 8 weeks. Subsequent sessions are then scheduled to allow sufficient time between sessions for "practice" with the helpful spouse. Throughout the treatment process, the behavioral goal remains the focus of the work, rather than the family dynamics. Discussion of termination must take into consideration the need to reinforce the family members' new ability to rely on one another rather than on the therapist in a new and helpful way.

Case Report

Mrs. M., a 40-year-old teacher's aide of developmentally disabled children, sought treatment for "one little phobia building up to a lot of other phobias." Six years before the current onset she had experienced her first panic attack when she was a passenger in a car and was ill with bronchitis. The current episode seemed to be triggered by a similar combination of circumstances—being ill and a passenger in a car. Mrs. M. did not know why her panics in the car had recurred.

The assessment interview was attended by Mr. and Mrs. M. Mrs. M. recounted the events that led her to seek therapy, while her husband listened intently. He was respectful of his wife's anxiety and added that she minimized the impact that their children have on her stress level. He thought that she was overly hard on herself. Mrs. M. responded that she tended to keep everything inside and did not want to burden the family with her problems. In addition, the family had recently moved to an old house, which Mr. M. himself was repairing. When asked what he did to be helpful with the phobic avoidance, Mr. M. replied that he was at a loss as to what to do. As a therapy goal, Mrs. M. specified her being able to relax when in the car, specifically when going to the shopping center.

The assessment was made that Mr. M. was in a neutral role in relation to his wife's phobia and thus in category 1. He believed her phobias were a result of maternal stress and he had no personal investment in her illness. The new house had made Mr. M. temporarily unavailable to his wife, which had exacerbated the family problem and resulted in their seeking treatment. In the initial sessions of therapy, the treatment was explained to the couple and Mr. M. was trained in the role as "coach." They were taught specific cognitive coping techniques to counteract the "fear of fear" cycle, and the importance of practice between sessions was emphasized. At each session, the practice that had occurred was reviewed and the next steps were determined.

Mrs. M. was able to accomplish her immediate goal of being comfortable as a passenger in the car when going to the shopping center in ten sessions over a 5-month period. A 6-month follow-up determined that continued progress had occurred, and the M. family were able to take a vacation trip by car over 200 miles from home.

A feature of this case worth noting is that Mr. M.'s beliefs about the phobia were based on his wife's minimizing her own stresses. He did not gain anything by her being phobic and thus would have nothing to lose if she were not. This factor is important, since it allowed the therapist to formulate a compliance-based treatment, directly influencing Mr. M. into a helpful "coach role." Of additional importance was the nature of the goal—it was a minimal, concrete, achievable goal that was a "first step" toward improvement. Goals created with these criteria establish that therapy is the beginning of the change process. Change then can occur, and certainly did in this case, beyond the end of the formal therapy process.

Category 2: The "other" enables the phobic behavior

In this category the nonphobic family member exhibits behaviors in relation to the phobia that enable phobic behavior. As previously described, these behaviors frequently take the form of "overprotecting" or "not insisting." These labels can be assigned on the basis of the belief on which the particular behavior is based. *Enabling* occurs when one believes he or she is helping another to avoid anxiety or discomfort or is helping to avoid an uncomfortable interpersonal conflict.

Family members in this category are unaware that the enabling behavior has been contributing to the maintenance of the phobia, and they are willing to be taught how to modify this behavior. They make themselves available for the assessment appointment, the therapy appointments, and the in vivo practices between appointments.

Once a family member's enabling behavior has been identified, therapy can be designed to instruct this member on what behaviors will not contribute to the maintenance of the phobia. When this shift in behavior has occurred, therapy proceeds in a fashion similar to that described for category 1.

Case Report

Mr. J., a successful self-employed insurance agent, had suffered from panic attacks and anxiety in social situations for 20 years. He called for an appointment after hearing a radio talk-show on phobias that discussed modern effective treatments. He identified with the symptoms described on the show, especially the loss of control that some people fear. He was sure, however, that his particular situation was stranger than what other people experience, so only his wife knew of it. He was obsessed with being near a bathroom whenever in a social situation. Social situations were most terrifying to him, causing him to fear loss of bowel and bladder control. He was becoming increasingly frantic as time drew closer to his first child's wedding date: "What if I lose control while sitting in the front pew of the church?"

At the assessment it was learned that Mr. J. was from a large, very close family; his parents, in fact, lived next door on one side and his sister on the other. Anxiety ran in the family. Mrs. J., a secretary at a local college, expressed perplexity at her husband's phobia, since he could attend social situations related to his work but not otherwise. Her pleasant manner masked a sadness about their restricted social life. When asked what she did to be helpful to her husband, she responded that she understood "he doesn't do it intentionally" (referring to his getting anxious and canceling social plans), so she felt she had to go along with what made him feel better. In regard to what would indicate improvement in his situation, Mr. J. said that he wanted to be comfortable at his son's wedding and that he'd like to be able to go out to dinner with his wife and another couple.

In the therapy, the first task was to explain that Mr. J. followed through with social plans in relation to his work because of the obligation he felt, while nonwork social situations he could easily arrange to avoid. The wife's acceding to her husband's desire to avoid was framed to her as being unwittingly destructive, an explanation she could readily understand. Mr. and Mrs. J. were then oriented to the treatment procedure. They were told about the nature of panic attacks, the "fear of fear" cycle, coping skills, and the role of in vivo practice sessions that would gradually move them toward their goal within the fifteen-session structure. Mrs. J.'s role would be to gently insist that her husband not avoid the graduated practice steps. She was told that her insisting would create anxiety for Mr. J., but he could get stronger only by confronting social events. When she realized that she could play an active role in her husband's recovery and that there was finally hope for them to enjoy social life, tears of joy and relief streamed down her cheeks.

Orienting the couple to the therapy process, establishing a goal, and shifting Mrs. J. from an enabling to a helpful role was accomplished in the first two therapy sessions. The subsequent eleven sessions dealt with questions and concerns and supported both

Mr. and Mrs. J. in their nonavoidance roles. The goal was accomplished 5½ months after therapy was initiated. At follow-up, 4 months later, Mr. and Mrs. J. reported continued progress as evidenced by repeated dinners out, movies, and successful attendance at their son's wedding.

Significant features of this case include, first, a determination of the nature of the spouse's enabling behavior. This behavior was assessed to be her hesitance to insist that her phobic husband confront nonwork social situations, based on her tenuous belief that she was helping him "feel better." Second, in formulating the strategy for the therapy, it was determined that Mrs. J. would comply with efforts to alter her interactions from enabling to insisting, based on her feeling about their current social life and her stated willingness to be involved in the therapy. Mr. J. was the complainant in this system but Mrs. J., because of her willingness to participate, could be considered a co-complainant. This case was therefore approached from a compliance base. Finally, the minimal, first-step nature of the goal was crucial in creating both a successful completion of therapy and further gains beyond therapy.

Category 3: The phobia enables the "other" to be "stronger"

This category is characterized by the feature that the nonphobic family member has something to lose by improvements in the phobia. In relation to the phobic individual, the nonphobic appears "stronger"—that is, more competent in life, less pathologic in regard to mental health, wiser, better, and so on. Also, the nonphobic person tends to derive a sense of usefulness in his or her role with the phobic. Compared with the spouse or "other" in the category 1 or 2 system, this individual will express a reluctance to be involved in the therapy process. Additionally, this person is often described by the phobic as controlling and "afraid to change." At times, from the therapist's perspective, this person only pays lip service to the stated willingness to be involved in the treatment. When action is expected, the resistance emerges.

Generally speaking, this family system will have reason to resist the efforts of treatment. Assessment often reveals numerous unsuccessful attempts at treatment. This system has been described (Rohrbaugh et al. 1981) as "defiant" or oppositional in nature, requiring approaches that use the reluctance to change in advantageous ways. These interventions are paradoxical and take the form of symptom prescription, raising the dangers of improvement, or suggesting the inadvisability of change (see, for example, Fisch et al. 1982, Frankl 1960, Haley 1973, 1976, Selvini-Palazzoli et al. 1978, Watzlawick et al. 1974, Weakland et al. 1974). Employing these methods "appears in opposition to the goals being sought in order to actually move toward them" (Weakland et al. 1974). Restraining measures are used throughout the course of treatment to keep the process moving; gains are framed as moving too quickly or as dangerous.

Case Report

Mrs. C. was a perky, talkative, government stenographer, age 34, married to a bus mechanic 15 years her senior. This marriage was her first and his second. Mr. and Mrs. C. had been married 5 years. His two young adult children lived with them in a hostile-dependent relationship. Mr. C.'s first wife died of morbid obesity; Mrs. C. had been a friend of hers.

Mrs. C. requested services for her phobias—"I don't mean just one, I have eight of them"—because of a growing fear of being alone and traveling alone. When arranging the assessment appointment, Mr. C. was invited to attend; the response was that he would probably come in, but just for the assessment.

At the assessment interview, Mr. and Mrs. C. sat close to each other with Mrs. C. responding to all the questions. She detailed her eight phobias and described how they were controlling her life. She reported getting confused when alone, therefore her husband couldn't go out. He drove her everywhere, including the daily ride to and from her job. When asked his thoughts on her situation, Mr. C. said she really didn't seem that bothered and that things in his life were fine. He expressed no complaints about his role with his phobic wife. She was not concerned about understanding the cause of these problems, but she did want to know a solution just in case she were to be alone.

In the formulation of the case plan, an oppositional strategy was selected. The reason was Mr. C.'s history of relationships with people who were overly dependent on him, and Mrs. C.'s basing of her complaint on an anticipated *future* fear. The plan would entail an explanation about her panic attacks, the "fear of fear" cycle of thinking, coping skills, and the apparent protective nature of her phobia in regard to her husband's need to have people strongly rely on him. A goal of therapy would be sought, but attaining the goal, it would further be explained, could carry great risks to her husband and their relationship. Her stated goal was to be able to venture a short distance from where her husband worked, on foot and alone. She understood the concern expressed about the negative consequences to her husband, but she said they would deal with this if the consequences developed.

Therapy progressed toward the goal, with each session focusing on both her progressive steps in walking alone and the effects of this change on her husband. In her obsessive manner, Mrs. C. would record, in a journal, her thoughts and actions during and after the in vivo practice sessions, as requested by the therapist. A verbatim entry follows:

10 p.m. took shower, thought about spending so much time evenings more or less away from Bob to get a hold on my phobia situation. Tough decision in my head—which is more important to me (a) spending that much time away from Bob in order to get control over the alone phobia (b) all the time Bob and I now share together—do I want to miss it (as I see it [and Bob has agreed] there is never enough time spent together when you consider all the time you both spend at work) (c) wouldn't it be better though to get better *just* in case I ever do have to be alone so I know how to handle it. (2)

The parenthetic "2" at the end of this journal entry is a determination by the client of the level of anxiety on a 0–10 rating scale, one of the coping techniques she was taught.

Mrs. C. attained her stated goal in thirteen sessions over a period of 8 months. She reported in each of the final three sessions that her husband seemed to be adjusting slowly to her increased independence. At follow-up 6 months later, Mrs. C. said that the situation was about the same as when therapy had terminated, "neither better nor worse," but that she felt more in control of her feelings.

In this family system, Mrs. C. was the complainant. Although the husband would not take an active role, owing to his motivation to maintain the status quo, interventions with Mrs. C. would gently confront the nature of their relationship as exhibited in their interactions. This case is an example of systems interventions with an individual client. The reluctant spouse is not required in the therapy as long as the complainant is present.

An oppositional strategy was formulated on a number of factors revealed in the assessment. Two prior therapies (with phobia-wise therapists) had not been successful, and both the husband and wife (he covertly and she overtly) expressed concerns about a successful completion of therapy. Weakland and his colleagues (1974) point out that patients seriously consider paradoxical interventions, since the message so closely fits their perspective. "Such warnings paradoxically promote rapid improvement, apparently by reducing any anxiety about change and increasing the patient's desire to get on with things to counteract the therapist's overcautiousness."

Of specific consideration in the use of paradox in phobia treatment is the weaving of this technique with the cognitive-behavioral technique. The therapist must be in the role of teacher, on the one hand, and that of cautious therapist, on the other. Stepwise progression toward the goal should be met with measured praise about the movement made and with cautious concern about the consequences of this progress.

Category 4: Mutually enabling behaviors (mutual protection)

Features similar to those in category 3 exist in the category 4 family system. Individuals here perceive that a change in behavior could make matters worse for their partner, for themselves, or for both. Positive change for each means negative consequences to the other.

The category 4 system is also characterized by each member's experiencing considerable psychological and/or physical (psychosomatic) distress. One member is phobic and the other is either anxious, phobic, obsessive-compulsive, depressed, physically ill (e.g., migraine, hypertension, ulcers, spastic colon), chemically dependent, or experiencing sexual dysfunction.

This system, then, has reasons to be reluctant to change, and assessments often reveal prior treatment failures. Assessments will need to be performed cautiously, uncovering motivations and beliefs without creating an expectation to change too much, too quickly. Experience with this system has shown that a helpful method for ascertaining individual beliefs and motivations in a cautious manner is to "split the session." Part of the assessment interview is spent with each member of the system, asking questions about the problem, about what would indicate improvement, and about what result this change would create for other members of the system.

Therapy for this system is paradoxical or restraining. Persistence may require hard restraints in order to produce the change requested. The therapist may be required to shift interventions from milder restraint (dangers of improvement) to a stronger restraint (advising no change) if therapeutic movement does not initially occur. As in category 3, each intervention is presented to the patient and others in the family in a carefully prepared manner, consistent with their beliefs and motivations.

Finally, in the category 4 system, the complainant may not be the person with the phobia. If the "other" has determined that his/her own situation or the phobia must be changed, then the "other" is more amenable to influence. At a minimum, then, this person must be present for the therapy. Usually, however, it is helpful if both (or all) members of the category 4 system are present for the therapy. If great reluctance is presented by noncomplainant members of the system, these individuals can be invited in on a limited basis or can be dealt with on the telephone.

Case Report

Mr. S., a 46-year-old career fireman, called for therapy for his wife, who was becoming increasingly more anxious about leaving the house to shop or do carpool driving for their three school-age children. She would experience palpitations and severe anxiety "spells" even when thinking about these responsibilities. Her phobia had recently worsened following a financial setback that Mr. S. had with a property investment. He was becoming increasingly frustrated about how to handle her reaction to his being called to the firehouse in an emergency, leaving her alone. He reported that his wife was not optimistic about therapy but would "give it a try."

At the assessment it was learned that Mrs. S. had been phobic in varying degrees for 20 years. She related that the phobia created problems for herself and her husband. Her inability to manage the shopping and the carpool made her feel terribly inadequate as a wife and mother and the phobia tied her husband close to home in ways that angered him. Arguments about her phobia were a daily event. Mrs. S. revealed that if her husband were more understanding and had less of a temper they might fight less, and she'd be calmer and be able to do more. She stated that his nightly six-pack of beer at home put him in a fighting mood.

Splitting the session gave each an opportunity to speak more freely. Mrs. S. expressed worry about her husband's drinking but added, "At least now he does it at home." She felt unable to confront this problem, because the beer did help him relax, and pushing him to stop drinking might drive him away. Mr. S. said that he could handle her phobia better when it was not so severe. He said that the situation was out of hand now, but at times he had enjoyed shopping with her—it gave them time together out of the house. He knew he was drinking more than he should, but he felt he would do something about this problem when the financial crisis passed. He said he felt stupid for getting into the property deal that he did. When asked further about his drinking, he responded defensively, saying he was here to talk about his wife's phobia, not his drinking.

It was postulated that, owing to the financial failure, Mr. S. was drinking more heavily and that consequently Mrs. S.'s phobia worsened. It was felt that through her "illness" (the phobia) she could help keep her husband's drinking "at home" and somewhat under control. By not confronting the drinking she was able to manage his problem to some degree and, in addition, she could feel that he wouldn't leave her. Additionally, the phobia was a problem to him now, but in the past it had actually afforded them time together.

This couple were embroiled in a vicious circle of interactions that included her not confronting his alcoholism and his acting hostile toward her phobia (or at times seeming to derive a sense of adequacy from being needed). Their beliefs and motivations prevented them from shifting their positions. Prior treatments, which had failed, attempted to influence Mrs. S. directly without regard to the consequences to her husband. Paradox or restraint was now selected as general treatment strategy.

The treatment phase was begun in such a way so as to not frighten Mr. and Mrs. S. out of therapy. Initially they were told that more information was needed to better understand this phobia, since there seemed to be more to it than what was apparent. Mr. S., in particular, was addressed in this regard. A goal of therapy was also established early in the therapy. Mr. S. wanted to be able to respond to emergency fire calls without his wife having a panic attack. Mrs. S. was asked if she wanted to explore the possibility of achieving this goal, or if she had another to suggest. She was told to think about her answer at home and not to respond immediately, since the therapist wanted to proceed with caution.

In the second session, Mrs. S. was asked about what she had thought. She agreed to her husband's goal and added that she might like to get out of the house more on her own. With a cautious note, the couple were then oriented to the treatment process. They were told of the general cognitive-behavioral approach and the need for in vivo practice between sessions. The second session was also used to begin to share the reasons for caution. Their protective roles vis-à-vis each other were explained, with more time being devoted to Mr. S.

Subsequent sessions focused on the practices and on their relationship. Missed practices and arguments were given a positive connotation; it was explained that these events were evidence of the dangers of improvement. In the sixth therapy session, however, a determination was made to restrain Mr. S. in a more forceful manner, since little movement toward the goal had occurred. He was told that what had occurred in the therapy indicated a need to maintain the status quo; he was offered an opportunity to learn to live with the current situation the way it was. The next session began with reports of far fewer fights, less drinking, and a number of helpful practices. To this movement, the therapist's response was caution. Therapy continued in this fashion to the goal. The goal was achieved in fifteen sessions over the course of a year's time. At follow-up, Mrs. S. was much more mobile and Mr. S. was not drinking.

An important technical consideration in the foregoing case is that while the identified problem was the phobia, the complainant was the nonphobic spouse. Interventions in such cases must be directed primarily at the complainant, at least initially. If the noncomplainant becomes a willing participant in the process at any point in the therapy, as she did here, interventions can be directed as needed.

Finally, the therapist, using this interactional model, must maintain a cautious restraining position throughout the therapy. Gains can be reversed with praise that is not tempered with caution. Experience has shown that category 4 systems are particularly entrenched in problem-maintaining behaviors, requiring a persistent position to which they can react.

TREATMENT OF CHILDREN'S PHOBIAS

Treating phobic children has traditionally used systems methods, even when the general approach is not systemic. Freud, for example, in 1909 treated Little Hans's horse phobia by altering an aspect of the boy's relationship with his father. Therapists who work with children interact with the parents, if it is simply to arrange the appointment. Frequently, however, in this practical age of psychotherapy, parents ask questions about what they can do about their child's phobia. Therapists, systemic and nonsystemic alike, are often in the position of involving the parents. A behaviorally oriented therapist, for example, would have the parent of an animal-phobic child involved in the development of the hierarchy and the in vivo desensitization.

For the most part, therapy for a child's phobia is initiated by a parent. Of special consideration for the approach presented in this chapter, then, is that the parent is the complainant. This factor dictates that if the child's phobia is to be ameliorated, the parent(s) must be involved in the therapy. Assessment interviews are conducted with parents present, and treatment proceeds on the assumption that the parents will be involved in an ongoing way.

Irrespective of the category of interaction, the parents, in the role of complainant, are used to help clarify the nature of the child's phobia. Parents can describe how the child may "language" his or her fears, using words that are particular to their family. One 8-year-old child, for example, invented a word for her panic attacks. Additionally, parents are necessary in the role of coach. With parents in the coach role, the therapy can be conceptualized as occurring through the parents to the child. Also, the therapy of a category 3 or 4 system, with a child phobic, will require the parents' presence to hear, and react to, restraining maneuvers.

Case Report of a Category 3 Child Phobia Treatment

The L. family was referred for family counseling after individual work with a child psychiatrist did not get 11-year-old Kenny back to school. The problem Mrs. L. called about was that her son was so fearful of attending the eighth grade that he had refused to go for the past 8 weeks. The school year was progressing, and they wanted him to get back to school as soon as possible.

Present at the assessment were Mr. and Mrs. L. and Kenny. Mr. L. did most of the talking, at times directing his wife and his son to speak their part. They described a daily, angry struggle to get their son to school; the parents and the school were demanding he attend, thus increasing his fear. The school, feeling manipulated by the youngster, took a firm position on his attendance. The parents, not knowing what else to do, threatened their son with hospitalization if he did not attend school.

Historical information obtained at the assessment was relevant to the current crisis. Mrs. L. reported that at birth Kenny had respiratory difficulties, inferring he was sickly. She described him as always being small, and she worried about him as he grew up. Mr. L.'s busy accounting career, coupled with his frequent evening civic responsibilities, left Mrs. L. with a vast majority of the child-rearing duties. Also, Mrs. L. described herself as a nervous mother who herself had been babied by her mother. Mrs. L. shared that at the time she met her husband, she was completing college, "but I never put my education to good use." In terms of a goal, everyone in the family was in agreement that getting Kenny back to school full time would be the only acceptable outcome.

It was postulated that the behaviors maintaining the problem were the parents' and school's high expectations and demands, coupled with Kenny's fearful avoidance. It was felt that the case plan would be to first confront their high expectations for rapidly getting their son back to school. The next task would be to detail the elements of a slow, progressive densensitization of Kenny's fearful reaction to school, and to introduce the dangers of improvement. Dangers were in the areas of Mrs. L.'s having to face her own independence and Mr. L.'s having to attend more to his husband role by being home more and being less critical of his wife. In addition, the school would need to be included in the case plan, since their role with Kenny was also problem maintaining.

The therapy was conducted along similar lines to the adult category 3 case described above. Each session was used to discuss the parents' progress (or lack of progress) in being able to coach Kenny in small steps. Angry interactions—"You aren't trying hard enough, Ken!"—were framed as indications that Mrs. L. was too fearful to face her own independence and Mr. L. might be unable to figure out (he was an accountant) how to be a more attentive husband. Simultaneously with this work, the school was regularly called by the therapist, who needed to shift and then maintain the school in a helpful role. The therapy required six sessions to begin to get the parents to lower their expectations for rapid change. Once this was accomplished, the process went smoothly. The therapy was successfully completed in twenty sessions over a 5-month period. The school year was nearing an end by the time the treatment was completed, but Kenny had kept pace academically with his classmates as a result of the school's providing home instruction during the course of the counseling. At the start of the new school year the following fall, additional sessions were held to help support the L. family, at their request. Kenny was able to travel to school on public transportation, with his friends, attending full-time. At follow-up, 6 months later, Mrs. L. stated that this crisis had been positive for all involved. She noted that she had begun to look for work and that she and her husband were closer than they had ever been.

Technical considerations for this case are that the school was an aspect of the system, and that the parents and the school, not the phobic child, were the complainants. Had the role the school played in problem maintenance not been successfully addressed, this youngster would not have had his phobia resolved. Finally, challenging this system by suggesting that there were reasons not to change allowed members of this family to reorganize their roles and interactions in ways that were helpful to all.

CONCLUSION

Phobia treatment has begun to incorporate the system within which the phobic person functions. The rationale for including the system has been discussed in the literature of phobia treatment, which finds lower dropout rates and progressive improvements beyond therapy when family members are involved. With these results, clinicians and researchers, in increasing numbers, are reporting on treatment approaches that focus on the system.

This chapter presents the Interactional Model first developed at the Mental Research Institute in Palo Alto, California, with specific application to treating adult and child phobias. The model postulates that problems, like phobias, are maintained by ongoing behaviors of the person with the phobia and the people with whom this person interacts. The model also holds that if these problem-maintaining behaviors can be altered, the phobia will be resolved.

Assessment procedures are outlined and treatment principles are delineated with regard to the nature of the interactions that maintain the phobia. Four categories of interaction and thus four treatment approaches are suggested. In general, the treatment strategy for each category is determined by the system's ability to comply with, or not comply with (oppose), direct methods of altering behaviors that contribute to the maintenance of the phobia. Direct approaches and paradoxical approaches, with case reports, are described.

The desire to understand phobias from a systems perspective is gathering steam. The knowledge that this perspective adds to current treatment approaches seems likely to create successful therapy outcomes for more phobic individuals and their families. Research must explore the questions this chapter should raise, since clearly there is much yet to be learned about treating phobias.

REFERENCES

Agulnik, P. (1970). The spouse of the phobic patient. *British Journal of Psychiatry* 117:59–67.

Barlow, D. H., and Mavissakalian, M. (1981). *Phobia: Psychological and Pharmacological Treatment.* New York: The Guilford Press.

Barlow, D. H., Mavissakalian, M., and Hay, L. R. (1981). Couples treatment of agoraphobia: Changes in marital satisfaction. *Behaviour Research and Therapy* 19:245–257.

Barlow, D. H., O'Brien, G. T., and Last, C. G. (1984). Couples treatment of agoraphobia. *Behavior Therapy* 15:41–58.

Chambless, D. L., and Goldstein, A. J. (1982). *Agoraphobia: Multiple Perspectives on Theory and Treatment.* New York: Wiley.

DuPont, R. L. (1983). Phobias in children. *The Journal of Pediatrics* 102:999–1002.

Emmelkamp, P. M. G. (1974). Self-observation versus flooding in the treatment of agoraphobia. *Behaviour Research and Therapy* 12:29–237.

Emmelkamp, P. M. G., and Van Der Hout, A. (1983). Failure in treating agoraphobia. In *Failures in Behavior Therapy*, ed. E. B. Foa and P. M. G. Emmelkamp, pp. 58–81. New York: Wiley.

Fisch, R., Weakland, J. H., and Segal, L. (1982). *The Tactics of Change: Doing Therapy Briefly*. San Francisco: Jossey-Bass.

Frankl, V. (1960). Paradoxical intention. *American Journal of Psychotherapy* 14:520–535.

Friedman, S. (1987). Technical considerations in the behavioral-marital treatment of agoraphobia. *The American Journal of Family Therapy* 15:111–122.

Goldstein, A., and Chambless, D. L. (1978). A reanalysis of agoraphobia. *Behavior Therapy* 9:47–59.

Haley, J. (1973). *Uncommon Therapy*. New York: Norton.

────── (1976). *Problem-Solving Therapy*. San Francisco: Jossey-Bass.

Hand, I., and Lamontague, Y. (1976). The exacerbation of interpersonal problems after rapid phobia-removal. *Psychotherapy: Theory, Research and Practice* 13:405–411.

Marks, I. M. (1978). *Living with Fear*. New York: McGraw-Hill.

Mathews, A. M. (1977). Recent developments in the treatment of agoraphobia. *Behavioral Analysis and Modification* 2:64–75.

Mathews, A. M., Gelder, M. G., and Johnston, D. W. (1981). *Agoraphobia: Nature and Treatment*. New York: Guilford Press.

Milton, F., and Hafner, J. (1979). The outcome of behavior therapy for agoraphobia in relation to marital adjustment. *Archives of General Psychiatry* 36:807–811.

Rohrbaugh, M., Tennen, H., Press, S., and White, L. (1981). Compliance, defiance, and therapeutic paradox: Guidelines for strategic use of paradoxical interventions. *American Journal of Orthopsychiatry* 51:454–467.

Ross, J. (1982). The role of the family member in the supported exposure approach to the treatment of phobias. In *Phobias: A Comprehensive Summary of Modern Treatments*, ed. R. DuPont, pp. 35–43. New York: Brunner/Mazel.

Selvini-Palazzoli, M., Boscolo, L., Cecchin, G., and Prata, G. (1978). *Paradox and Counterparadox: A New Model in the Therapy of the Family in Schizophrenic Transaction.* New York: Jason Aronson.

Stedman, J. M., and Murphy, J. (1984). Dealing with specific child phobias during the course of family therapy: An alternative to systematic desensitization. *Family Therapy* 11:55-60.

Watzlawick, P., Weakland, J., and Fisch, R. (1974). *Change: Principles of Problem Formation and Problem Resolution.* New York: Norton.

Weakland, J., Fisch, R., Watzlawick, P., and Bodin, A. M. (1974). Brief therapy: Focused problem resolution. *Family Process* 13:141-168.

19 Psychoanalytic Psychotherapy

Dr. Abend presents in this chapter a brief outline of the fundamental assumptions of psychoanalytic psychotherapy concerning the dynamic structure of a phobia. He then presents an illustrative case report in which the interpretive sequence enables the patient to overcome her phobia.

The relationship between psychoanalysis and phobia therapy is remote, because the fundamental assumptions underlying the two schools are contradictory. The phobia therapists point to the research showing their techniques are more efficient and expedient. The psychoanalysts consider that they are treating the person as a whole, rather than allowing the symptom to define the person. Further, the psychoanalyst has a basic mistrust of behaviorism as simplistic and violating the principle of "neutrality." The phobia therapist believes that when a patient comes to him seeking symptom relief, the patient has made the decision to change that behavior and the therapist should use all his skill to effect that change. The psychoanalyst would reply that the patient's desire to change is often complicated by unconscious factors, which might prove to be quite contradictory to his or her announced intention.

As so often occurs in developing sciences, there has been a gradual shift of both positions toward the center. Psychoanalysts are more frequently making referrals for symptom relief, either concurrent with, or preceding, more intensive therapy. Phobia specialists are finding that a psychodynamic understanding may inform all phases of treatment, and such psychotherapy techniques may be important in managing other aspects of the therapist's interaction with the phobic patient, even when symptom-focused techniques are being employed.

Psychoanalytic Psychotherapy

Sander M. Abend

The treatment of phobias by psychoanalysis, or by psychodynamic psychotherapies derived from psychoanalysis, rests on the assumption that all phobias are defensively altered representations of underlying unconscious conflicts. The essence of the treatment consists in the uncovering and working through of these unconscious determinants; if successfully accomplished, this can alleviate their surface manifestations, the phobic symptoms themselves.

Thus, just as the analytic therapies regard the contents of dreams reported in a session as a perfect point of departure for analytic investigation, the surface texts of phobic concerns are similarly understood as the starting points for exploration of unconscious concerns and the fantasies that express them. Often, to begin with at least, the suffering patient may have no awareness of the existence of these underlying conflicts, much less of their relationship to the phobic symptoms to which they have given rise. The resolution of these unconscious stresses will often result in the disappearance of the phobia to which they are related.

Perhaps the best-known case of phobia every reported in the psychoanalytic literature was that of Little Hans, a 5-year-old boy who developed a paralyzing fear of horses. The monograph in which the unraveling of his phobias is described, entitled *Analysis of a Phobia in a Five-Year-Old Boy* (1909), is one of five famous lengthy clinical reports published by Sigmund Freud. Psychoanalytic theory and practice have evolved since the case of Little Hans first appeared in print, hence some of Freud's observations and explanations have been superseded by later findings and modifications. For our present purposes two points are worthy of note:

1. Freud classified phobias as closely related to what he called at the time *anxiety hysteria*, noting that the little boy's phobia only began some time after a more generalized anxiety state had made its appearance.

2. The "phobia" was not a single consistent fear of horses, but instead turned out to be a set of different, rather specific ideas, all involving horses, that frightened the little boy. These included (a) that a horse would bite him, (b) that only a big white horse was likely to bite him, (c) that a horse would fall down dead in the street, (d) that a horse would enter his room at night, and (e) that horses were to be feared only if they were pulling heavily laden carts or wagons. These individual variations, or refinements, of the patient's fears gradually came to light as the treatment progressed.

Freud did not conduct Little Hans's treatment himself. The boy was "analyzed," after a fashion, by his own father, with some help from Freud, at a time when no organized technique for psychoanalysis or psychotherapy of children had yet been developed, and when even the treatment of adults by psychoanalysis was at a very early stage of development. Even so, the material of the case led Freud to state with some confidence that many layers of unconscious meaning were all *condensed*, thus contributing in conjunction to the form of the phobic symptoms, and that in phobias the fearful situation was *projected* outside the individual's mind and onto an aspect of the environment that could then be avoided, thus enabling the patient to substitute a degree of constriction of life for what might otherwise be an intolerable and unavoidable subjective state of psychic discomfort. Although he did not use the precise term *displacement* at that time to explain the formation of the phobic symptoms, it is clear from his clinical descriptions that the horses, wagons, and so forth all stood for other persons or objects associated with them only by unconscious connections.

Freud's explanatory formulations in the Little Hans case stressed childhood sexual wishes and the conflicts stemming from them. His main purpose in writing up and publishing the case, however, was to lend support to his thesis about the potential pathogenic significance of infantile sexual concerns and theories. One can find, in the detailed clinical descriptions, hints of what analytic theory would only much later incorporate more explicitly: the role played by aggressive wishes and conflicts in phobia formation. One may also detect, in the explication of the case material, evidence of the contribution of pre-oedipal constellations and issues, of unconscious need for punishment, and of the secondary gains obtainable by manipulation of persons in the patient's environment.

It is also important to keep in mind that Freud's first theory of anxiety held sway when this report was written. At that time, anxiety was believed to be the end product of some quasi-biological alteration in the libido, conceived of rather concretely as if it were a physical substance. The transformation of libido into anxiety was somehow caused by the repression of the forbidden sexual wishes that were thought to be energized by this mysterious libido. Since anxiety was thought to be produced by repression, treatment was aimed at restoring health through the lifting of the repressions, which was gradually to be achieved by the psychoanalytic work.

Although theories and schools of psychoanalytic thought have multiplied since Freud's day, any statement of the current psychoanalytic understanding of the treatment of phobias would certainly include the principle that the symptom itself is overdetermined—that is to say, that a number of levels of meaning are likely to be found in the course of its successful unraveling.

Accordingly, no matter what general description of a phobia is obtained at the outset of treatment from a patient, analytic therapists expect that it will be revised in the course of treatment into several, perhaps even many, more specific subtexts, each of which will be related to some aspect or aspects of the unconscious significance of the symptom.

The assumption that phobic symptoms all do have unconscious underpinnings still characterizes the psychoanalytic theory of phobias. In pursuit of the sources of specific phobias analytic therapists are likely to seek associative evidence indicating the nature of their linkage to the unconscious wishes, fears, and fantasies they have come to represent, rather than to pursue a cognitive elaboration of the reality situation that obtained when the symptoms first appeared. It would be anticipated, as a matter of course, that sexual and aggressive wishes and their associated conflicts, stemming from all developmental levels, invariably including certain manifestations of guilt such as restitution or punishment, will combine to contribute to the establishment and maintenance of any phobia.

It is often stated that separation anxiety is likely to play an important role in phobia. It should be realized that *separation anxiety* does not refer merely to the real or imagined loss of an attachment. It is instead a kind of shorthand term for anxiety associated with a whole variety of real or fantasied losses. The complexity of unconscious mental activity is such that any perceived or dreaded loss may represent symbolically any or all the varieties of childhood danger situations and is not to be understood invariably to refer to loss of the mother or other primary caretaker.

As is well known, the therapeutic emphasis on discovering the unconscious meanings behind the surface phobic symptoms leads to a specific technical posture on the part of the analytic therapist. Efforts are directed toward uncovering the unconscious conflicts that give rise to the phobic concerns, rather than focusing primarily on the manifest descriptions and consequences of the phobias themselves or on efforts at reassuring, educating, or otherwise encouraging patients to combat or overcome their problems. It is no longer even considered appropriate analytic technique to urge patients to enter the avoided phobic situations, although that was at one time accepted practice, even among psychoanalysts of the most traditional stripe. The change in technique reflects strongly the accumulated and more accurate understanding arrived at in the recent period of psychoanalytic theory, which holds that the patients' defenses, manifested in treatment as resistance to progress, cannot merely be swept aside or overpowered. Resistance, too, like the forbidden wishes for sexual or aggressive gratification, and like the multiple influences of the patient's internalized moral system, must all receive equal and careful attention from the therapist in order to determine their respective roles on the symptoms and other aspects of the patient's psychological functioning.

In summary then, psychoanalytic therapists regard symptoms as providing a variety of manifest texts that one must attempt to understand and interpret. Treatment consists of as thorough an uncovering of their unconscious significance as is possible to achieve. The hidden significance will in all cases turn out to be complex; many levels of conflict, elaborated into unconscious fantasies, are likely to be incorporated into the formulation of phobic symptoms.

Perhaps the clearest and most comprehensive way to understand matters is to think of the phobias as compromise formations. This means the symptoms are the psychological result of the interplay between (1) certain sexual and aggressive wishes of childhood mental life, (2) the anxiety to which these give rise, (3) various expressions of superego reaction to these forbidden wishes, in the forms of punishment, undoing, restitution, and placation of the internalized moral authority, and (4) a panoply of defenses that may be mobilized against either the forbidden wishes, the anxiety, the superego influences, or some combination of all these forces in concert.

Among the ego mechanisms that are used defensively, those most commonly associated with the formation of phobic symptoms are condensation, displacement, and projection, but many other aspects of psychological functioning can also serve defensive ends.

The tracing out of these unconscious elements and their interrelationships is likely to take many months, even years, and if the effort is successful, the potential benefits of the treatment usually go far beyond the relief of the specific phobia or other symptoms. Patients today generally recognize both the longer time frame and the broader goals of psychoanalysis and psychoanalytic psychotherapy, so it would be unusual for a patient to seek such treatment or accept a recommendation for it, solely for the relief of even the most troublesome phobia. These days, the analytic understanding of phobic symptoms most often comes about during the course of a treatment that was initially undertaken for other reasons, or at least for reasons in addition to the phobic complaints themselves. Conversely, patients who are solely interested in the relief of a specific phobia, and who have no apparent awareness of other coexistent problems, as a rule do not seek psychoanalytically oriented treatment.

Only therapists with a thorough grounding in psychoanalytic conceptualization and techniques are likely to utilize this therapeutic approach to the treatment of patients' phobias. Such therapists and their patients will be prepared for the possibility that, even in successful therapies, improvement may come very slowly and gradually. This is not invariable, however, and in some cases improvement may be quite rapid. It is impossible to predict the rate and degree of change in a given symptom at the outset of analytic treatment, especially since the unconscious determinants of the problems often cannot be guessed at, nor can the patient's genuine motivation for change be accurately assayed from what he or she says to the therapist at the beginning of therapy.

The following brief clinical vignette will serve to illustrate some of the points mentioned.

> A divorced woman in her early thirties, a successful junior executive in a multinational corporate enterprise, sought treatment

because a flying phobia threatened to limit her career advancement. She revealed to the consultant who evaluated her that she had also had a bout of severe anxiety associated with flying some years earlier; this had subsided in the course of a limited psychotherapy that was a mixture of support and exploration. The symptoms had returned about a year ago, but this time a brief course of treatment similar to her earlier, successful, limited-goal therapy did not bring relief. If anything, the anxiety associated with flying seemed to be worsening. The patient added that she had an ongoing relationship with a man she valued highly; she wanted some help to try to assure that problems of hers that she thought had contributed to her previous marital failure did not spoil her present prospects for happiness. Both the patient and the consultant thought that a more intensive psychoanalytically oriented therapy was indicated at this time.

Despite many difficulties in immersing herself freely in the treatment, the patient's persistent and conscientious work gradually permitted a progressive unfolding of the many levels of meaning of her phobia about flying, accompanied by relief to the point of full recovery. (Certain other dimensions of her treatment were also successful but will not be described in the context of this illustration.)

The first level of understanding to emerge was that the patient used her anxiety before and during flights as a way of tormenting and punishing herself unmercifully. This punishment came to be seen as related to her career ambitions, which she imagined would necessarily involve intense and deadly competition, especially with men. As this configuration became clearer, the patient became able to report a more precise description of her anxiety about flying. She was terrified that in the course of a flight her discomfort would grow so intense that she would lose control of herself and become hysterical. Such an outburst would be intensely humiliating to her, especially if it were to occur in the company of a male co-worker. Eventually she was able to elaborate her view that such a hysterical loss of control as she imagined and dreaded would characterize her as a weak, contemptible female, destroying the image of the competent, firm, rational, and composed person (qualities she attributed to men) that she wished to present to the world. This disgrace would be a fit punishment for her ruthlessly defeating the males she competed with, which she imagined humiliated them terribly. In time it also became clear how these conflicts resonated with issues in her childhood relationship to her father, a successful businessman.

After this was worked out, she was able to recall that the current outbreak of flying phobia had commenced after a particular flight during which a male co-worker accompanying her party had regaled them with "war stories," consisting of harrowing tales of his heroism while in military service as a flyer. She had responded to his boasting with a mixture of inner fury, envy, and the conviction that she would not have been able to stand such experiences.

By this time in the therapy she was able to fly without experiencing much, if any, anxiety, but she still had considerable anticipatory dread. She noted the dread was much worse before flights home than it was when going elsewhere on business or vacation. This observation ushered in an elaboration of a new level of meaning of her phobic anxiety. She now had thoughts of panic and loss of control as a consequence of being confined within the plane with no way to get out, even if she became upset. Claustrophobic feelings led to a fuller exploration of her ambivalent relationship with her mother and to rivalrous feelings toward siblings of both sexes. In one session she described a fantasy that the airplane she was in might break apart, spilling her to her death. This led to associations about pregnancy, delivery, and abortion.

These subjects were also on her mind as she was considering alternatives to her business career, since she and her boyfriend were contemplating marriage. In the course of exploring these issues she revealed she had long held a conviction that her mother had come to wish she had aborted the patient, who had been a troublesome and difficult child. This idea about her mother, which was never confirmed, was expressed symbolically in the patient's fear that the plane would open up, dropping her to her death. With this reconstruction, the flying phobia improved still more.

One last level remained to be clarified. It came up in the course of the patient's description of her preflight ritual. Whenever she noted stirrings of anxiety, she thought of the therapist and usually experienced immediate relief. When she was asked why she though she needed to evoke his image, since she had obviously done much of the work of overcoming her problem herself, she became flustered and angry. She revealed that she believed she would always need treatment, and she berated her therapist for seeming to take away her comfort and undermining her peace of mind. It took some further time to clarify that she liked the idea of not being alone, especially when she felt possible danger to be present. This meant to her that the therapist had assumed the role of the wished-for benevolent and protective mother, in place of her real mother, with whom she had so unsatisfactory a relationship. When the therapist questioned her need for this fantasy relationship, the patient experienced this questioning as tantamount to rejecting her. The thought of ever ending treatment also carried that connotation. After a mild and brief regression, however, her phobic symptoms again disappeared as work toward termination proceeded.

The foregoing case demonstrates a number of features described in the introductory material. Several different specific versions of fear were incorporated in this woman's flying phobia. Various conflicts contributed to it, and these could only gradually be teased out of the material as treatment progressed. The transference dimension of her phobic structure came to light at the last, but it was clearly essential to be included in the treatment, or else the potential for another serious relapse in the future, after termination, would obviously have been much greater.

It should be added that this patient at all times considered her phobia to be irrational, and she clearly remembered her earlier success in overcoming it. Only in retrospect could she see that her lack of confidence in being able to maintain mastery over her symptoms on her own was itself a symptom, having a specific unconscious meaning, and one that had to be worked through in its turn. Only then could she begin to see the future more optimistically, with some sense that she now possessed the capability for mastering her phobia herself.

20 Medication

As noted in the introductory chapter, the biochemical understanding and psychopharmacology of anxiety disorders have become crucial aspects of treatment. Major innovations and improvements in pharmacotherapy continue to occur. The contributions of Dr. Klein and his collaborators, especially their original research on psychotropic medication in the anxiety disorders, eminently suit them to provide this survey chapter, which gives us an up-to-date, practical orientation to the medications currently in use.

Medication

Eric Hollander
Donald F. Klein

INTRODUCTION

Pharmacological treatment of the anxiety disorders can be a gratifying experience for the informed psychiatrist. Rarely does a group of disorders have such a clear response to medication, or is there such dramatic relief in the patients' subjective distress.

This chapter will summarize current approaches to the pharmacological treatment of panic disorder and generalized anxiety disorder, social phobia, and obsessive-compulsive disorder. Rather than an exhaustive review of controlled studies, it describes practical approaches and common pitfalls.

GENERAL PRINCIPLES

Treatment approaches differ for different types of anxiety disorders. This makes precise differential diagnosis crucial prior to treatment. Treatments highly effective for one type of anxiety may be ineffective for another. In addition, it is imperative to rule out underlying medical conditions that might masquerade as anxiety disorders. These include, but are not limited to, thyroid and parathyroid disease, pheochromocytoma, cardiac abnormalities and arrhythmias, temporal-lobe epilepsy, alcohol and substance abuse (cocaine in particular), and caffeinism.

Since anxiety patients are often extremely sensitive to medication, and may actually experience a paradoxical exacerbation of symptoms early in treatment, especially if initial doses are too high, one must begin with very low doses, and the patient should be warned about this possibility. Another treatment problem frequently encountered is the use of inadequate doses of medication or duration of treatment. Patients should receive an "adequate trial" of a given medication prior to the decision to change medication. Thus the maxim "Start low, go high, and persist" is appropriate.

MEDICATION TREATMENT OF PANIC DISORDERS

Pharmacological treatment of panic disorder is based on the three-stage model of panic developed by Klein (1981). The core symptom is recurrent, spontaneous panic attacks. Repeated experience of unexpected panic attacks leads to anticipatory anxiety or dread about when or where the next one will occur. Many patients then begin to avoid situations in which help might be unavailable or escape difficult if a panic attack occurs. This is the agoraphobic complication of panic disorder.

The initial goal of treatment is to block the spontaneous panic attacks with medication. Achieving this usually takes several weeks. Patients are then encouraged to re-enter phobic situations. Re-entry will confirm that the patient no longer panics in the feared situation, and this assurance will help extinguish the avoidance behavior. Persistent absence of panic in spite of return to normal activity extinguishes the anticipatory anxiety as well.

It is important that the patient learn to distinguish between panic and anticipatory anxiety, since the medication will block panic but not anticipatory anxiety. In measuring effects of drug treatment, it is necessary to specifically inquire about spontaneous panic attacks, anticipatory anxiety, and phobic avoidance. It is helpful for the patient to keep a daily diary of anxiety symptoms and episodes during the course of treatment. Often patients will state that they are unimproved because of persisting anticipatory anxiety, but a diary review shows sharp improvement in panic experience.

A central feature of panic is fear of loss of control. It is helpful to give reassurance that medication specifically tailored for panic attacks will not affect the patient's ability to control himself or the environment. It is also important to discuss possible early side effects of the medication, so that the patient does not interpret somatic sensations as signs of imminent panic.

Before initiation of treatment, it is important to conduct an individualized medical evaluation. This is necessary to rule out other illnesses masquerading as panic or anxiety, as discussed above. It is also important to determine if there are existing medical illnesses that might be exacerbated by treatment, such as cardiac conduction defects and narrow-angle glaucoma. Other illnesses may preclude specific treatments, such as asthma precluding MAO inhibitors.

Antidepressants

Tricyclics

The central feature in treatment of panic disorder is the pharmacologic blockade of the spontaneous panic. Several classes of medication are effective in accomplishing this. The most widely used and studied are the tricyclic antidepressants, especially imipramine, desipramine, and clomipramine. Other tricyclics, including nortriptyline and amitriptyline, have not been systematically studied. Monoamine oxidase inhibitors (MAOIs) are effective antipanic drugs but are usually reserved for patients who do not respond to tricyclic antidepressants. The presence of depressed mood is not a requirement for any of these drugs to be effective in blocking panic attacks.

Imipramine has been the most extensively studied tricyclic. Klein (Klein and Fink 1962, Klein 1964) first noted the antipanic effects of imipramine in studies of hospitalized phobic anxiety patients. Imipramine blocked panic but had little effect on anticipatory anxiety or phobic avoidance. Subsequent double-blind studies confirmed the superiority of imipramine compared to placebo (Ballenger et al. 1977, Klein 1967, Mavissakalian and Michelson 1986a, Sheehan et al. 1980, Zitrin et al, 1978, Zitrin et al. 1980). Patients with panic attacks who do not have agoraphobia do equally as well as agoraphobics with panic (Garakani et al. 1984, Liebowitz et al. 1984). The antipanic effect of imipramine has been shown to be independent of depression (Mavissakalian and Michelson 1986b, Zitrin et al. 1983). There is some evidence that higher doses yield better outcome (Mavissakalian and Perel 1985, Zitrin et al. 1983).

When initiating a drug regimen, it is crucial for the patient to understand that the drug will block the panic attacks but not necessarily decrease the amount of intervening anticipatory anxiety. Patients may need also to take a benzodiazepine for a short time to reduce the level of anticipatory anxiety.

Some patients with panic disorder display an initial hypersensitivity to tricyclic antidepressants and monoamine oxidase inhibitors in which they complain of jitteriness, agitation, a "speedy" feeling, and insomnia. This is transient, but it is recommended that patients with panic disorder be started on lower doses of tricyclics or monoamine oxidase inhibitors than would be given to depressed patients.

One regimen is to start the patient at a dosage of 10 mg daily, at night, of imipramine and increase the dose by 10 mg every other night until 50 mg is reached. The dosage can be given all at once. Since imipramine tends to be sedating, bedtime dosing is helpful for insomnia and reduces daytime drowsiness. The occasional patient who is overstimulated can take the medication in the morning. If 50 mg is inadequate for full-panic blockade, the dosage is raised by 25 mg increments every 3 days or by 50 mg weekly to as high as 300 mg. Most patients need at least 150 mg daily of tricyclics. Unfortunately, underdosage commonly occurs. In some cases a dosage of imipramine over 300 mg is necessary. This requires monitoring of the electrocardiogram. Panic patients not responding to 300 mg/day of imipramine should have blood tricyclic levels measured. Often, blood levels will be disproportionately low for the dose, suggesting rapid metabolism or excretion, malabsorption, or noncompliance.

Patients who experience excessive anticholinergic side effects to imipramine can be given desipramine instead. Desipramine treatment is often accompanied by less dry mouth, blurred vision, and constipation. In addition, there is less sedation, so that daytime drug administration is possible.

Once full remission of panic attacks has been accomplished, it is recommended that the patient be kept on medication for a full 6 months to a year to prevent early relapse. After this, it is reasonable to taper the patient from medication. Although for many, panic disorder tends to be a recurrent condition, several studies suggest that up to two-thirds of patients will not relapse immediately after cessation of medication (Cohen et al. 1984, Zitrin and Klein 1983). Further studies in this area are needed.

Preliminary studies have indicated that tricyclic antidepressants may also be effective in treating chronically anxious patients who have neither depression nor panic. To date, the findings of tricyclic utility in nonpanic anxiety are still preliminary, and we do not recommend this as a primary treatment.

MAO Inhibitors

Since monoamine oxidase inhibitors (MAOIs) have the additional rare side effect of hypertensive crisis, they are regarded as a second-line treatment for panic disorder. To prevent the possibility of hypertensive crisis, it is important to review a list of foods and medications that must be avoided. Foods that contain tyramine are avoided, since with the blockade of intestinal monoamine oxidase, the enzyme that normally degrades tyramine, the blood pressure may rise to dangerous levels. These foods include, but are not limited to aged cheeses, smoked or processed meats or fish, and red wine. Tyramine is a product of protein fermentation. Other medications that are sympathomimetic should also be avoided. These include epinephrine, often used in dental procedures, or phenylpropanolamine, an over-the-counter stimulant. Illicit drugs such as cocaine, and the marketed analgesic medication Demerol also must be avoided.

However, MAO inhibitors are quite effective and should be considered for those patients who do not respond to tricyclics, cannot tolerate them, or have coexistent atypical depression or social phobia, for which MAOIs may be the treatment of choice. Available MAOIs include phenelzine (Nardil), isocarboxazid (Marplan), and tranylcypromine (Parnate). In our experience the antihypertensive pargyline (Eutonyl) is also effective.

In a double-blind placebo-controlled comparison of imipramine and phenelzine in agoraphobic patients, phenelzine was slightly better than imipramine and had fewer side effects (Ballenger et al. 1977, Sheehan et al. 1980).

Phenelzine, is often the MAOI used first. However, if sedation and weight gain are of great concern, tranylcypromine, which is less sedating and decreases appetite, can be given. Phenelzine may be initiated at 15 mg daily, in a morning dose. The dose may be raised by 15 mg every 4 to 7 days, as tolerated, to a maximum dose of 90 mg. Tranylcypromine (Parnate) is begun at 10 mg in the morning. The dose may be raised by 10 mg every 3 to 4 days, as needed, to a maximum of 80 mg per day.

After informing the patient about the common side effects, as well as the rare but potentially life-threatening side effect of hypertensive crisis, treatment with monoamine oxidase inhibitors may begin. Common side effects include daytime sedation, nighttime insomnia, and orthostatic hypotension. These side effects, if they arise, may be managed by reduction of the dosage. Daytime sedation may be effectively treated with the addition of caffeine in moderation or methylphenidate. Nighttime insomnia can be managed by adding 25 to 50 mg of trazodone at bedtime.

Orthostatic hypotension is treated by adding salt to food, using salt tablets, or adding the mineralocorticoid florinef, 0.1 mg, 1 to 3 times per day. Other possible side effects include dry mouth, constipation, blurred vision, sweating, tremor, palpitations, urinary hesitancy, sexual side effects, anorgasmia, and liver toxicity. Pyridoxine (vitamin B6 deficiency) has also been reported, presenting with numbness and tingling, and may be treated by adding B6, 100 to 300 mg per day.

The hypertensive reaction may present with a severe throbbing headache, nausea, vomiting, and high blood pressure. While the incidence of paroxysmal headaches is about 2%, progression to intracranial bleed or myocardial infarction is very rare, with the fatality rate less than one in 100,000 (Klein et al. 1980). A patient who experiences the symptoms described should proceed to an emergency room to have their blood pressure monitored. If blood pressure is elevated, treatment with intravenous phentolamine, an alpha antagonist, is the treatment of choice. Patients may also be advised to carry around a 20-mg capsule of the antianginal medication nifedipine (Procardia). At the first sign of a hypertensive reaction they chew on the capsule, which rapidly lowers blood pressure. It is important to note that the risk of hypertensive crisis continues for 2 weeks after discontinuation of an MAOI, so the diet must be continued during this time. Also, different MAOIs are incompatible, so on switching from one to the other, a 2-week washout is required. The serotonin reuptake blocker fluoxetine (Prozac) is also contraindicated for 2 weeks following discontinuation of a MAOI.

Benzodiazepine Derivatives

The high-potency benzodiazepine alprazolam (Xanax) is an effective antipanic drug. There is less data about the efficacy of the other high potency benzodiazepines, clonazepam (Klonopin) and lorazepam (Ativan), but what exists is promising. Long-term efficacy and possible physiological dependency are still under investigation. These medications have fewer initial side effects than tricyclic antidepressants and monoamine oxidase inhibitors but require longer periods for withdrawal (25 mg every 7 days is a safe regimen). Doses as high as 10 mg daily may be required, although 3 mg to 5 mg given in divided doses daily are generally sufficient. Alprazolam may occasionally cause mania and clonazepam depression.

The major drawback of these medications is the substantial risk of withdrawal symptoms during taper (Fyer et al. 1987). In severe cases, delirium and seizures have been reported with abrupt withdrawal. Alprazolam's short duration of action often necessitates every-4-hour dosing. Because of this short half-life, the phenomenon of "clock-watching" has been reported. The patient may notice an increased level of anxiety prior to his next dose. This is less of a problem with clonazepam, which has a longer half-life. Another early side effect of these agents is sedation.

Generalized anxiety disorder (GAD), features persistent anxiety and worrisomeness lasting at least 6 months. Symptoms include motor tension, autonomic hyperactivity (sweating, heart pounding, and frequent urination), apprehensive expectation, and vigilance and scanning (insomnia, difficulty concentrating). The pharmacologic treatment of GAD is less well established. Traditionally, chronically anxious patients have been placed on benzodiazepines. However, no study has yet shown benzodiazepines to be more effective than other drugs or treatment methods in patients specifically diagnosed with GAD. One study suggests that benzodiazepines such as chlordiazepoxide may peak in effectiveness after 4 weeks of treatments, and that tricyclics such as imipramine may be more effective for patients with generalized anxiety over the longer term (Kahn et al. 1986). But the study may have included panic patients and requires replication.

Although generally safe, with side effects limited mainly to sedation, there is growing concern that some patients may become tolerant or even physiologically dependent on benzodiazepines. Available data indicate that most patients are able to stop taking them without serious sequelae and that the problem of frank addiction is substantially overestimated. It is probably limited to an addiction-prone population (e.g., past history of alcoholism) or to patients with panic disorder who often escalate standard benzodiazepine usage in unsuccessful attempts at self-medication. Withdrawal symptoms of insomnia, agitation, irritability, and sensory disturbances can occur and are considerably lessened by gradual tapering of the medication. The distinction between actual withdrawal and a simple recrudescence of the original anxiety symptoms when the benzodiazepine is stopped remains controversial. However the onset of insomnia is a useful clue to withdrawal. A few preliminary studies have shown continued efficacy of these drugs at the same dose level up to 6 months after beginning treatment.

A new drug, buspirone, is a nonbenzodiazepine antianxiety agent that appears to have less sedative property than the benzodiazepines and less potential for abuse. It has been shown clinically efficacious in GAD but not in panic disorder. The problem is a slow onset of action and a lack of subjective feeling of relaxation. More investigation is required.

Serotonin Reuptake Blockers

There has been a great deal of interest lately in the use of serotonin reuptake blockers for the treatment of panic disorder. Studies with a specific serotonin receptor agonist, m-CPP, have shown that panic patients have greater anxiety reactions than controls in response to this challenge (Kahn et al., unpublished observations), suggesting some level of serotonergic dysregulation. Early studies with fluoxetine (Prozac) reported that many panic patients could not tolerate the 20-mg initial dose (Gorman et al. 1987). However, those that could tolerate this initial dose often showed improvement. Recent studies report that the experimental serotonin reuptake blockers fluvoxamine and clomipramine are equally effective in panic disorder, but that clomipramine has a better antidepressant effect (Den Boer 1988.) A controlled comparison of experimental selective serotonergic (fluvoxamine) and noradrenergic (maprotiline) antidepressants in panic disorder reported superiority for the serotonergic agent fluoxetine (Den Boer 1988). In a double-blind placebo-controlled study of fluvoxamine and ritanserin (a specific 5HT-2 receptor antagonist) in panic disorder, fluvoxamine resulted in a profound reduction in the number of panic attacks, followed by a subsequent decrease in agoraphobic avoidance behavior. Treatment with ritanserin appeared ineffective (Den Boer 1988). In our clinical experience, panic-disorder patients have a good response to fluoxetine (Prozac) if treatment is initiated at a low dose of 5 mg. The 20-mg capsule may be dissolved in water to attain this dose.

Other Medications

Beta-adrenergic blocking drugs, such as propranolol, are said by some to be useful in a variety of anxiety disorders (Munjack et al. 1985), but there is no proof that they are specifically effective in blocking spontaneous panic attacks. Our impression is that they are only occasionally active and work less well than tricyclic antidepressants, monoamine oxidase inhibitors, or alprazolam. They are not to be used as primary, first-choice drugs.

Clonidine, which quiets locus ceruleus discharge, would seem for theoretical reasons to be a good antipanic drug. Although in a small series two-thirds of patients responded (Liebowitz et al. 1981), for several the therapeutic effect was lost in a matter of weeks despite continuation of dose. This, plus a number of bothersome side effects, makes clonidine a poor initial choice for panic disorder. One controlled 2-week crossover study found clonidine to be efficacious for both panic disorder and GAD (Hoehn-Saric 1981). However, Hoehn-Saric agrees that the effects are lost with time.

MEDICATION TREATMENT OF PHOBIC DISORDERS

Agoraphobia

The clinical picture in agoraphobia consists of fears and avoidance behaviors that center around three main themes: (1) fear of leaving home, (2) fear of being alone, and (3) fear of being in a situation where one cannot escape or help is not available. There is some disagreement as to the best method of treatment of agoraphobia with panic attacks. One widely employed strategy is the use of medication to block panic attacks followed by a psychoeducational intervention that encourages the patient to re-enter phobic situations. (For a discussion of the pharmacotherapy of panic attacks, see the panic-disorder section of this chapter.) A second strategy uses behavioral psychotherapy alone in treatment of these patients. Lately there has been a shift from exposure to phobic situations to exposure to paniclike sensations, in an attempt to prevent catastophizing. Comparative controlled trials are needed.

The treatment for agoraphobia without panic attacks is behavioral psychotherapy that includes or encourages exposure to phobic situations. Limited symptom attacks, however, should be treated like panic attacks, and in our experience are almost uniformly present in so-called agoraphobia without panic.

Social Phobia

In social phobia, the central fear is of humiliation or embarrassment in front of others. This may be generalized (occurring in most social situations) or discrete (occurring only in performance situations, such as public speaking). Medication studies in social phobia are few. Analogue (nonclinical samples with performance or social anxiety) studies suggest beta-blocker efficacy, particularly when used acutely prior to a performance (Liden and Gottfries 1974, Brantigan et al. 1982, Hartley et al. 1983). Many performing artists or public speakers find that propranolol 10-20 mg p.o. 1 hour before stage time reduces palpitations, tremor, and "the butterfly feeling."

The MAO inhibitor phenelzine was found effective in mixed agoraphobic-social phobic samples (Tyrer et al. 1973) and in an open trial of social phobics (Mountjoy et al. 1977). In this trial a number of patients with generalized social phobia (also meeting criteria for avoidant personality) became much more socially comfortable and outgoing within 6 weeks on phenelzine 45-90 mg/day. Cessation within 6 months was followed by relapse, and more chronic treatment requires study. Liebowitz et al. (1988) conducted a double-blind, placebo-controlled comparison of phenelzine and the beta blocker atenolol in a large sample of carefully diagnosed social phobics. Phenelzine was superior in the vast majority of patients with generalized social phobia. Atenolol was helpful for subjects with discrete social phobia, such as public speaking. Further studies are needed to compare the efficacy and possible synergism of medications and behavioral treatments of social phobia.

Simple Phobia

Simple phobias are circumscribed fears of specific objects, situations, or activities. The fear is usually not of the object itself but of some dire outcome that may result from contact with the object. Examples are fear of snakes, heights, driving, and enclosed spaces. In the limited number of studies available to date, tricyclics, benzodiazepines, and beta blockers generally do not appear useful for simple phobics. Exposure therapy is often effective.

MEDICATION TREATMENT OF OBSESSIVE-COMPULSIVE DISORDER

Recent advances in the pharmacotherapy of obsessive-compulsive disorder (OCD) have generated a great deal of excitement in the study of this disorder and have led to a re-evaluation of the etiology of OCD.

Because of OCDs chronic, refractory nature a wide variety of medications have been used in its treatment. There have been case reports documenting a response to lithium, trazadone, alprazolam, phenelzine, tranylcypromine, imipramine, amphetamine, and tryptophan in individual OCD patients, without the use of controls. Uncontrolled series have also demonstrated improvement with MAO inhibitors only in those patients with coexistent panic attacks (Jenike et al. 1983) and an improvement during acute exacerbations with neuroleptics (Ananth 1976). There are also reports of improvement in OCD symptoms following oral (Knesevich 1982) and intravenous (Hollander et al. 1988a) clonidine, although this effect appears to be transient.

The most promising development has been with the tricyclic antidepressant clomipramine (Anafranil) (CMI). This drug is not yet easily available in the United States but is widely used in treating OCD in Canada and Europe. Since the 1970s, a number of uncontrolled studies from these countries have documented improvement in primary OCD patients with clomipramine.

More recently, a series of well-controlled double-blind studies have documented that clomipramine is more effective than placebo in reducing OCD symptoms (Ananth 1976, Flament et al. 1985, Insel et al. 1983, Montgomery 1980, Thoren et al. 1980a, Volavka et al. 1985). Clomipramine is equally effective for OCD patients with pure obsessions and those with rituals, in contrast to behavioral treatments, which are less useful for patients with obsessions not accompanied by rituals.

In a review of all seven CMI studies with a total of 106 patients, two-thirds were found to be significantly improved on blind ratings (Insel and Zohar 1988). Some patients show an almost complete remission, others little or no improvement. Overall, there appears to be an average reduction of OCD symptoms of more than 40%. There is a relatively slow improvement with CMI, with a maximum improvement occurring after 5 to 12 weeks of treatment. While one study found a greater effect of CMI compared to placebo only in the most depressed subgroup (Marks et al. 1980), the majority of studies find specific antiobsessional effects irrespective of depressive symptoms (Flament 1985, Insel et al. 1983, Montgomery 1980, Thoren et al. 1980, Volavka 1985). Controlled studies also suggest CMI is more effective than other antidepressants.

Studies with one specific serotonin reuptake blocker zimelidine report mixed results, but others such as fluvoxamine and fluoxetine have also demonstrated specific antiobsessional effects in uncontrolled and controlled trials. Intravenous clomipramine has met with success in some patients refractory to oral clomipramine (Warnecke 1985). Other strategies for treating partially refractory OCD patients include addition of lithium, clonidine (Hollander et al. 1988b), and especially fenfluramine (Pondimin) (Hollander and Liebowitz 1988c) to existing serotonin reuptake blocker treatment.

It is of great interest that oral M-CPP (*m*-chlorophenyl piperazine), a selective 5HT antagonist, has been found to increase obsessions in OCD patients when given acutely (Zohar et al. 1987, Hollander 1988). This effect has been shown to decrease after chronic treatment with clomipramine (Zohar et al. 1988) or fluoxetine (Hollander et al., unpublished observations), suggesting that chronic treatment may correct the serotonin dysregulation.

Case Management Approach

Patient cooperation is an invaluable aid to treatment with psychotropic agents. A common cause of treatment failure is noncompliance, or not taking the medication. One reason for resistance is that accepting medication forces the patient to admit that he is sick. Some patients also fear loss of control to the medication.

Building of rapport between doctor and patient is of great importance. Empathy, reassurance, and clarification from the physician will enable most patients to take medication regularly and without undue anxiety. However, severe cases may require added interventions. Arranging for the patient to talk with another anxiety-disorder patient who has previously taken the medication is helpful. Participation in a short-term educational support group with other patients who are currently starting medication is also helpful.

A psychoeducational approach involves describing to the patient the entire course of treatment as envisioned. This includes the period of time before clinical improvement is expected, the frequency in changes of drug dosage, the eventual dose that probably will be attained, and the expected length of drug treatment. Possible and expected side effects should be described to help prevent catastrophizing as a result of new somatic sensations and to build confidence in the treatment.

The patient should be instructed to notify his doctor immediately of any unusual side effects. The physician should be available during the initial phases of treatment. We routinely provide 24-hour telephone coverage. This is an extremely reassuring experience, and most patients do not abuse this practice.

Sometimes problems arise if the psychotherapist is covertly competitive with the effectiveness of drug treatment. This may lead to low dose and premature termination of medication. Therefore, there must be good rapport between psychotherapist and psychopharmacologist.

For most patients, the combination of medication, education about the illness, and supportive encouragement are sufficient. For others, adjunctive treatment (behavioral or cognitive exercises) may be required. Treatment failures are most commonly due to inadequate dose, insufficient medication trial, or misdiagnosis of concomitant psychiatric disorder, rather than the refractory nature of the illness.

REFERENCES

Ananth, J. (1976). Treatment of obsessive-compulsive neurosis: pharmacological approach. *Psychosomatics* 17:180–184.

Ananth, J., Solyom, L., Bryntwich, S., et al. (1979). Clorimipramine therapy for obsessive-compulsive neurosis. *American Journal of Psychiatry* 136:700–701.

Ballenger, J. C., Sheehan, D. V., and Jacobson, G. (1977). Antidepressant treatment of severe phobic anxiety. In *Abstracts of Scientific Proceedings of the 130th Annual Meeting of the American Psychiatric Association, Toronto.*

Brantigan, C. O., Brantigan, T. A., and Joseph, N. (1982). Effect of beta blockade and beta stimulation on stage fright. *American Journal of Medicine* 72:88–94.

Cohen, S. D., Moneiro, W., and Marks, I. M. (1984). Two-year follow-up of agoraphobics after exposure and imipramine. *British Journal of Psychiatry* 144:276–281.

Den Boer, J. A. (1988). Serotonergic mechanisms in anxiety disorders: An inquiry into serotonin function in panic disorder. *Cip-Gegevens Koninklijke Bibliotheek, Den Haag.*

Flament, M. F., Rapoport, J. L., Berg, C. J., et al. (1985). Clomipramine treatment of childhood obsessive compulsive disorder: A double blind controlled study. *Archives of General Psychiatry* 42:977–986.

Fyer, A. J., Liebowitz, M. R., Gorman, J. M., et al. (1987). Discontinuation of alprazolam treatment in panic patients. *American Journal of Psychiatry* 144:303–308.

Garakani, H., Zitrin, C. M., and Klein, D. F. (1984). Treatment of panic disorder with imipramine alone. *American Journal of Psychiatry* 141:446–448.

Gorman, J. M., Liebowitz, M. R., Fyer, A. J., et al. (1987). An open trial of fluoxetine in the treatment of panic attacks. *Journal of Clinical Psychopharmacology* 7:329–332.

Hartley, L. R., Ungapen, S., Davie, I., and Spencer, D. J. (1983). The effect of beta adrenergic blocking drugs on speakers' performance and memory. *British Journal of Psychiatry* 142:512–517.

Herman, J. B., Rosenbaum, J. F., Brotman, A. W. (1987). The alprazolam to clonazepam switch for the treatment of panic disorder. *Journal of Clinical Psychopharmacology* 7:175–178.

Hoehn-Saric, R., Merchant, A. F., Keyser, M. L., et al. (1981). Effects of clonidine on anxiety disorders. *Archives of General Psychiatry* 38:1278–1282.

Hollander, E., Fay, M., Cohen, B., et al. (1988a). Serotonergic and noradrenergic sensitivity in obsessive-compulsive disorder: Behavioral findings. *American Journal of Psychiatry* 145:1015-1017.

Hollander, E., Fay, M., and Liebowitz, M. R. (1988b). Clonidine and clomipramine in obsessive-compulsive disorder. *American Journal of Psychiatry* 145:388-389.

Hollander, E., and Liebowitz, M. R. (1988c). Augmentation of antiobsessional treatment with fenfluramine. *American Journal of Psychiatry* 145:1314-1315.

Insel, T. R., Murphy, D. L., Cohen, R. M., et al. (1983). OCD: A double blind trial of clomipramine and clorgyline. *Archives of General Psychiatry* 40:605-612.

Insel, T. R., and Zohar, J. (1988). Psychopharmacological approaches to obsessive compulsive disorder. In *Psychopharmacology, vol. I, A Generation of Progress*, ed. H. Meltzer. American College of Neuropsychopharmacology.

Jenicke, M. A., Surman, O. S., Cassem, N. H., et al. (1983). Monoamine oxidase inhibitors in obsessive compulsive disorder. *Journal of Clinical Psychiatry* 44:131-132.

Kahn, R. J., McNair, D. M., Lipman, R. S., et al. (1986). Imipramine and chlordiazepoxide in depression and anxiety disorders. *Archives of General Psychiatry* 43:79-85.

Klein, D. F. (1964). Delineation of two drug responsive anxiety syndromes. *Psychopharmacologia* 5:397-408.

────── (1967). Importance of psychiatric diagnosis in prediction of clinical drug effects. *Archives of General Psychiatry* 16:118-126.

────── (1981). Anxiety reconceptualized. In *Anxiety: New Research and Changing Concepts*, ed. D. F. Klein and J. G. Rabkin. New York: Raven Press.

Klein, D. F., and Fink, M. (1962). Psychiatric reaction patterns to imipramine. *American Journal of Psychiatry* 119:432-438.

Klein, D. F., Gittleman, R., Quitkin, F., et al. (1980). *Diagnosis and Drug Treatment of Psychiatric Disorders: Adults and Children*, 2nd ed. Baltimore: Williams & Wilkins.

Knesevich, J. W. (1982). Successful treatment of obsessive-compulsive disorder with clonidine hydrochloride. *American Journal of Psychiatry* 139:364-365.

Liden, S., and Gottfries, C. G. (1974). Beta-blocking agents in the treatment of catecholamine-induced symptoms in musicians. *Lancet* 2:529.

Liebowitz, M. R., Fyer, A. F., Gorman, J. M., et al. (1984). Lactate provocation of panic attacks. I. Clinical and behavioral findings. *Archives of General Psychiatry* 41:764-770.

Liebowitz, M. R., Fyer, A. J., McGrath, P., and Klein, D. F. (1981). Clonidine treatment of panic disorder. *Psychopharmacology Bulletin* 17:122-123.

Liebowitz, M. R., Gorman, J. M., Fyer, A. J., et al. (1988). Pharmacotherapy of social phobia: An interim report of a placebo controlled comparison of phenelzine and atenolol. *Journal of Clinical Psychiatry* 49:252-257.

Liebowitz, M. R., Quitkin, F., Stewart, J. W., et al. (1984). Phenelzine versus imipramine in atypical depression: A preliminary report. *Archives of General Psychiatry* 120:669-667.

Marks, I. M., Stern, R., Mawson, D., et al. (1980). Clomipramine and exposure for obsessive compulsive rituals. *British Journal of Psychiatry* 136:1-25.

Mavissakalian, M., and Michelson, L. (1986a). Agoraphobia: Relative and combined effectiveness of therapist assisted in vivo exposure and imipramine. *Journal of Clinical Psychiatry* 47:117-122.

Mavissakalian, M., and Michelson, L. (1986b) Two year followup of exposure and imipramine treatment of agoraphobia. *American Journal of Psychiatry* 143:1106-1112.

Mavissakalian, M., and Perel, J. (1985). Imipramine in the treatment of agoraphobia: Dose-response relationships. *American Journal of Psychiatry* 142:1032-1036.

Montgomery, S. A. (1980). Clomipramine in obsessional neurosis: A placebo controlled study. *Pharmaceutical Medicine* 1:189-192.

Mountjoy, C. Q., Roth, M., Garside, R. F., and Leitch, I. M. (1977). A clinical trial of phenelzine in anxiety depressive and phobic neuroses. *British Journal of Psychiatry* 131:486-492.

Munjack, D. J., Robal, R., Shaner, R., et al. (1985). Imipramine versus propranolol for the treatment of panic attacks: A pilot study. *Comparative Psychiatry* 26:80-89.

Sheehan, D. V., Ballenger, J., and Jacobsen, G. (1980). Treatment of endogenous anxiety with phobic, hysterical, and hypochondriacal symptoms. *Archives of General Psychiatry* 37:51-59.

Thoren, P., Asberg, M., Cronholm, B., et al. (1980). Clomipramine treatment of obsessive-compulsive disorder: A controlled clinical trial. *Archives of General Psychiatry* 37:1281-1289.

Thoren, P., Asberg, M., Bertilsson, L., et al. (1980). Clomipramine treatment of obsessive-compulsive disorder. II. Biochemical aspects. *Archives of General Psychiatry* 37:1289-1294.

Tyrer, P., Candy, J., and Kelly, D. (1973). A study of the clinical effects of phenelzine and placebo in the treatment of phobic anxiety. *Psychopharmacology* 32:237-254.

Volavka, J., Neziroglu, F., Yaryura-Tobias, J. A. (1985). Clomipramine and imipramine in obsessive-compulsive disorder. *Psychiatry Research* 14:83-91.

Warneke, L. B. (1985). Intravenous chlorimipramine in the treatment of obsessional disorder in adolescence: Case report. *Journal of Clinical Psychiatry* 46:100-103.

Zitrin, C. M., Klein, D. F., Woerner, M. G. (1980). Treatment of agoraphobia with group exposure in vivo and imipramine. *Archives of General Psychiatry* 37:63-72.

Zitrin, C. M., Klein, D. F., Woerner, M. G., and Ross, D. C. (1983). Treatment of phobias. I. Comparison of imipramine and placebo. *Archives of General Psychiatry* 40:125-138.

Zitrin, C. M., Klein, D. F., Woerner, M. G., et al. (1978). Behavior therapy, supportive psychotherapy, imipramine, and phobias. *Archives of General Psychiatry* 35:307-316.

Zohar, J., Mueller, E. A., and Insel, T. R. (1987). Serotonergic responsivity in obsessive-compulsive disorder: Comparison of patients and healthy controls. *Archives of General Psychiatry* 44:946-951.

Zohar, J., Insel, T. R., Zohar-Kadouch, R. C., et al. (1988). Serotonergic responsivity in obsessive-compulsive disorder: Effects of chronic clomipramine treatment. *Archives of General Psychiatry* 45:167-172.

Index

Agoraphobia, 41-82
 anger, 67-68, 78-80
 bibliotherapy for, 329-337
 complex, 76-81
 interpersonal maneuvers, 343-345
 in vivo exposure, 56-60
 onset of, 46-47
 panic-management strategies for, 60-71, 332-334
 prevalence of, 45, 76
 problems associated with, 47-48
 psychopharmacological intervention for, 68-71, 417-418
 treatment planning for, 48-56
Agras, W. S., 358
Agulnik, P., 342
Alprazolam (Xanax), 70, 119, 217, 414
Amies, P. L., 98-100
Analysis of a Phobia in a Five-Year-Old Boy (Freud), 396
Ananth, J., 419-420

The Anatomy of Melancholy (Burton), 18
Andrasik, F., 213
Anticipatory anxiety, 7-8
 contextual therapy, 240
 coping techniques, 256-257, 273
 generalized anxiety disorder, 120-121
 flying phobia, 174-175
Antidepressants, 69, 409-416
Anxiety, 94
 anticipatory, *see* anticipatory anxiety
 chronic, 47-48
 endogenous, 23
 evaluation, 89-112
 exogenous, 23
 feelings mislabeled as, 67-68
 normal, 61-62
 physiology of, *see* physiology of anxiety
 public-speaking, 105-108
 and repression, 397

427

Anxiety (*continued*)
  separation, *see* separation anxiety
  social, 48
  stranger, 148-149
  test, 109-111
Anxiety coping techniques, 245-258
  flying, *see* in vivo desensitization
Anxiety disorders
  diagnosis of, 17-34
  Interview Schedule (ADIS), 212-213. *See also* individual disorders
  myths and misinterpretations, 233-236
Apotrepic therapy, 187
Arnow, B. A., 358
Assertiveness, 80, 88
Attention manipulation, 62-63
Automatic inhibition, 93-94
Aversion therapy, 186-187
Avoidance, 212, 262
  cognitive therapy for, 65-66
  diagnosis, 22-23, 24, 26
  generalized anxiety disorder, 121-123
  in vivo exposure for, 56-60, 77
  obsessive compulsive, 195-196
  systems theory, 370
Avoidant disorder, 148-150

Ballenger, J. C., 30, 410, 412
Bandura, A., 273, 295, 296
Barlow, D. H., 27, 36, 41, 59, 82, 125, 142, 209-216, 211-221, 222-236, 298, 341-342, 367-368
Beck, A., 10, 87-88, 112, 113, 120, 143, 210, 215
Beech, H. R., 186
Behavioral approach, 5-6, 10
  marital therapy and, 341-343
  for obsessive-compulsive disorder, 186-187
Benzodiazepines, 413-415
Bernstein, D. A., 127, 215
Beta-adrenergic blockers, 416

Bibliotherapy, 329-337
Birmaher, B., 30
Black, A., 185
Boisvert, J. M., 59
Borkovec, T. D., 66, 127, 215
Bowlby, J., 6-7, 345
Boyd, J. H., 25
Brantigan, C. O., 417
Breathing, 64-65, 126, 170, 229, 298, 299-325, 335. *See also* hyperventilation
  abdominal, 322-324
  and flying phobia, 70
  and generalized anxiety disorder, 119-120, 126
  and panic management, 64-65
  and relaxation, 293-295
  retraining, 319-324
Breier, A., 29
Breitner, C., 185
Buglass, D., 7, 43
Burton, R., 18
Buspirone, 415

Cameron, O. G., 26-27
Cardiac illnesses, 32. *See also* symptoms, cardiac
Cartledge, G., 150
Cerny, J. A., 342, 360
Chambless, D. L., 39-86, 188, 204, 341
Checkers, checking, 184, 200
Childhood phobias, 146, 147-157, 386-389
Clancy, J., 30
Clomipramine (Anagranil), 155, 409, 411
Clonidine, 416
Cobb, J. P., 59, 342
Cognitive-behavioral therapy, 211-220
  assessment, 212-214
  treatment, 214-216
Cognitive set, *see* public speaking anxiety
Cognitive therapy, 10, 60-64, 65-66, 215. *See also* A. Beck
  alternative conclusions, 130-121
  attention manipulator, 62-63

catastrophizing, 129, 137–138
generalized anxiety disorder, 113–114, 120–123, 127–134
logic, 129
overgeneralizing, 129
paradoxical intention, 63–64, 65
rational responses, 133–134
reattribution, 131–132
social phobias, 87–112
Cohen, S. D., 411
Compernolle, T., 310, 317
Compromise formation, 399
Condensation, 396
Contextual therapy, 238–241, 245–258. See also in vivo desensitization, exposure
goal setting, 246–247
practice, 250–258
six points, 239–241
Cooper, J. E., 186
Crowe, R. R., 44
Curie, M., 179

Da Costa syndrome, 18
Dalton, J. W., 299
Deep-muscle relaxation, 127
Defenses, 97–98
Den Boer, J. A., 416
Depersonalization, 28–29. See also symptoms
Depression, 29–30, 47
GAD and, 141
medication and, 409
severe, 55
Desensitization, 5
Diagnosis, 17–34
DSM-II, 19–20, 115
DSM-III, 2, 19–21, 25, 95, 98, 115–116, 213
DSM-III-R, 2, 17, 20–22, 25, 115–117, 142, 147, 213
of GAD, 115–117
of hyperventilation, 310–318
Diagnostic classification, 2–3
Diazepam (Valium), 70

Dietch, J. T., 31
Di Nardo, P. A., 212–213
Displacement, 397
Dunn, P., 4, 7
DuPont, R. L., 174, 368
Dysfunctional thought record, 137–138

Einstein, A., 168
Emery, G., 120, 215
Emmelkamp, P. M. G., 57, 59, 65, 188, 191, 196, 341, 343, 367
Ericksonian techniques, 269–270
Esquirol, J. E. D., 183
Evaluation anxieties, 89–112
Exposure to anxiety cues, 186, 216
in obsessive-compulsive disorder, 196–198

Faint, 94. See also symptoms
Fear
management of, 240–241
reactions caused by, 261–262
Fensterheim, H., 298, 309, 311
Fight/flight response, 226
Fink, M., 6
Fisch, R., 380
Flament, M. D., 155, 419
Fluoxetine (Prozac), 155, 413, 416
Flying phobia, 159–160, 161–179
case example, 400–403
imaginal desensitization of, 273–274, 277–283
Flying seminars
first, 162–164
graduation flight, 175–179
preparing for graduation flight, 172–175
preseminar procedure and first session, 164–172
safety information, 166–168
Foa, E. B., 24, 181–206
Frankl, V. E., 189, 380
Frances, A., 4, 7
Freud, S., 3, 19, 386, 396–397
Freudian orientation, 2–4, 393–403

Fried, R., 300, 317
Friedman, S., 339, 341-363, 368-369
Fry, W., 342
Fyer, A. J., 414

GAD (generalized anxiety disorder), 113-114, 115-142
  and benzodiazepines, 414-415
  and depression, 141
  diagnosis of, 115-117
  and panic disorder, 118-119, 139-140
  prevalence of, 117-118
  treatment of, 123-135
Gamsu, C. V., 142
Garakani, H., 410
Gelder, M. G., 41, 98-100, 342
Gittelman-Klein, R., 151-152
Gliebe, P. A., 299
Going crazy, 233-234
Goldstein, A., 39, 41, 56, 63, 74, 82, 83, 84, 188, 204, 341-342, 343, 367, 368
Gorman, J. M., 415
Grayson, J. B., 188
Grimshaw, L., 186
Gruen, G. E., 154
Grunhaus, L., 30
Guidano, V. F., 344
Gurney, C., 29

Hafner, R. J., 74, 342, 360, 367
Haley, J., 380
Hall, R. C. W., 31
Hamilton Anxiety Scale, 213
Hamilton Depression Scale, 213
Hand, I., 342, 345, 360, 367
Hardy, A. B., 259-267
Harris, E. L., 46-47
Hartley, L. R., 417
Heart attacks, 235-236. *See also* symptoms, cardiac
Heide, F. J., 66
Himle, J., 26
Hodgson, R., 188, 196, 202
Hoehn-Saric, R., 416

Hofbauer, L., 299
Hoodguin, K., 310
Huey, S. R., 303
Hyperventilation, 229, 298, 299-326, 335
  breathing retraining, 315-316, 319-324
  definition of, 300-302
  diagnosis of, 310-318
  and generalized anxiety disorder, 119-120
  physical symptoms of, 303-306
  psychological and behavioral symptoms of, 307-310
  rebreathing, 318-319
  treatment of, 318-325
  voluntary exertion, 319. *See also* breathing
Hypnosis, 269-270, 277-278
  and option-oriented language, 288-292, 295
  resistance to, 274-276
  and success imagery, 276-287
  and visualizations, 273-276

Imaginal desensitization, 269-270, 271-296
Imipramine (Togranil), 6, 69, 152, 409, 411
Implications, 291-292
Implosive therapy, 187
Insel, R. R., 419
Insight therapy, 265-267
  agoraphobia, 66-67, 72
  cognitive therapy, 128
Integrative approach, 10-11, 53-56, 71-74
Interactional categories, 372-374
In vivo desensitization, 5, 56-60, 238-267. *See also* contextual therapy, exposure
  action and talking therapy, 261-267
  anxiety coping techniques, 245-258
  for avoidance, 56-60, 77
  in groups, 78-79
  in marital therapy, 356-357

for obsessive-compulsives, 186-193, 196-200
for panic disorder, 216
practice, 250-258
record keeping, 72, 214, 247-250

Jackson, D., 263-264
Jacobson, E., 5
James, W., 10
Janet, P., 19
Jannoun, L., 66
Jannson, L., 56
Jenike, M. A., 419
Joele, L., 310
Johnston, D. W., 41, 342

Kahn, R. J., 414-415
Katon, W., 31
Kerr, W. J., 299
Klein, D. F., 6, 8, 20, 27, 36, 68, 151-152
Knesevich, J. W., 419
Kraanen, J., 188
Kringlen, E., 185
Kuipers, A. C. M., 341

Lader, M., 31
Lamontague, Y., 342, 345, 360, 367
Lang, P. J., 192, 216
Language
  option-oriented, 287-292
  visual rehearsal with, 292-295
Last, C. G., 59, 368
Lesser, I. M., 17, 29-30, 36, 38
Levis, D. J., 187
Lewis, A. J., 183
Lewis, B. I., 304-305
Liberthson, R., 32
Liden, S., 417
Liebowitz, M. R., 27, 68, 150, 410, 416, 418
Lindsay, W. R., 142
Liotti, G., 344
Little Hans case (Freud), 3, 386, 395-397
Losing control, 234, 257-258, 274
Loss of love, 104-105
Lum, C., 298, 300, 304, 317, 324

Madden, J., 162
MAO (monoamine oxidase) inhibitors, 27, 69, 119, 150, 409, 411-413, 419
  and agoraphobia, 69-71
  and childhood disorders, 150
Marital therapy, 339-340, 341-361
  and agoraphobia, 73-74, 265
  and behavioral treatment, 341-343
  couple tasks in, 357-359
  education, 352-356
  family interview, 348-352
  initial family contact, 346-348
  in vivo exposure group, 356-357
  results of, 359-361
Marks, I., 9, 43, 45, 74, 187-188, 191, 335, 368, 420
Mather, M. D., 188
Mathews, A. M., 41, 58, 341-343, 353, 367
Mavissakalian, M., 65, 367, 410
Mawson, D., 74
McClure, J. N., 305
McLaughlin, E., 142
Medical disorders, 31-34, 409
Medical workup, 33-34
Mellman, T. A., 27
Mental Research Institute, 263, 369
Merbaum, M., 187
Merikangas, K. R., 117
Meyer, V., 187
Michaelson, L., 410
Milburn, J. F., 150
Mills, H. L., 188
Milton, F., 342, 367
Montgomery, S. A., 419-420
Mountjoy, C. Q., 29, 418
Movement, 170-171
Munjack, D. J., 416
Murphy, J., 347, 368

Nervous collapse, 234-235
Neurologic symptoms, 33
Nichols, K. A., 101
Noyes, R., 26
Nunes, J. S., 188

O'Brien, G. T., 59, 368
Obsessive-compulsive disorder, 155, 181–182, 183–203
  checking, 184–185
  cleaning, 198–199
  exposure and response prevention, 187–193
  failures and relapses, 202–203
  and familial patterns, 201–202
  and functioning without symptoms, 202
  information-gathering period, 194–196
  medication treatment of, 418–421
  and noncompliance, 201
  treatment of, 193–200
Ollendick, T. H., 154
Option-oriented language, 287–295
Organic anxiety disorder, 31
Öst, L. G., 56
Overanxious disorder, 153–154

Panic attacks, 22, 43–45, 231–233
  blocking of, 7
  coping with, 333–334
  spontaneous, 8–9, 25–26, 67–68, 271, 408
Panic disorder
  and childhood phobias, 152
  diagnosis of, 17–34
  GAD and, 118–119
  and medical disorders, 31–34
  medication treatment of, 408–416
  and other psychiatric disorders, 25–30, 55, 233–234
Panic-management strategies, 60–71, 123–127
Paradoxical intention, 63–64, 358–359
Pavlov, I. P., 5
Perel, J., 410
Performance feedback, see public speaking
Phenelzine (Nardil), 6, 9, 150, 412
Phenothiazines, 68

Phobia(s)
  acceptance of, 239–240
  childhood, 147–157, 386–389
  as compromise formations, 399
  flying, 161–179
  Little Hans case, 3, 386, 395–397
  school, 45
  simple, 153
  social, 94–95
Phobia therapy
  development of, 1–11
  psychopharmacological, 417–418
Physiological arousal management, 124–127
Physiology of anxiety, 225–233
  behavioral system, 230
  cardiovascular effects, 228
  fight/flight response, 226
  mental system, 230–231
  nervous and chemical effects, 227–228
  panic attacks, 231–233
  respiratory effects, 229
  sweat-gland effects, 229
Pitts, F. N., 305
Practice, 250–258
  motivation in, 252–253
  versus testing, 253
Progressive relaxation, 215
Projection, 396
Proper breathing, 64–65, 126
Propranolol (Inderal), 69–70, 416, 417–418
Psychiatric disorders, 27–30
Psychobiological approach, 6–9
Psychoeducation, 215, 223–224, 225–236
  couples, 352
  medication, 421
Psychopharmacological intervention, 6–9, 68–71, 407–421
  general principles of, 407–408
  for obsessive-compulsive disorder, 418–421
  for panic disorders, 408–416
  for phobic disorders, 417–418

Psychotherapy, 265–266
  for panic management, 60–68
  psychoanalytic, 395–403
  resistance in, 271–272
Public-speaking anxiety, 105–108
  cognitive set, 107–108
  performance feedback, 107

Qualifiers, 289
Questions, 288–289

Rabavilas, A. D., 196
Rachman, S., 188, 191, 196–197, 202
Raj, A., 31
Ramm, L., 74
Ramsey, R. W., 74
Rayner, P., 5
Reattribution technique, 131–132
Reciprocal inhibition, 5
Regier, D. A., 17
Reich, J., 30
Relaxation, 164
  example induction, 279–281, 288–289, 293–295
  fear of, 274–275
  generalized anxiety disorder, 124–125
  Jacobson technique, 5
  progressive relaxation, 66, 215
Repression, 397
Resistance, 274–277, 347, 358, 399
Respiratory disorders, 32–33. *See also* hyperventilation
Roberts, A. H., 41
Robins, L. N., 17
Rohrbaugh, M., 371, 380
Rosa, J., 368
Ross, M. W., 74
Roth, M., 29
Rubin, R. D., 187
Rules and formulas, 93
Russell, B., 174

Sarason, I. G., 111
Scanning, 126

Schapira, K., 29
Schneider, K., 183
School phobia, 45
Sechrest, L., 303
Seif, M. N., 72
Self-confidence, 91–93
Self-efficacy, 273, 277–278, 295
Selvini-Palazzoli, M., 358, 380
Sensitization, 330–331
Separation anxiety, 6–7, 104–105, 398
  agoraphobia, 73–74, 79–80
  and anaclytic depression, 6–7
  disorder, 150–152
  and infantile sexuality, 4
  social phobia, 104–105
Separation-anxiety disorder, 150–152
Serotonin reuptake blockers, 415–416, 420
Shame, 102–104
Shaw, P. M., 98–100
Shear, M. K., 32
Sheehan, D. V., 23, 31, 44, 152, 410, 412
Sheehan, K. H., 23
Simple phobia, 153, 418
Skinner, B. F., 10
Social anxiety, 48, 89–112
  childhood, 148–150
  differentiating from agoraphobia, 98–100
  medication for, 417–418
  paradoxes of, 95–98
  phenomena of, 101–111
  social phobias and, 94–95
Social image, 102–104
Stampfl, T. G., 181, 187, 189
Status, 91–92
Stavrakaki, C., 29
Stedman, J. M., 347, 368
Steketee, G., 26, 192
Stoops, R., 111
Stranger anxiety, 148–149
Studies in Hysteria (Freud and Breuer), 3
Substance abuse, 55–56, 165–166, 415
Success imagery, 19, 21–22, 28, 231–232, 278–287

Symptoms, 334-335
  cardiac, 18, 31-32, 70, 119, 228-229, 235-236
  depersonalization, 28-29, 64, 229
  dizziness, 64, 229
  fainting, 94
  functioning without, 202
  of GAD, 119-123
  of hyperventilation, 303-310
  neurologic, 33
  social phobia and agoraphobia compared, 100-102
  somatic, 100
  unconscious underpinnings of, 4, 398-400
Systems therapy, 367-390
  assessment procedures, 372
  for children's phobias, 386-389
  interactional categories of, 372-374
  principles of, 371
  treatment of the interaction, 374-386

Taylor, C. B., 358
Telch, M. J., 70, 358
Terrap program, 264-267
Test anxiety, 109-111
Therapy, see individual types of
Thoren, P., 419-420
Thyer, B. A., 26
Tranquilizers, 68-69, 413-415
  and generalized anxiety disorder, 27, 118-119, 414
  and panic disorder, 27
Treatment
  failures, 201-203, 336
  limitations of, 74-81
  process of, 71-74
Tricyclic antidepressants, 69, 119, 409-411
Turner, S. M., 189
Tyrer, P., 23, 418

Uhde, T. W., 27

Van Der Hout, A., 343, 367
Van Valkenberg, C., 30
Vargo, B., 29
Vaughan, M., 186
Ven Katesh, A., 32
Visual rehearsal, 292-295. *See also* hypnosis, desensitization
Volavka, J., 420
Vulnerability, 91

Walton, D., 188
Warnecke, L. B., 420
Washers, 184, 198-199
Watson, J. B., 5
Watzlawick, P., 369, 380
Weakland, J., 369-370, 380
Weekes, C., 63, 328, 329-337
Weissman, M. M., 45, 76, 117, 152, 158
Wessels, H., 191, 196
Williams, S. L., 58
Wolfe, B. E., 41, 341
Wolpe, J., 5, 191

Zane, M. D., 62, 72, 86, 238, 239-241
Zitrin, C. M., 71, 86, 410-411
Zohar, 419-420